OECD Health Policy Studies

Who Cares? Attracting and Retaining Care Workers for the Elderly

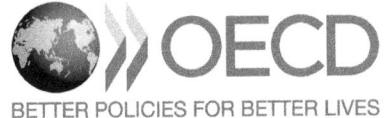

This work is published under the responsibility of the Secretary-General of the OECD. The opinions expressed and arguments employed herein do not necessarily reflect the official views of OECD member countries.

This document, as well as any data and any map included herein, are without prejudice to the status of or sovereignty over any territory, to the delimitation of international frontiers and boundaries and to the name of any territory, city or area.

Please cite this publication as:
OECD (2020), *Who Cares? Attracting and Retaining Care Workers for the Elderly*, OECD Health Policy Studies, OECD Publishing, Paris, https://doi.org/10.1787/92c0ef68-en.

ISBN 978-92-64-38857-4 (print)
ISBN 978-92-64-38374-6 (pdf)

OECD Health Policy Studies
ISSN 2074-3181 (print)
ISSN 2074-319X (online)

The statistical data for Israel are supplied by and under the responsibility of the relevant Israeli authorities. The use of such data by the OECD is without prejudice to the status of the Golan Heights, East Jerusalem and Israeli settlements in the West Bank under the terms of international law.

Photo credits: © Diego Cervo/Shutterstock.com

Corrigenda to OECD publications may be found on line at: *www.oecd.org/about/publishing/corrigenda.htm*.
© OECD 2020

You can copy, download or print OECD content for your own use, and you can include excerpts from OECD publications, databases and multimedia products in your own documents, presentations, blogs, websites and teaching materials, provided that suitable acknowledgement of OECD as source and copyright owner is given. All requests for public or commercial use and translation rights should be submitted to *rights@oecd.org*. Requests for permission to photocopy portions of this material for public or commercial use shall be addressed directly to the Copyright Clearance Center (CCC) at *info@copyright.com* or the Centre français d'exploitation du droit de copie (CFC) at *contact@cfcopies.com*.

Foreword

Elderly people and their care workers have been disproportionately affected by the COVID-19 pandemic. Older adults and those with multiple chronic conditions or health risk factors are at a significantly higher risk of severe complications from the disease than other groups, and indeed most of the deaths have been among the elderly. Across the OECD, more than one in six people are older than 65, with 60% of them living with multiple chronic conditions. In addition to the added health risks, certain elderly people significantly struggle to access social support, or to cope with the mental strains provoked by the COVID-19 crisis.

Many OECD countries have taken measures to contain the spread of the infection and mitigate its impact on vulnerable groups. Yet the health crisis is highlighting and exacerbating pre-existing structural problems in the long-term care (LTC) sector. In many OECD countries, recruiting enough workers in LTC remains a challenge and care workers experience difficult working conditions. Skills mismatch, poor integration with the rest of health care and inadequate or poorly enforced safety standards in LTC lie at the root of preventable hospital admissions even in normal times. During a pandemic, the structural shortcomings in the LTC sector are becoming even more visible: care workers are under huge strain in delivering their services in often very difficult conditions and limited support. This in turn is affecting the management of the infection and exposing elderly people to further risks.

Looking forward, the evident challenges in the LTC sector are likely to become ever more acute if no further action is taken to address these structural shortcomings. Demand for LTC is expected to grow in the coming decades, with the proportion of the population over 80 years-old projected to double by 2050 in the OECD. Also by 2050, there will be only two persons of working age for every one person over 65 years old. This large increase in the old-age dependency ratio can constrain the supply of both informal and formal long-term care workers (LTC). In short, demand for care is going up, the supply pool is dwindling. As more people live a longer life, complex health and care needs and multiple comorbidities are becoming more common, particularly among the oldest old. As no two elderly have the same needs, LTC systems need to move towards a model of care that is more tailored, person-centred and better integrated with the rest of health care.

This new report provides a detailed picture of LTC workers: 90% are women, over 20% are foreign-born and over 70% of LTC workers are personal carers with low entry requirements into the job, with 56% of workers being in institutions and the rest working in individual homes. The report highlights the main functions and tasks of LTC workers and finds that care is often more complex than generally portrayed and that LTC workers are often not well-equipped with the right skills. In more than two-thirds of countries, personal care workers' tasks go well beyond activity of daily living provision (i.e. help with dressing or hygiene) and involve cooperation with other professionals. In more than three-quarters of countries, nurses working in the LTC sector perform case management tasks, and they lack sufficient geriatric and interpersonal skills training. Most workers do not stay long in a LTC sector that is characterised by a high labour turnover because of poor working conditions. Pay is 35% lower than the hospital sector for workers in the same occupation; the rate of part-time work is often twice as high as in the overall labour force and more than 60% of workers are exposed to physical risk factors.

This report examines different recruitment policies across countries, in particular those focusing on unemployed people and on improving the image of LTC. It finds that only half of the countries have implemented recruitment policies or reforms since 2011. In evaluating country progress, this report draws attention to the importance of policies to improve working conditions, especially providing better wages, improving workers' autonomy, and addressing occupational health challenges. The report also highlights the role of social dialogue in achieving such policy changes. Task delegation can help to address some skills mismatches and increase efficiency, as long as workers are adequately trained. Leveraging productivity gains through appropriate use of technology, for example by promoting the use of sensors and alarms and facilitating the sharing of information electronically, will help LTC workers to focus more on personal attention to the elderly. Enhancing prevention and ensuring that the elderly stay healthy and independent for as long as possible will also help to ensure that they can stay safely at home if they wish to. This can be done, for example by improving the collaboration between LTC workers and other health professionals such as GPs and those in hospital care and improving the expertise of LTC workers to detect health risks and manage health conditions.

Acknowledgements

This report is the outcome of a collective effort with contributions from a team of policy analysts from the OECD Health Division of the Directorate for Employment, Labour and Social Affairs (ELS). Ana Llena-Nozal led the team and co-ordinated the project and the publication. The overview Chapter 1 was written by Ana Llena-Nozal, drawing on the analyses carried out in other chapters, who benefited from in-depth comments by Francesca Colombo. Principal authors of the chapters were Ana Llena-Nozal: Chapters 4 and 5; Liliane Moreira (OECD at the time of writing): Chapters 5 and 6; Thomas Rapp (OECD at the time of writing): Chapters 2, 3 and 4; Eileen Rocard: Chapters 2 and 4. Sarah Nedjar-Calvet (OECD at the time of writing) provided research assistance to Chapter 6. Jacob Wright (McMaster University) contributed to Chapters 2, 3 and 4. Other contributors to the report include Kate Cornford, Akiko Maeda, Gaetan Lafortune, Alberto Marino, Karolina Socha-Dietrich, and Elina Suzuki.

The authors would like to thank the country delegates and experts who provided responses to the scoping survey and questionnaire, as well as those who participated in interviews for the report. The report benefited from information gathered through interviews from various experts during fact-finding missions to France, Germany, Norway, the Netherlands and Portugal. The report also benefited from the very helpful comments received by delegates from the OECD Health Committee meeting.

We are grateful to Jonathan Chaloff and Jean-Christophe Dumont for comments on Chapter 2, to Annelore Verhagen for comments on Chapter 3, to Christopher Prinz and Andrea Garnero for comments on Chapter 4. Thanks also go to Lucy Hulett, Eileen Rocard and Lukasz Lech for their administrative support and help in preparing the manuscript for publication. We are very grateful to Francesca Colombo, Head of the Health Division, for supervising the preparation of this report and providing useful comments on various drafts. We also thank Stefano Scarpetta and Mark Pearson, Director and Deputy Director of Employment, Labour and Social Affairs at the OECD for their guidance and extensive comments on various versions of the report.

This document was produced with the financial assistance of the European Union. The views expressed herein can in no way be taken to reflect the official opinion of the OECD member countries or the European Union.

Table of contents

Foreword	3
Acknowledgements	5
Executive summary	10

1 Overview — 13
- 1.1. How to tackle current and future demand for care workers — 13
- 1.2. More carers will be needed — 16
- 1.3. Poor job quality limits recruitment and retention in LTC — 20
- 1.4. Attracting and retaining LTC workers requires a comprehensive policy package — 25
- 1.5. Conclusion — 30
- References — 30
- Notes — 31

2 Addressing the shortfall in workers — 32
- 2.1. Where do countries stand in terms of recruiting long-term care workers? — 33
- 2.2. LTC workforce supply is not increasing enough to meet demand — 34
- 2.3. LTC workers' profiles are unchanged — 42
- 2.4. Policies have been implemented to attract more people into LTC careers — 47
- 2.5. Conclusion — 54
- References — 54
- Annex 2.A. Definitions and data sources — 59
- Notes — 65

3 Tasks, qualifications and training of long-term care workers: reducing the skills gap — 66
- 3.1. A better skills match is needed — 67
- 3.2. While many tasks are low skilled, LTC jobs are more complex than often portrayed — 68
- 3.3. Current training requirements may not always ensure care quality — 76
- 3.4. Better training policies can address the shortfall in skills — 84
- 3.5. Conclusion — 90
- References — 91

4 Addressing retention by creating better-quality jobs in long-term care — 94
- 4.1. Many more quality jobs are needed — 95
- 4.2. LTC workers do not stay long in the sector — 96
- 4.3. Low pay and poor job quality prevail in LTC — 101
- 4.4. Improving working conditions will contribute to reducing turnover — 115

4.5. Conclusion	123
References	123
Annex 4.A. Country abbreviations	129
Notes	130

5 Improving care pathways for elderly people — 131

5.1. More integrated care is needed	132
5.2. Some countries are developing integrated health and care pathways	134
5.3. LTC workers will benefit from additional skills for integrated care	142
5.4. Informal carers are also key actors in LTC services	145
5.5. Conclusion	153
References	154
Note	159

6 Shortfall in innovation: how technology, skill mix and self-care can change long-term care — 160

6.1. Increasing productivity and delaying long-term care needs will increase quality of care	161
6.2. Technologies can help LTC professionals improve their productivity	164
6.3. Improving the skill mix is another way to improve productivity in LTC	171
6.4. Engaging elderly people to help themselves can delay LTC needs	174
6.5. Conclusion	183
References	184

FIGURES

Figure 1.1. Trends in the share of the population aged over 80 years, 1990-2050	16
Figure 1.2. In over three-quarters of OECD countries growth in LTC workers per 100 elderly people has stagnated or decreased	17
Figure 1.3. Over 70% of LTC workers are personal carers across OECD countries	18
Figure 1.4. LTC workers are mostly middle-aged women with a high share of foreign-born workers in some countries	19
Figure 1.5. An additional 60% LTC workers are needed by 2040	20
Figure 1.6. Median hourly wages are lower in the LTC sector than in hospitals	21
Figure 1.7. A substantial share of LTC workers have non-standard contracts	22
Figure 1.8. Numerous physical and mental risk factors at work can lead to health problems and accidents for LTC workers	23
Figure 1.9. About two-thirds of LTC workers have a medium level of education	24
Figure 1.10. LTC workers perform several care tasks well beyond basic care	25
Figure 2.1. The population aged 65+ grew at the same pace or faster than LTC workforce supply in most countries	36
Figure 2.2. More than half of countries have started to move LTC out of residential facilities and into the community	38
Figure 2.3. Home-based workers and nurses often represent a small share of carers	39
Figure 2.4. The median age of LTC workers is 45 years old across OECD countries	42
Figure 2.5. Women represent the overwhelming majority of LTC workers in all countries	44
Figure 2.6. Over 20% of LTC workers are foreign-born in OECD countries	45
Figure 2.7. Migrants report being overqualified more frequently in the LTC sector	46
Figure 2.8. Foreign-born workers' regions of origin vary widely	46
Figure 2.9. In most surveyed countries, the policy challenge associated with recruitment of new LTC workers is high	48
Figure 3.1. Basic care, monitoring and communication are the most common functions of personal care workers	69
Figure 3.2. Most common tasks of personal care workers involve hygiene, lifting and transporting elderly people	70

Figure 3.3. Beyond care provision, monitoring, care co-ordination and communication are also key functions for nurses 73
Figure 3.4. Most common tasks for nurses include health monitoring and co-ordinating care 74
Figure 3.5. Most LTC workers hold high school diplomas or vocational degrees 76
Figure 3.6. Personal carers are more likely to have lower education levels than nurses 77
Figure 4.1. Many countries rank retention as a challenge of high importance within the LTC agenda 97
Figure 4.2. More workers are looking for another job in the LTC than in the hospital workforce 98
Figure 4.3. Tenure is lower in the LTC workforce than in the overall workforce 99
Figure 4.4. The median tenure in the LTC workforce varies across OECD countries 100
Figure 4.5. Tenure and size of the workforce differ across countries 101
Figure 4.6. Salaries in the LTC workforce tend to be low 102
Figure 4.7. Workers are paid less in the LTC than the hospital sector 102
Figure 4.8. About 45% of LTC workers hold part-time positions across OECD countries 104
Figure 4.9. Half of carers work shifts on average in OECD countries 104
Figure 4.10. Temporary contracts are more common in the LTC than the hospital sector 106
Figure 4.11. Over 15% of LTC workers report work-related health problems 107
Figure 4.12. Accidents at work leading to injuries are higher in LTC than in hospitals 108
Figure 4.13. Work-related health problems and accidents at work tend to be correlated 109
Figure 4.14. About 64% of LTC workers report exposure to physical risk factors across OECD countries 110
Figure 4.15. About 46% of LTC workers report exposure to mental well-being risk factors across OECD countries 111
Figure 4.16. Association between mental and physical risk factors is strong for LTC workers 112
Figure 4.17. The majority of LTC workers have children 114
Figure 5.1. Co-ordination is the number one policy in countries' workforce agendas 132
Figure 5.2. There are gaps in hospital discharge planning 135
Figure 5.3. TCN's impact on total health care costs (in USD) 139
Figure 5.4. Receiving informal care alone is predominant but 30% of elderly people receive both formal and informal care 146
Figure 6.1. Productivity ranks as a medium/high priority for the majority of countries 162
Figure 6.2. Four categories of technology are available to support LTC workers 165
Figure 6.3. The likelihood of health and personal care worker positions being automated is low 167
Figure 6.4. There are six areas of action in which health and social workers can support elderly people to age healthily and remain autonomous 174
Figure 6.5. LTC expenditure will increase, but less so in conjunction with healthy ageing 175
Figure 6.6. Health professionals do not discuss nutrition and physical activity with elderly people 176
Figure 6.7. The proportion of people aged 65 and over receiving flu shots is decreasing in the majority of countries 176

TABLES

Table 2.1. The numbers of LTC workers grew in most OECD countries 35
Table 2.2. Public spending on LTC home-based LTC care increased 40
Table 2.3. Age at which LTC work participation is highest 43
Table 2.4. Foreign-born workers are more likely to work more hours and stay longer in the LTC sector 47
Table 2.5. Many countries implemented recruitment measures targeting underrepresented profiles of workers 49
Table 2.6. Men tend to work more than women once in the LTC workforce 51
Table 3.1. In most countries, personal care workers' tasks are diverse 72
Table 3.2. Nurses' tasks show little variation across OECD countries 75
Table 3.3. Requirements for personal carers are low 78
Table 3.4. Some countries provide certification for personal care workers 79
Table 3.5. Personal care workers' top ability needs are comprehension and communication 80
Table 3.6. Social and interpersonal skills are in demand for personal carers 80
Table 3.7. Customer service, language and psychology are the top knowledge requirements for personal carers 81
Table 3.8. Personal care workers are asked to use many technical tools 83
Table 3.9. Several measures could improve initial training for nurses 86
Table 3.10. Enhanced training for personal care workers is available in some countries 90
Table 4.1. Managerial issues explain in part low workforce retention in LTC 113

Table 4.2. Correlation between the number of children and LTC workforce participation	115
Table 4.3. Policies improving quality of earnings in the LTC workforce have been implemented since 2011 in some countries	116
Table 5.1. More countries have leave entitlements to care for the sick than ten years ago	151
Table 5.2. Most countries have cash benefits for informal care	152
Table 6.1. Four core digital skills are needed by care workers in the United Kingdom	169
Table 6.2. Guidelines and toolkits improve LTC workers' communication with elderly people	181
Annex Table 2.A.1. Industry and occupation codes for European countries	62
Annex Table 2.A.2. Result of cross-checking for European countries	63
Annex Table 2.A.3. Industry code and occupation code for the United States	64
Annex Table 4.A.1. Abbreviations used for countries in Figures 4.5 and 4.13	129

Follow OECD Publications on:

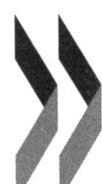

 http://twitter.com/OECD_Pubs

 http://www.facebook.com/OECDPublications

 http://www.linkedin.com/groups/OECD-Publications-4645871

 http://www.youtube.com/oecdilibrary

 http://www.oecd.org/oecddirect/

Executive summary

The COVID-19 crisis is hitting the long-term care (LTC) sector very hard, both because of the large numbers of people dependent on care falling ill and because of the added exposure of LTC workers to infections. The pandemic is highlighting LTC's structural problems in terms of insufficient staffing, poor job quality and insufficient skills, all of which have a toll on quality of care and safety.

The LTC sector suffers from shortages of workers, and this is likely to get worse in the future. In three-quarters of OECD countries, growth in the number of LTC workers has been outpaced by the growth in numbers of elderly people between 2011 and 2016. Demand for care will likely keep going up and put more pressure on the LTC sector. The number of people aged over 80 years will climb from over 57 million in 2016 to over 1.2 billion in 2050 in 37 OECD countries. Keeping the current ratio of five LTC workers for every 100 people aged 65 and older across OECD countries would imply that the number of workers in the sector will need to increase by 13.5 million by 2040.

Low job quality leads workers to leave the elderly care sector

LTC workers are often dissatisfied with pay, working conditions and career prospects, adding to the physical and mental stress of the job. That, in turn, leads to low recruitment and retention and an overall shortage of workers in elderly care.

LTC workers earn much less than those working at hospitals in similar occupations. The median wage for LTC workers across European countries was EUR 9 per hour, compared to EUR 14 per hour for hospital workers in broadly similar occupations. There are also more career promotion prospects in hospitals than in the LTC sector.

Non-standard employment, including part-time and temporary work, is common in the sector. Almost half (45%) of LTC workers in OECD countries work part-time, over twice the share in the economy as a whole. Temporary employment is frequent: almost one in five LTC workers have a temporary contract, compared to just over one in ten in hospitals. Furthermore, jobs are physically and mentally very demanding. For example, half of LTC workers do shift work, which is associated with health risks such as anxiety, burnout and depression.

Insufficient training and skills can pose risks to the quality of care

Personal care workers and those providing routine personal care who are not qualified or certified as nurses, account for 70% of the LTC workforce across the OECD. The vast majority of LTC workers are middle-aged women. One in five are foreign-born.

In more than two-thirds of OECD countries, their tasks go well beyond help with basic activities, such as washing, lifting out of bed, helping with feeding. They are often involved in monitoring health, participating in the implementation of care plans and maintaining health records. However, less than half of the surveyed countries require that personal care workers pass or hold a licence or certification. Low qualifications relative to the tasks required can raise the risk of substandard care, particularly to elderly people with more complex care needs.

Policies to attract workers, retain them, and improve productivity

Attracting more workers

Despite the mounting need for more recruitment into the sector, only half of OECD countries have implemented policies or reforms to boost recruitment since 2011. Most initiatives focussed on incentives to (re)enter the LTC sector or on improving its image.

Supporting LTC training programmes for students or the unemployed can be effective: Japan managed to increase in the number of LTC workers by 20% between 2011 and 2015. Other countries such as Israel, the Netherlands and the United States are providing financial support for such training. Belgium, Portugal and the United Kingdom have also tried to improve the perception of LTC jobs by using public image campaigns. Other policy options include recruiting beyond the traditional pool of women, though only a few countries have tried to attract men, notably Norway and the United Kingdom.

Enhancing retention

Increasing retention rates through better job quality and training is a top policy priority to develop an adequate LTC workforce. Low wages, stress, a heavy workload and onerous working conditions all make it hard to keep people in the LTC sector. The poor record in protecting care workers from COVID-19 is likely to make more people question whether working in the sector is for them. More than half of OECD countries implemented measures to improve working conditions and address retention in the past decade.

Evidence from the United States and France shows that wage increases in LTC are associated with greater recruitment of workers, longer tenure and lower turnover. However, wage increases need to be financed and regulated. Otherwise, wage increases that are not matched by increases in resources lead to increased workload and duties.

Collective bargaining can be used to improve working conditions and wages in the sector. The extent of unionisation levels and social dialogue is uneven across and within countries in the LTC sector, limiting its reach. For example, in Germany and Portugal, the profit sector is not covered by social dialogue. In other countries, such as the Czech Republic and Poland, collective agreements are conducted at the enterprise level.

Beyond wages, promoting a healthier work environment and prevention of work-place accidents and illness can reduce absenteeism, turnover and poor workers health. Few countries report nation-wide programmes in this area. The Netherlands has developed coaching programmes, while Japan has workplace counselling services to promote prevention of accidents and burnout. It is to be expected that, post COVID-19, these issues will need more attention than they have received up to now.

Giving workers more flexibility and control can also boost job satisfaction and reduce turnover. Self-managed teams, such as in the Netherlands, Australia and Japan, have given nurses more autonomy. A few countries such as Denmark and Korea promote training and career options for personal care workers.

Improving productivity and outcomes for the money spent

Better use of technology to assist care workers in their job and improved care coordination across home, institutional and hospital care settings are critical to raise efficiency in the sector, particularly for communicating with, and monitoring, patients, as well as improving data records. Assistive technology such as the use of alarms and sensors, for example, in Estonia, Norway and the Netherlands, remote care such as *Helix* in Australia, monitoring and self-management solutions such as CanAssist in Canada hold potential to increase productivity, improve working conditions and enhance care quality.

As for co-ordination, one-third of OECD countries have implemented task delegation (transferring responsibility for the performance of an activity while retaining accountability for the outcome) between LTC workers since 2011. For instance, Australia and the United States, trained and supervised care workers to assist nurses with medicine management.

Closer integration and coordination among formal care workers, and with informal carers such as family and friends, is also essential. One third of OECD countries have in place policies to support better co-ordination of services more integrated care across and health and social sectors. In some countries, such as Portugal and the United States, multidisciplinary teams care help co-design and co-decide care plans to support the elderly. Less than half of countries (45%) have implemented policies to strengthen co-ordination of care provided by formal and informal long-term care workers. In Australia, for instance, family carers have access to shared care planning tools.

Finally, very few countries invest in activities that help elderly people age well or recover their autonomy when disabled. Nordic countries have rehabilitation or re-ablement embedded as part of the LTC needs assessment and this approach helps to delay long-term care needs. Japan is putting a stronger emphasis on prevention and healthy ageing. Following the COVID-19 epidemic, countries will likely ask LTC workers to place a stronger emphasis on prevention and safety to reduce infections and injuries.

1 Overview

This introductory chapter provides an overview of the entire report, drawing on the analyses carried out in the five subsequent chapters. It documents the difficult working conditions many workers in the sector face and the training gaps, given the relatively complex tasks they have to perform. It also highlights the likely shortfall in the long-term care (LTC) workforce, given the rising in demand and little attractiveness of the sector. The chapter also stresses how these structural shortcomings have been fully exposed during the COVID-19 pandemic. It also looks at policies implemented across OECD countries to improve recruitment, training and retention. The report discusses how improvements to working conditions and skills are important to attract and retain workers while improving the quality of care, particularly to address safety. Strengthening co-ordination and increasing effectiveness will also help OECD countries to face the rising demand for LTC while ensuring early recognition of infections and other safety risks.

1.1. How to tackle current and future demand for care workers

The COVID-19 crisis has put the spotlight on the workforce shortcomings of the long-term care[1] (LTC) sector. Estimates indicate that up to 50% of deaths related to COVID-19 are in long-term care (LTC) facilities. Older adults needing LTC often have a compromised immune system or chronic conditions and are at a significantly higher risk of severe complications from the disease. Yet, some of those safety failures could have been prevented with more investment in LTC workforce and infrastructure to ensure suitable levels of trained staff, with decent working conditions and prioritising care quality and safety. Lessons would have to be learned on how LTC institutions have coped with the spread of the virus in order to better equip them to face similar emergencies, both from a personnel and an infrastructure points of view.

Looking forward, rapid population ageing is adding pressure on the long-term care (LTC) workforce to step up efforts to have sufficient workers to meet the growing demand. This chapter highlights the challenges to ensuring an adequate LTC workforce and the policies to address them – in particular, how poor job quality discourages workers from entering and staying in the sector. Beyond the sheer rising total numbers of workers needed, the elderly population is changing: more people have multiple chronic conditions and/or dementia. The skills profile of LTC workers does not yet reflect these new needs of the elderly population, and their training should be adapted accordingly.

Facing these challenges requires a comprehensive policy approach, focusing on three elements. First, improving working conditions and training is crucial. Second, better use of appropriate technology and improved care co-ordination could also help increase the effectiveness of services provided. Finally, greater use of prevention policies could contribute to delaying LTC needs by helping older people age well, while containing growth in LTC expenditure. Without policy changes in all these areas, recruitment efforts to find new workers are not likely to be fruitful, as LTC worker numbers will not be sufficient, and they will not be working at their full potential.

Key findings

There will be not enough long-term care (LTC) workers without further policy effort to recruit and retain them

- The long-term care workforce is not keeping pace with the growth in the number of older adults who require LTC services. In the past decade, population ageing has outpaced the growth of LTC workers in three-quarters of OECD countries.
- In the coming decades, countries will need additional skilled long-term care workers to respond effectively to growing needs. The number of LTC workers will need to increase by 60% by 2040 or 13.5 million workers across the OECD to keep the current ratio of carers to elderly people. Using technology and changing work arrangements to increase effectiveness of service delivery could halve the additional workers needed by 2040, helping to alleviate the pressures.
- In spite of future forecasted shortages, only half of OECD and EU countries implemented policies or reforms to enhance LTC workers' recruitment since 2011.

Workers in LTC are often not well equipped to do their care job well

- Personal care workers[2] constitute the bulk of the LTC workforce (70%), and have very low entry requirements into the job. Less than half of the OECD countries require that personal care workers hold a minimum education level or provide official certificates, and few guarantee that personal care workers received sufficient training.
- Despite low-skilled workers being the main care providers, LTC requires workers to spend significant time delivering more complex tasks than basic care, including helping with washing, eating and moving. In more than two-third of OECD countries, workers perform activities such as health condition monitoring, communication with families and professionals, and case management.
- LTC workers do not always have enough training on geriatric conditions, interpersonal skills, care after hospital discharges, and management of emergencies or bereavement. This can hamper the quality of care delivered.

Low-pay and stressful jobs limit recruitment and retention in LTC

- Almost two-thirds of OECD countries identify LTC workers' retention as a one of the highest policy challenge. The average tenure is two years lower in the LTC workforce than in the overall workforce. There are more workers looking for another job in the LTC sector than in the hospital workforce, reflecting either dissatisfaction with the work or lack of job prospects.
- Non-standard and often precarious contracts are sizeable in LTC. More than half of LTC workers work in shifts, which has a toll on work-life balance. Part-time employment is on average twice higher than the average rate in the economy. Temporary contracts represent almost 20% of employment in LTC (representing a share that is 25% higher than the average rate) and other new forms of employment raise concerns for job security. Undeclared work, while unknown in size, is also present in the LTC workforce.
- LTC is predominantly a low-paid sector. On average, LTC workers (nurses and personal carers) receive EUR 9 per hour (median wage), compared to EUR 14 for workers in the same occupation in the hospital sector.
- The LTC workforce has a high rate of health problems. The prevalence of health issues related to work is higher than in the hospital sector. More than half (64%) of LTC workers suffer from physical risk factors across OECD countries. In addition, on average just under half (46%) of LTC workers are exposed to mental health risks.

More efforts are needed to improve the effectiveness of care, delay autonomy loss and promote integrated care

- Innovative technologies are slowly making their way into LTC in a few countries such as Japan and Scandinavian countries. While most technologies currently are simple ones, such as smartphones, alarm systems, sensors, and GPS monitors, more sophisticate devices such surveillance and companionship robots or comprehensive technologies such as self-sufficient smart homes are starting to appear.
- Nurses often perform work for which they are overqualified (e.g. dressing elders). Yet, only one third of countries allow task delegation from doctors to nurses, and from nurses to personal care workers.
- Healthy ageing can lead to a reduction in care needs, thereby resulting in better quality of life for the elderly person, and mitigate pressure on spending. For instance, approximately 28-35% of people aged 65 or over fall each year around the world generating unnecessary suffering, and a deteriorating health, all which could be prevented. Similarly, health-care associated infections are common in LTC institutions.
- Co-ordination of workers is the most important LTC policy concern among countries. Yet, only one third of OECD countries have in place policies to support better co-ordination of services provided by caregivers and promote more integrated care across health and social sectors, and even within different parts of the health sector.
- Many countries rely heavily on informal carers to provide help to the elderly and are expanding formal care provision. Others are considering enhancing informal care given financial pressures or difficulties to expand the formal workforce. At the same time, co-ordination between formal and informal carers ranks low as a priority for countries. Less than half of countries (45%) have implemented policies to strengthen the co-ordination of care provided by formal and informal long-term care workers.

1.2. More carers will be needed

1.2.1. Population ageing will increase demand for LTC services and workers

Over the coming decades, all countries will undergo significant demographic changes due to ageing. On average across OECD countries, by 2050, the proportion of those aged 80 and above will increase from nearly 5% to almost 10% of the population. Population ageing is particularly pronounced in Japan, where the share of the population aged 80 years and older was already nearly 8% in 2015 and is expected to double by 2050 (Figure 1.1). In Korea, the population remains relatively young, but is expected to age rapidly in the coming decades, so that by 2050 the share of the population over 80 will be nearly the same as in Japan. In European countries, such as Italy, Spain, Portugal and Germany, the proportion of the population aged over 80 is expected to more than double between 2015 and 2050.

Figure 1.1. Trends in the share of the population aged over 80 years, 1990-2050

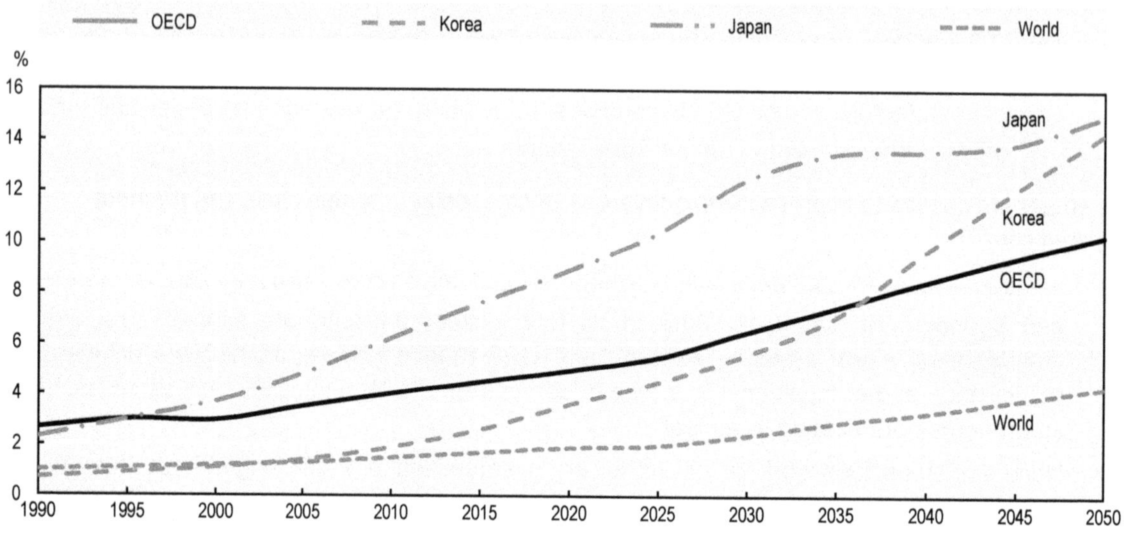

Source: OECD (2019[1]), *Health at a Glance 2019: OECD Indicators*, https://dx.doi.org/10.1787/4dd50c09-en.

As the number of elderly people increases, population ageing also leads to a decline in the potential supply of labour in line with a reduction in the working age population. On average across OECD countries, there were slightly more than four people of working age (15-64 years) for every person aged 65 years and over in 2012. This rate is projected to halve, from 4.2 in 2012 to 2.1 on average across OECD countries over the next 40 years (OECD, 2017[2]).

1.2.2. The numbers of carers relative to elderly people has stagnated in recent years

With coming demographic changes, many countries will need to strengthen the supply of formal LTC workers who provide care to recipients at home or in institutions, such as nurses and personal care workers (see Box 1.1 for the definition of LTC workers). While in a number of countries, the total number of LTC workers has increased, it has not kept pace with population ageing. As a result, the supply of LTC workers per 100 elderly people (aged 65 and over) has stagnated in most countries since 2011 (Figure 1.2).

In several countries, the numbers of carers relative to the population aged 65 and over is far lower than the OECD average, raising concerns about capacity. There are, on average, five LTC workers per 100 people aged 65 and over across 28 OECD countries. Numbers are much lower in France and several southern European (Italy, Portugal, Greece) and central European countries (Slovak Republic, Poland), leading to waiting lists for access to care and insufficient capacity to meet needs (Figure 1.2).

Figure 1.2. In over three-quarters of OECD countries growth in LTC workers per 100 elderly people has stagnated or decreased

Number of LTC workers per 100 individuals aged 65 and over, in 2011 and 2016 (or nearest year)

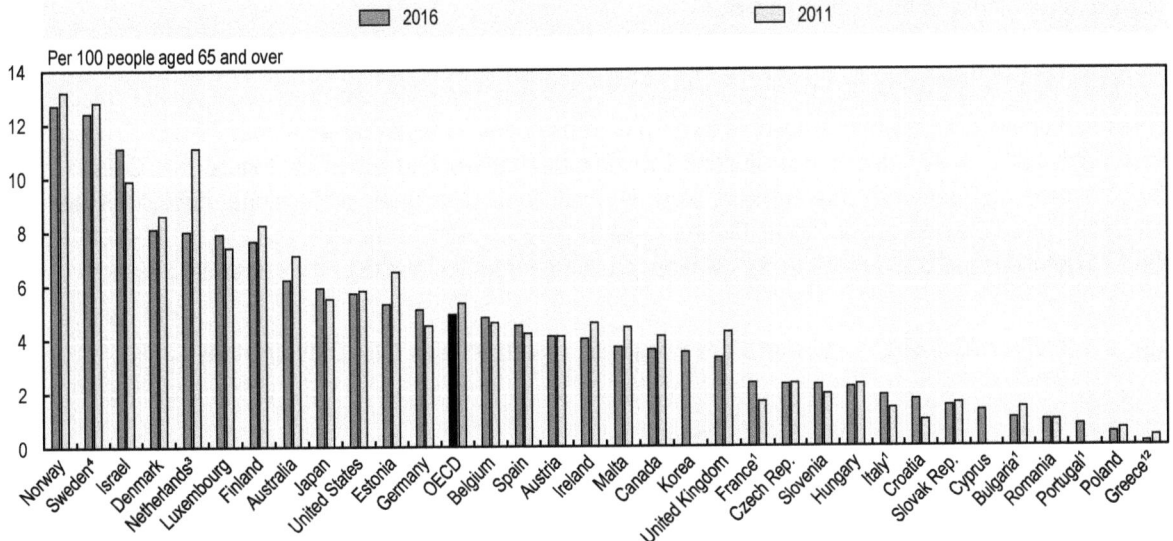

Note: The OECD data point is the unweighted average of the 28 OECD countries shown in the chart. EU-Labour Force Survey data are based on specific 4-digit codes of the international standard classification of occupations (ISCO) and the 2-digit codes of the classification of economic activities (NACE).
1. Data are based on ISCO 3-digit and NACE 2-digit codes. 2. Data must be interpreted with caution, as sample sizes are small. 3. The decrease in the Netherlands is partly due to a methodological break in 2012 as well as reforms. 4. Data refer only to the public sector in Sweden.
Source: EU-Labour Force Survey and OECD Health Statistics 2018, with the exception of the Quarterly Labour Force Survey for the United Kingdom and ASEC-CPS for the United States; Eurostat Database for population demographics (data refer to 2011 and 2016 or nearest year).

Box 1.1. Defining LTC workers

LTC is a highly labour-intensive sector, which consists of a range of medical, personal care and assistance services that are provided with the primary goal of alleviating pain and reducing or managing the deterioration in health status for people with a degree of long-term dependency, assisting them with their personal care (through help for activities of daily living, such as eating, washing and dressing) and assisting them to live independently (through help for instrumental activities of daily living, such as cooking, shopping and managing finances).

LTC workers are individuals who provide care to LTC recipients at home or in LTC institutions (other than hospitals). Following the OECD definition, formal LTC workers comprise two main professional categories: nurses and personal care workers. Over 70% of LTC workers are personal carers across 19 OECD countries, with roughly half of them working in institutions and the other half working at homes (Figure 1.3). Overall, over half of nurses and personal care workers work in institutions. The other professional categories are not included in the LTC workforce definition. For instance, the OECD definition does not consider that doctors who work in institutions are LTC workers. LTC workers can come from the health or the social care branch.

Figure 1.3. Over 70% of LTC workers are personal carers across OECD countries

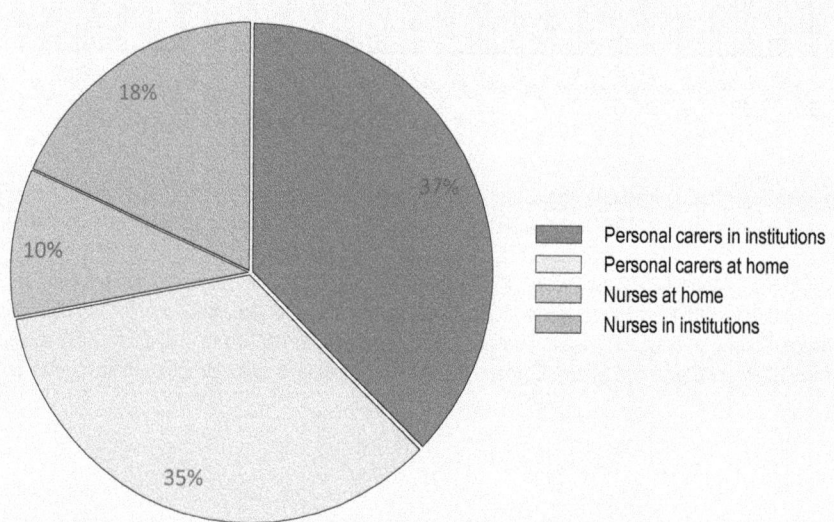

Note: Data are the unweighted averages of the country-specific shares in 19 OECD countries.
Source: EU-Labour Force Survey and OECD Health Statistics 2018 (data refer to 2016 or nearest year).

The overwhelming majority of LTC workers are women in all OECD countries and most of them are middle-aged (Figure 1.4). While the share of foreign-born LTC carers is substantial on average, it varies widely across OECD countries.

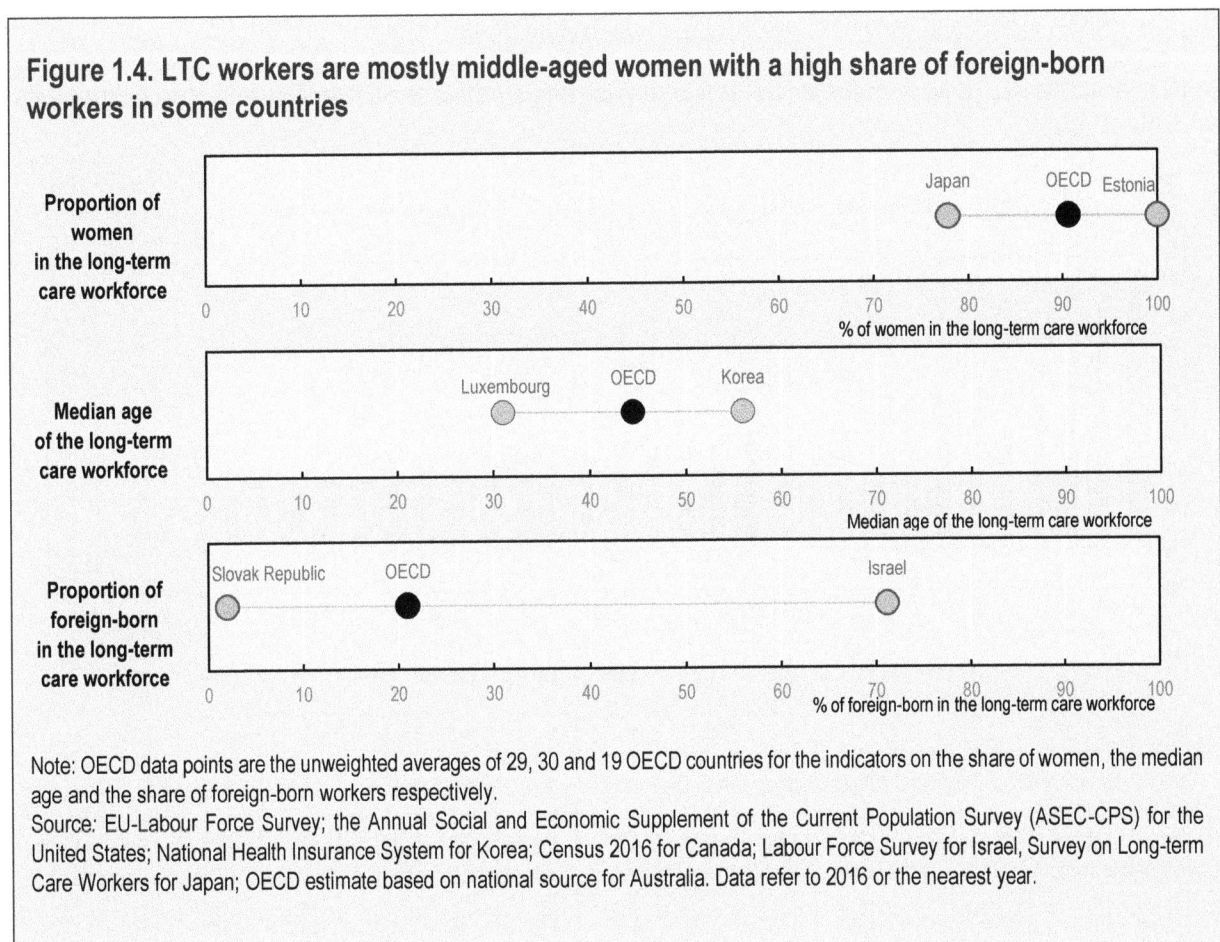

Figure 1.4. LTC workers are mostly middle-aged women with a high share of foreign-born workers in some countries

Note: OECD data points are the unweighted averages of 29, 30 and 19 OECD countries for the indicators on the share of women, the median age and the share of foreign-born workers respectively.
Source: EU-Labour Force Survey; the Annual Social and Economic Supplement of the Current Population Survey (ASEC-CPS) for the United States; National Health Insurance System for Korea; Census 2016 for Canada; Labour Force Survey for Israel, Survey on Long-term Care Workers for Japan; OECD estimate based on national source for Australia. Data refer to 2016 or the nearest year.

1.2.3. Shortages of LTC workers are expected in most countries

OECD countries need to increase their pool of LTC workers significantly by 2040 to care for their ageing populations (Figure 1.5). If countries wish to keep the current ratio of caregivers to the elderly population, they need to more than double the current number of LTC workers, on average. For some countries, the increase in relative terms would be small such as Bulgaria (4%); in others, such as Luxembourg and Korea, LTC worker numbers need to increase by 100% or more. A more optimistic estimate, factoring in productivity improvements, which would lead to each care workers being able to look after more elderly people without compromising care quality[3], suggests that the number of LTC workers will still need to increase by 30% to keep the same ratio of caregivers to the elderly population.

Figure 1.5. An additional 60% LTC workers are needed by 2040

Number of additional LTC workers needed by 2040 to keep the ratio constant as a share of the total number of workers in 2016

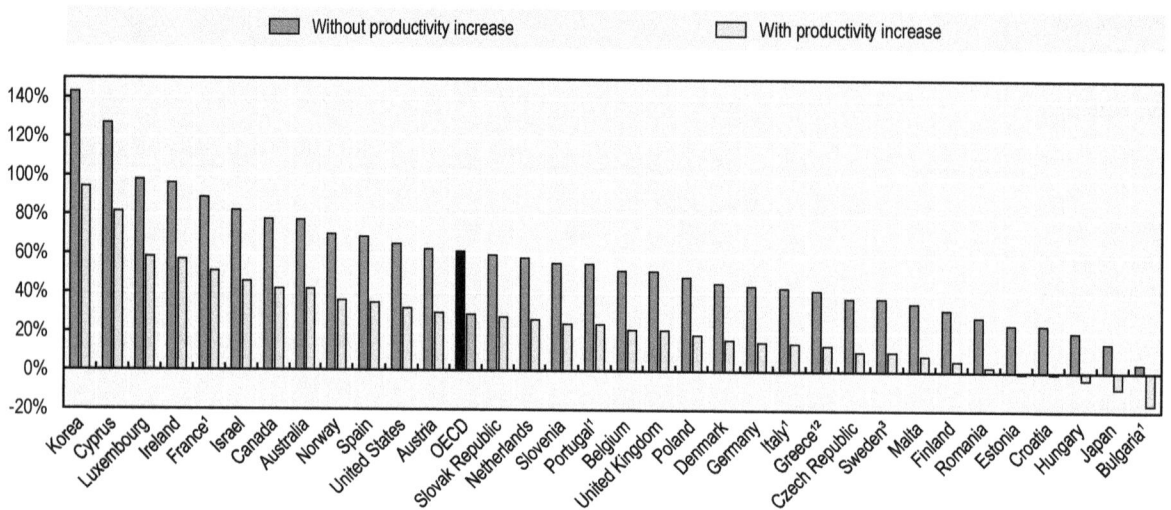

Note: OECD is the unweighted average of the 28 OECD countries shown in the chart.
1. Data are based on ISCO 3-digit and NACE 2-digit codes. 2. Data must be interpreted with caution, as sample sizes are small. 3. Data refer only to the public sector.
Source: EU-Labour Force Survey and OECD Health Statistics 2018, with the exception of the Quarterly Labour Force Survey for the United Kingdom and ASEC-CPS for the United States; Eurostat Database for population demographics (data refer to 2016 or nearest year).

1.3. Poor job quality limits recruitment and retention in LTC

In many countries, the LTC sector is struggling to attract and retain sufficient numbers of workers. In the United States, for example, less than one in five workers stay in the LTC workforce over two consecutive years.

1.3.1. Low pay and poor promotion prospects discourage workers

LTC workers are among the lowest-paid and earn much less than those working with similar qualifications in other parts of the health care sector. The median hourly wage for LTC workers across 11 OECD countries was EUR 9 per hour, compared to EUR 14 for hospital workers in the same occupation (Figure 1.6). In a number of countries, such as Estonia and Portugal, LTC workers earn an hourly rate similar to the minimum wage. In the United Kingdom, the Low Pay Commission has flagged social care as a sector of concern in terms of compliance with the national minimum wage. Low pay also has implications for gender equality, as this is a heavily dominated female sector (see Figure 1.4 in Box 1.1).

Figure 1.6. Median hourly wages are lower in the LTC sector than in hospitals

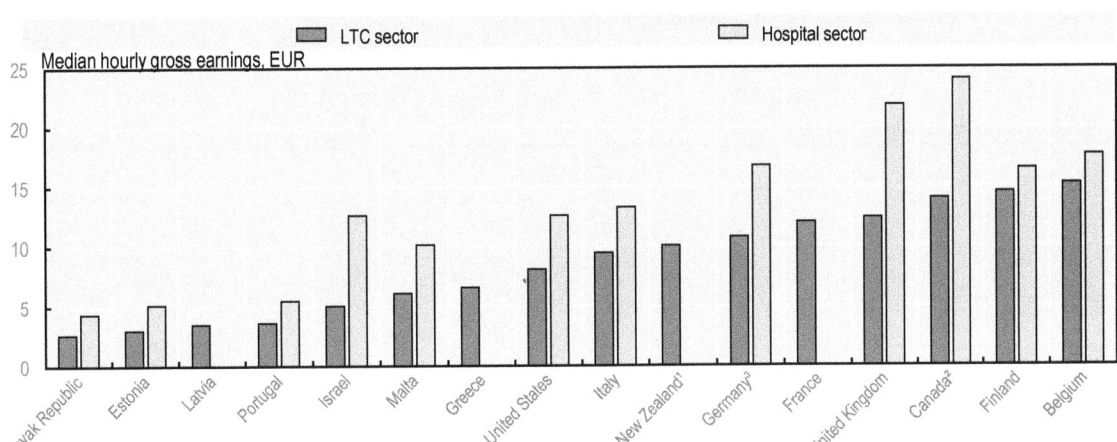

Note: Wages are compared for workers with the same occupation for different industry codes (hospital and LTC).
1. Data refer only to personal carers. 2. Data cover those working full time, full year. 3. Data on the hospital sector cover those working full-time and assume an equal distribution of nurses and personal carers.
Source: Structure of Earnings Survey (2014), OECD questionnaire (2018) for Latvia, national source for Germany, ASEC-CPS (2015) for the United States, Census 2016 for Canada, OECD estimate based on national source for New Zealand (2016); data refer to 2014 or nearest year).

LTC workers are often devoted to their job but dissatisfied with pay and career prospects. Because jobs involving the same types of worker (i.e. nurses and personal carers) in LTC pay less, workers tend to leave the sector to work in hospitals as opportunities arise. Similarly, there are more promotion opportunities in the hospital sector than in LTC. OECD estimates for Europe show that tenure[4] is low in the LTC sector, two years lower than in the overall working population.

1.3.2. Non-standard work generates lower social protection, job insecurity and unpredictable hours

Non-standard employment (e.g. shift, part-time or temporary work) is common in the LTC sector (Figure 1.7). Close to 45% of LTC workers in OECD countries work part time. This is twice the average rate in the economy. Short working weeks are attractive to some, but unattractive to others because of difficulties in obtaining a decent income. As noted in Section 1.3.1, hourly wages are relatively low in the LTC sector, so annual income can be particularly low, especially for personal care workers. Part-time workers are more likely to be poor, often have fewer promotion opportunities and, in some countries, have less access to employment benefits and social protection (OECD, 2018[3]).

Figure 1.7. A substantial share of LTC workers have non-standard contracts

Share of LTC workers with non-standard contracts, in 2016

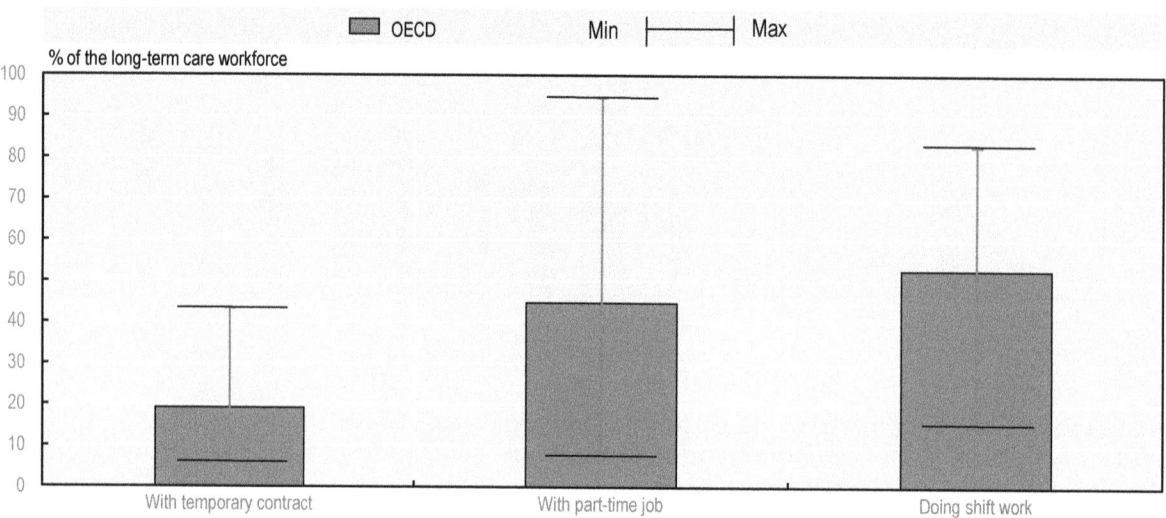

Note: The OECD data points are the unweighted averages of the 22, 25 and 20 OECD countries for which data are available for respective indicators on temporary contract, part-time job and shift work[5]; the lines represent the countries with the minimum and maximum shares. The bars represent the country-specific lowest and highest values. EU-Labour Force Survey data are based on ISCO 4-digit and NACE 2-digit codes.
Source: EU-Labour Force Survey; ASEC-CPS for the United States; Census 2016 for Canada; Labour Force Survey for Israel; Survey on Long-term Care Workers for Japan; National Health Insurance System for Korea; OECD estimate based on national source for Australia. Data refer to 2016 (or nearest year).

Temporary employment is also frequent and new forms of employment, such as casual work[6] and zero-hours contracts,[7] are common in some countries, contributing to job insecurity in the sector. Almost 20% of LTC workers have a temporary contract, a much higher share than in the hospital sector (11%). Workers under this type of contract typically have less access to training, do not always have benefits such as paid annual leave, suffer from low job security and have less access to social protection. In France, for example, one-third of institution-based LTC workers were temporary agency workers. In England, United Kingdom, the share of zero-hours contracts in the sector is high compared to the average in the economy. Lack of continuity in staffing also affects quality of care.

On average, half of LTC workers engage in shift work[8] across 25 OECD countries. A large body of evidence suggests that shift work is associated with a wide range of health risks, such as anxiety, burnout and depressive syndromes. While dependent elderly patients require care 24 hours a day, irregular shifts and the lack of choice about the work schedule can be problematic for care workers and recipients. Workers cannot provide high-quality care unless they have reasonable working conditions.

1.3.3. Jobs in LTC are among the most physically and mentally demanding

Care work is demanding, and the LTC sector suffers from high levels of absenteeism owing to sickness. More than 60% of LTC workers report being exposed to physical risk factors at work, across OECD countries (Figure 1.8). Among physical health problems, those related to musculoskeletal conditions, such as back pain when lifting patients and bending over a bed while providing care, are widespread.

In addition, on average under half (46%) of LTC workers are exposed to mental well-being risk factors, which generate high psychological stress. They may be subject to stressful behaviour from care recipients, in particular from people with dementia who might exhibit aggressive behaviour. Some LTC workers report suffering from violence and harassment, or threats thereof. Many have also experienced severe time pressures and constraints, an overload of work and reduced opportunities to use their professional skills and knowledge. Care workers often have high caseloads and limited time with patients, which generates a feeling of frustration and overload.

At the same time, workers report that they do not always have the autonomy to meet patient needs, and have high administrative and reporting requirements. In a number of countries, care work has become increasingly standardised, generating a heavier administrative burden and a feeling of lack of control. In addition, care workers often work alone with the care recipient, especially in home care settings, and have to make difficult professional decisions on their own. Having a supportive manager can bring relief to the strain.

Figure 1.8. Numerous physical and mental risk factors at work can lead to health problems and accidents for LTC workers

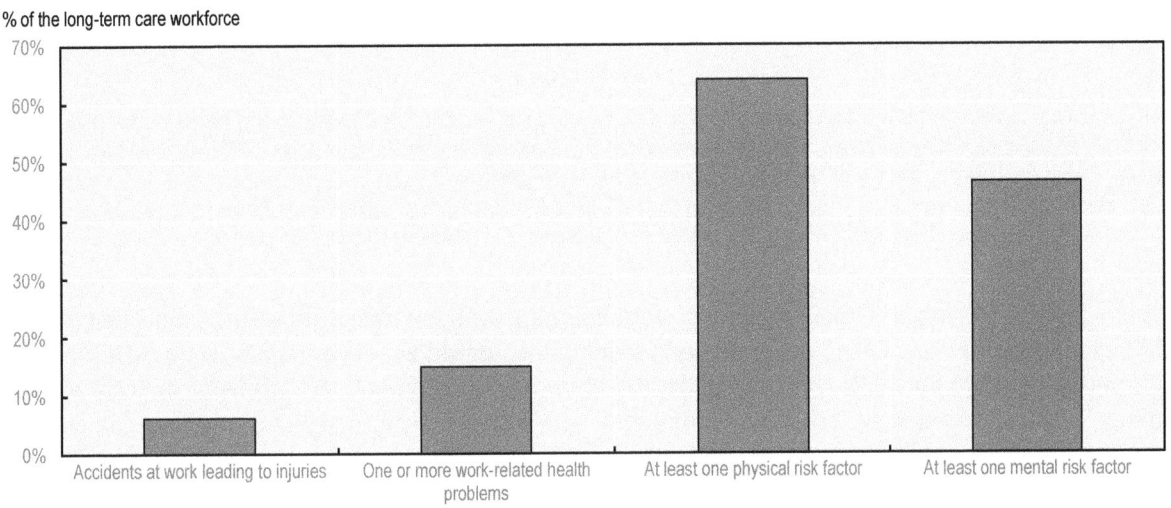

Note: Data refer to the unweighted averages of 21, 23, 19, 18 OECD countries for accidents at work, work-related health problems, exposure to physical risk factors and exposure to mental risk factors. Mental well-being risk factors cover severe time pressure or overload of work, violence or threat of violence, harassment or bullying. Physical risk factors cover difficult work postures or work movements, handling of heavy loads, noise or strong vibration, chemicals, dust, fumes, smoke or gases, strong visual concentration and risk of accidents.
Source: Ad hoc module EU-Labour Force Survey (data refer to 2013); Survey on Long-term Care Workers for Japan.

1.3.4. Training is insufficient for the tasks performed

Personal care workers – people providing routine personal care who are not qualified or certified as nurses – represent 70% of the LTC workforce across OECD countries. The vast majority hold medium levels of educational qualifications: the equivalent of high school or upper secondary schooling. Most workers have obtained a high school diploma or attended vocational schools, while 16% have low education or the equivalent of less than upper secondary schooling (Figure 1.9). LTC workers generally have lower qualifications than health workers.

Figure 1.9. About two-thirds of LTC workers have a medium level of education

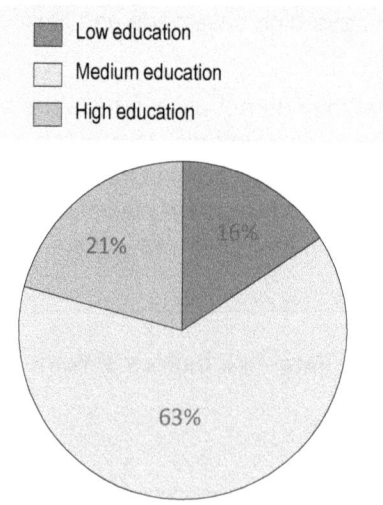

Note: Low education corresponds to a lower secondary education (international standard classification of education (ISCED) 0-2), medium education to an upper secondary education or a post-secondary non-tertiary education – vocational schools (ISCED 3-4), and high education to tertiary level of education – university (ISCED 5-8). Data refer to 2016 or nearest year.
Source: EU-Labour Force Survey; ASEC-CPS for the United States; Census 2016 for Canada; Labour Force Survey for Israel; Survey on Long-term Care Workers for Japan. Data are the unweighted averages of the shares of LTC workers by education level across 21 OECD countries.

In more than two-thirds of OECD countries, personal care workers' tasks go well beyond helping with activities such as washing, lifting out of bed and feeding – so-called activities of daily living (ADL). Helping older people perform their ADL still represents the core of what personal care workers do: their six most common tasks are centred on ADL and instrumental activities of daily living (IADL)[9] provision. In addition, personal care workers are also involved in health condition monitoring, participating in the implementation of care plans and maintaining records of health status and response to treatment (Figure 1.10). The identification of distress situations is a central aspect of their monitoring role, as they are often the first professionals to encounter patients in distress.

In more than three-quarters of OECD countries, nurses working in the LTC sector can be involved in case management tasks, which often involve the management of complex interactions between the older person, families and care professionals. Supervising and co-ordinating care with other health care professionals is the most frequent co-ordination task provided by nurses (in 19 out of 26 countries).

Both personal care workers and nurses are also heavily involved in communication tasks, especially providing psychological support, as they are usually one of the principal people interacting with the person being cared for. Providing psychological support through conversation is the third most common task reported for personal care workers. This task requires soft skills – for example, when talking about death with informal care providers.

The LTC sector suffers from skill mismatches. Most LTC workers do not have sufficient geriatric care knowledge, understanding of safety procedures or caring needs after hospital discharge, stress management skills or soft skills. They could also usefully be equipped with skills to manage chronic diseases and complex needs such as dementia. Communication and soft skills are usually not taught in general training, but LTC workers increasingly need to master these skills. At the same time, nurses are in some cases overqualified for some of the basic tasks they perform, frequently providing help with personal care in addition to health care.

Figure 1.10. LTC workers perform several care tasks well beyond basic care

The most common tasks provided by the LTC workforce (personal care workers and nurses) within each function

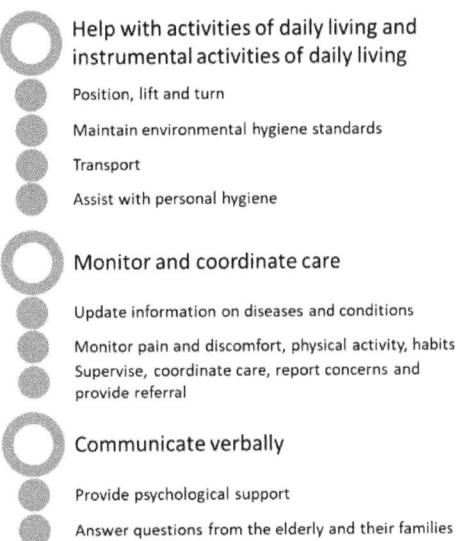

Note: Functions and tasks are ranked by their occurrence among OECD countries (i.e. functions and tasks presented at the top are the most recurrent tasks). This figure provides a summary of tasks, and aggregates nurses and personal care workers' tasks.
Source: OECD Long-term Care Questionnaire, 2018.

Educational and training requirements for personal care workers are low, which can be problematic if they need to maintain treatment or implement care plans. Less than half of the surveyed countries require that personal care workers hold a minimum education level. Among those that do, it varies from vocational training (Hungary, Luxembourg, the Netherlands and Latvia) to a high school degree (Belgium and Sweden) or a technical degree after high school (Canada/Ontario, Malta and Estonia after 2020). Less than half of the surveyed countries require personal care workers to pass or hold a licence or a certificate showing that they have sufficient competencies and skills.

On-the-job training is not sufficiently available in LTC. Only a few OECD countries provide official certificates to guarantee that personal care workers have received sufficient training (Australia, Canada, Korea and the United States). In addition, because of the prevalence of shift work, difficulties with replacing workers during training explain low take-up of training. Both workers and employers need more incentives to follow training.

1.4. Attracting and retaining LTC workers requires a comprehensive policy package

Over the past decade, OECD countries have implemented policies to prevent future shortages and improve the quality of LTC supply. Three main policy categories have been followed, aiming to widen recruitment efforts to attract new workers, improve retention by enhancing job quality and training, and increase the effectiveness of the services provided – through better use of technology and care co-ordination – while postponing elderly people's needs for LTC.

Challenges in the sector and successful examples from some countries provide insight into future priorities. Given the extent of poor job quality and the high costs generated by turnover, improved working conditions and training prospects are the first policy priority, while a safe work environment should remain the foundation of LTC systems. At the same time, in Scandinavian countries, the Netherlands and Japan, enhancing productivity in the workforce through the use of technology and better allocation of tasks is perceived as important – possibly even more so than improving working conditions. Both types of intervention will yield better results in the long run than focusing solely on recruitment measures. For instance, the Dutch plan of action for the care sector estimates that future shortages in care sector in the Netherlands will be addressed as follows: 38% via improved working conditions, 16% via better use of technology and 26% via better task allocation (and reduced administration), but only 20% via recruitment (Dutch Ministry of healthcare, well-being and sports, 2018[4]).

1.4.1. Addressing future shortages requires widening recruitment efforts

While improving LTC worker recruitment ranks high in policy priories, only half of countries have implemented policies or reforms to enhance it in recent years. Where recruitment initiatives have occurred, priority has been placed on providing incentives to (re)enter the sector or on improving its image. A third type of policy – recruiting beyond the traditional pool, such as targeting recruitment of men into the LTC workforce – is less prevalent.

Providing financial support for LTC training is an effective policy option, as its impact on recruitment can be large. Japan has sponsored basic training programmes for both new students and experienced workers willing to return to work after a long break. These initiatives led to an increase in the number of LTC workers of around 20% between 2011 and 2015. In the United States, the Health Resources and Services Administration has funded the Geriatrics Workforce Enhancement Program, which is an inter-professional education and training programme. Other countries (e.g. Israel, Romania) have provided financial support and perseverance grants for LTC education to train unemployed people or to assist people to come back into the sector.

Several countries (including Belgium, Portugal and the United Kingdom) have tried to increase the share of students entering the LTC sector – for example, using image campaigns to help make the sector more attractive among young workers and students. In the United Kingdom, the Proud to Care initiative seeks to improve the sector's image, while efforts have been made to improve information for those who provide social care career advice (teachers, staff in job centres and so on) with initiatives such as the Care Ambassadors, who visit schools and job centres to talk about their jobs.

A few countries are expanding recruitment pools, particularly to attract unemployed men. The Norwegian Men in Health Recruitment Programme was set up to recruit (unemployed) men aged 26-55 to the health and care sector. It entails eight weeks of guided training as health recruits in a regional health institution or health care service. The Programme has been very effective in the Norwegian context to motivate men for a job in LTC. In the United Kingdom, Skills for Care commissioned two Men into Care programmes to attract more men into the LTC workforce. Incentivising male recruitment can be a promising avenue, as men tend to stay longer in the sector and work more hours than women, and breaking down gender stereotypes about "male jobs" and "female jobs" serves a wider social and economic purpose.

1.4.2. Enhancing job quality and training are the foremost priorities to improve retention

Retaining LTC workers is not straightforward because of the multiplicity of factors. Low wages present a challenge for staff retention, especially because there are few opportunities for pay progression. However, wages are not the only factor driving low retention: workers also point to working times, stress, heavy workload, and poor support; and addressing these factors is similarly important. Better jobs will mean better quality of care and reductions in the high staff turnover and related costs.

Addressing the poor quality of LTC jobs will help retain more workers

Increasing entry wages and offering opportunities for career progression helps motivation to stay in the sector. There is evidence that wage increases in LTC have led to employment of more workers, longer job tenure and lower turnover. When higher wages have led to an increase in skilled workers, they have contributed to more consumer value than they cost (Hackmann, 2017[5]). Several countries have tried to improve wages in the sector. For instance, the United States extended the right to the minimum wage to unlicensed home care workers in 2015 and Korea introduced allowances to increase personal care workers' wages. Wage increases need to be properly financed and regulated to prevent a decline in working hours, an increase in non-standard work or higher workloads.

Beyond wages, promoting a healthier work environment by focusing on prevention of workplace accidents and illness linked to the job, and on coaching, can reduce absenteeism and turnover. Stress management programmes (the Netherlands), mentoring programmes (the United States) and counselling services promotion (Japan) are interesting solutions to improve employment conditions. Environmental interventions (Norway, the Netherlands) to assist with sit-to-stand transfers and behavioural management are also useful.

Protecting workers from infections, injuries and severe psychological distress is key to retain workers but also ensure appropriate care delivery to patients. Safety standards related to appropriate and sufficient skill-mix workforce could be developed and enforced to ensure that minimum standards are met. There are numerous innovative models of safety standards, from legislation on staffing ratios to advanced accreditations that may be effective for improving the quality and safety of care provided. Moreover, policies that encourage the accountability of care of patients across the LTC and acute care settings can enhance the safety and quality of LTC care. Several countries, including Denmark, Finland, Norway, Portugal, and Sweden have created national indicators with the objective of increasing quality and safety of LTC residents (de Bienassis, Llena Nozal and Klazinga, forthcoming[6]).

Changing the organisation of work in LTC is a promising strategy to improve LTC worker satisfaction and reduce turnover. In Australia, management models in nursing homes that allow greater flexibility in scheduling and choice over shifts led to a reduction in turnover. Given the high rate of part-time work, especially for low hours of care per week, additional solutions to give workers the option to increase working hours would be suitable. These could involve combining work in LTC with work in other aspects of health care or offering work between various LTC settings, such as home care and day care. Self-managed teams, such as those in the Netherlands, Australia and Japan, provide examples of good practice whereby nurses have more autonomy to decide on not only the type but also the amount of care needed by each client.

Better enforcement in labour contracts through collective bargaining agreements and addressing undeclared work are also essential elements of good working conditions. In a number of countries, providers are not covered by collective agreements; in others, firm-level bargaining is the norm. Such firm-level bargaining, without co-ordination within and across sectors, tends to be associated with somewhat poorer labour market outcomes in terms of productivity and wages (OECD, 2018[3]). Better organised social partners in the sector or, where national legislation and practice permits, well tailored administrative extensions of collective agreements would be likely to have an impact on improving wages and working conditions. Addressing undeclared work is important both for carers and for the quality of the care provided. The provision of service vouchers or tax credits to buy LTC services in France, Finland and Sweden is a measure that has been successfully used to reduce undeclared work.

Reducing the skills mismatch should improve care quality and job satisfaction

Better training for both young and experienced workers would help to achieve a better mix of positions and competencies in LTC settings. While in the future most LTC needs are likely to continue to be addressed by personal care workers providing many low-skilled tasks, LTC workers equipped with more advanced geriatric care and co-ordination care competencies as well as soft communication skills will also be needed. Skills mismatches reduce the ability of LTC workers to provide high-quality and people-centred care.

A few countries have redesigned initial training to address shortcomings in geriatric knowledge and place greater emphasis on communication and interpersonal skills. This includes, for instance, the introduction of scholarships for nurses specialising in geriatric care (Germany, Japan and Israel), the implementation of dual-track programmes in general care and geriatric care for nurses (the Netherlands and Germany), the development of excellence programmes in LTC for nurses and care workers (Canada, Bulgaria) and the promotion of internship opportunities for nurses in LTC (Canada). France and Israel are considering better initial training for personal care workers.

A number of countries have implemented measures to provide better on-the-job training by using telecommunication technologies to increase the flexibility of training delivery (the United States) or improving the modularity of training (Korea). Modular training for personal carers is also under development in other countries, as it provides career perspectives for those seeking to access managerial roles or for nurse aides wanting to become nurses (Denmark, Germany, Korea).

Task delegation can help to address some skills mismatches and increase efficiency, as long as workers are adequately trained. In Belgium, the Wallonia region allows personal care workers to perform nursing tasks when the elderly person needs them and no other care options are available. New technologies will provide increasing opportunities for task delegation. For instance, digital aids assist personal care workers performing tasks such as taking a care recipient's temperature or blood pressure (Israel). Finland and the Netherlands have redesigned competencies for professionals in the LTC sector to ensure better division of tasks.

1.4.3. Increasing effectiveness and promoting healthy ageing will be necessary

Making better use of technology should reduce the work burden and improve quality

LTC is a labour-intensive sector, but greater use of technology could help increase productivity. Because of the relational nature of LTC work, technology in the care sector is more likely to supplement and complement workers rather than replace them. New technologies hold enormous potential to support LTC workers, particularly when it comes to improving communication and monitoring of elderly patients, helping to record and process patient data and improving professionals' working conditions.

The greatest potential of technological use in LTC lies in better networking and communication, easier information gathering and processing. Recording of data on elderly people is a laborious task that is still done by hand in many countries, and nurses and personal care workers spend up to one-third of their time on administrative reporting. For instance, the lack of a uniform electronic record that connects health and social care reduces continuity of care and can lead to poorer care quality, as well as inefficiencies. The Netherlands has implemented new legislation on electronic health records that will lead to LTC professionals being able to use direct electronic recording for medication and the care plan, reducing paperwork for care workers. Germany is also moving towards sharing patient records electronically. This would help to facilitate electronic billing and communicating with doctors and other health professionals.

Beyond communication, new technologies in the areas of assistive technology, remote care, monitoring and self-management hold enormous potential to increase productivity, improve working conditions and enhance care quality. In Norway and the Netherlands, the use of cameras and sensors at night in care homes for elderly people has led to reductions in emergency visits and reduced staff needs. Telecare or remote care assistance can also lead to a reduction in travel time and hospitalisations (Estonia, Israel). Home devices (like intelligent fridges) and medication dispensers can promote self-care and allow better management of elderly people's basic needs. Remote care can also help address shortages of LTC staff, particularly in geographical areas that are difficult to access or rural areas.

The use of technology in the sector has been growing recently, but it remains limited owing to financing barriers, low IT literacy among workers and lack of buy-in from LTC workers. Japan and Germany are supporting the introduction and development of technology in the sector with government grants. In

Germany, the Nursing Practice Centre is testing the application of technology and the transfer of technical support in nursing practice for issues such as pressure ulcers, incontinence and other needs. In Norway, a new nationwide strategy has been introduced to improve the digital skills of care workers during initial education. However, the proper handling of new technologies is often currently neglected in education, training and further education of caregivers.

Enhancing integration between health and LTC and with informal carers will create synergies

Elderly people, many of whom endure several chronic conditions, require attention from multiple providers across often fragmented and poorly co-ordinated health and social care systems. Poor co-ordination increases the risk of unnecessary hospitalisation, long hospital stays and readmission, increasing overall costs. This can be particularly harmful because older patients' health and functional well-being can deteriorate rapidly in hospital settings (OECD, 2018[7]).

Some countries are seeking to increase integration across hospitals and home care. Prompt discharge from hospital requires appropriate follow-up, and "step-down" alternatives can ensure continuity of care at lower cost. There is scope for expanding the role of nurses and personal care workers to perform more duties in monitoring health conditions among elderly people, health coaching and assisting transitions from hospital to home. In Portugal, for example, trained nurses can perform both care and cure, and receive a good level of training, including training in hospital-based management of medical conditions. In the Netherlands, Spain and the United States, nurses are given a key role to ensure timely discharge from hospital and ensure appropriate care at home.

With care becoming more complex as people suffering from combinations of multiple chronic conditions, mental health problems and social problems on top of LTC needs, workers in the sector are asked to do more co-ordination and case management, and such roles require training. Quebec (Canada), the United Kingdom and the United States are encouraging multidisciplinary teams working in communities to enable elderly people to stay at home for longer.

Given the potential shortage of LTC workers, facilitating the work of informal carers and collaboration between formal and unpaid carers, as well as integration of informal networks and associations into the team, is essential. Some OECD countries include carers as part of the care team. In Australia, for instance, family carers have access to shared care planning tools. Professional carers are also increasingly asked to collaborate with family carers, providing skills training and directing family carers to the services available for them.

Several OECD countries have improved the recognition of family carers and their dual role as workers and carers, but better support is still needed to reduce the risks of physical and mental harm. More than three-quarters of countries (30 countries) provide some leave from work to care for a family member – either paid or unpaid. This figure has risen from two-thirds of counties 10 years ago. Few countries, however, have made access to overnight respite care a right for family carers, although Germany offers legal entitlement to a minimum number of respite care and short-term care days per year. There is recent evidence that education, training and information interventions are effective policy interventions to improve the well-being of informal carers. Beyond training, carers who spend a substantial amount of time out of the labour force would also benefit from recognition and certification of skills acquired as carers.

Promoting healthy ageing and rehabilitation will help to postpone LTC needs

Several OECD countries are promoting "healthy ageing" campaigns, aiming to reduce the number of years of disability among the elderly and promoting living independently as long as possible. Japan has implemented an LTC prevention project, which aims to strengthen social connections of older people in their communities, irrespective of their age and condition (mental or physical). Australia has introduced the Commonwealth and Home Support Programme to help frail elderly people living in the community to maximise their independence through delivery of timely, high-quality entry-level support services, taking into account each person's needs.

LTC workers will be increasingly required to detect health risks and manage health conditions for elderly people. For instance, LTC home care nurses in the Netherlands are also case managers as part of the SamenOud or Embrace model; they provide advice on health conditions, housing adaptation and both health and social care.

1.5. Conclusion

Ensuring that the LTC needs of elderly people are met will contribute to the much needed comprehensive response to population ageing, and will help to improve social outcomes. An effective policy package requires measures to increase the attractiveness of the sector as a source of employment and to improve the productivity of LTC workers through better use of technology, for instance, and care co-ordination.

Retention through better job quality and training is a top policy priority to develop an adequate LTC workforce. Improving the status of care workers, providing stable jobs with suitable hours and a reduction of mental and physical risks will be important to reduce the high costs of staff turnover. The changing characteristics of OECD countries' populations increase the urgency to enhance the LTC workforce's competencies, and governments need to address several challenges as priorities. In the future, LTC workers will increasingly have to master specific skills. Therefore, training efforts need to be pursued across OECD countries to provide sufficient skills in geriatric knowledge, care management, communication and use of technology. The LTC workforce will be able to focus increasingly on outcomes (e.g. disability prevention, re-enablement and healthy ageing) rather than on outputs (e.g. day-to-day tasks that cover the immediate needs of elderly people).

There is a need for providing adequate resources in the sector by having a greater number of workers and with better-quality jobs. As this is likely to put pressure on LTC spending, improving efficiency and co-ordination will also be necessary. Making good use of appropriate technology will increase quality of care and allow workers to make better use of their care time. Increased co-ordination between professionals and between formal and family carers, as well as greater promotion of self-care and healthy ageing, will also lead to greater efficiency and better social outcomes.

References

de Bienassis, K., A. Llena Nozal and N. Klazinga (forthcoming), "The Economics of Patient Safety Part III: Long-Term Care", *OECD Health Working Papers*, OECD Publishing, Paris. [6]

Dutch Ministry of healthcare, well-being and sports (2018), *Actieprogramma werken in de Zorg*. [4]

Hackmann, M. (2017), *Incentivizing Better Quality of Care: The Role of Medicaid and Competition in the Nursing Home Industry*, National Bureau of Economic Research, Cambridge, MA, http://dx.doi.org/10.3386/w24133. [5]

OECD (2019), *Health at a Glance 2019: OECD Indicators*, OECD Publishing, Paris, https://dx.doi.org/10.1787/4dd50c09-en. [1]

OECD (2018), *Care Needed: Improving the Lives of People with Dementia*, OECD Health Policy Studies, OECD Publishing, Paris, https://dx.doi.org/10.1787/9789264085107-en. [7]

OECD (2018), *OECD Employment Outlook 2018*, OECD Publishing, Paris, https://dx.doi.org/10.1787/empl_outlook-2018-en. [3]

OECD (2017), *Pensions at a Glance 2017: OECD and G20 Indicators*, OECD Publishing, Paris, https://dx.doi.org/10.1787/pension_glance-2017-en. [2]

Notes

[1] Long-term care consists of a range of medical, personal care and assistance services that are provided with the primary goal of alleviating pain and reducing or managing the deterioration in health status for people with a degree of long-term dependency, assisting them with their personal care (through help for activities of daily living, such as eating, washing and dressing) and assisting them to live independently (through help for instrumental activities of daily living, such as cooking, shopping and managing finances).

[2] Personal care workers include formal workers providing LTC services at home or in institutions (other than hospitals) and who are not qualified or certified as nurses.

[3] The projection assumes that less workers will be needed to take care of the same number of elderly based on technological improvements and changing work arrangements as assumed by similar projections in the Netherlands (Dutch Ministry of healthcare, well-being and sports, 2018[4]).

[4] Tenure is defined by the number of years LTC workers spend with their employer.

[5] Shift work refers to work comprising recurring periods in which different groups of workers do the same jobs in relay.

[6] Casual employees are employees who do not have regular or systematic hours of work or an expectation of continuing work.

[7] A zero-hours contract is a type of contract between an employer and a worker in which the employer is not obliged to provide any minimum working hours.

[8] Shift work refers to work comprising recurring periods in which different groups of workers do the same jobs in relay.

[9] IADL include activities such as doing laundry, shopping, transportation, meal preparation and housekeeping. They are not considered to be essential for basic functioning but are regarded as important for independent living.

2 Addressing the shortfall in workers

This chapter explores recent trends in the long-term care (LTC) workforce and the demographic characteristics of LTC workers, and outlines recruitment policies to attract LTC workers in OECD countries. It shows that in most countries the LTC workforce supply has increased more slowly than the number of people aged over 65, and that countries expect shortages of workers in the future. The chapter highlights the predominance of female workers and personal care workers and the important of foreign-born workers in some countries, together with the relative importance of institution-based workers. Several policies could be implemented to find new workers and address the shortfall: widening the pool of applications to recruit younger workers, unemployed people and men; targeting the traditional pool; and improving the image of LTC. However, only half of the countries studied have implemented policies or reforms in any of these directions since 2011.

2.1. Where do countries stand in terms of recruiting long-term care workers?

A previous OECD publication, *Help Wanted? Providing and Paying for Long-Term Care*, drew a comparative picture of the LTC workforce (Colombo et al., 2011[1]). It underlined some of its main characteristics: the overwhelming importance of women, the lack of home-based workers, the limited number of young workers and the importance of personal care workers, who represent most of the LTC workforce. It also raised the urgent need to implement policies to increase the size of the LTC workforce in most OECD countries, especially targeting specific profiles who may represent large sources of new workers: young/old workers, men and foreign-born workers.

Where do OECD countries stand today? The objectives of Chapter 2 are to explore recent trends in countries' LTC workforce supply and characteristics and to review policies implemented in the past decade to target the recruitment of new profiles of workers to LTC. The chapter adds three main contributions to the existing international knowledge. First, it identifies the LTC workforce with better levels of accuracy and validity than previous work. Second, it provides a detailed update on its composition, characteristics and recent recruitment policies. Third, it provides a broader international comparison, extending the coverage to a larger group of countries.

The remainder of the chapter is organised as follows. Section 2.2 shows that demand for LTC has not grown as fast as population ageing in most countries, raising concerns about shortages. Section 2.3 shows that the profile of LTC workers has remained unchanged since 2011, indicating some inertia among countries in the recruitment of new profiles. Section 2.4 shows that less than half of countries implemented recruitment measures to recruit new profiles of workers, and none pursued a strategy of recruiting foreign-born workers from abroad through labour migration channels. Section 2.5 provides a brief conclusion.

Key findings

- The LTC workforce has not increased enough since 2011. Population ageing outpaced the growth of LTC workforce supply in three-quarters of countries.
- Many countries have low numbers of carers relative to the elderly population. The situation is most concerning in eastern and central European countries such as Poland, Romania and the Slovak Republic, where the number of LTC workers represents less than half the OECD average, and where there has been no growth (or sometimes a decrease) in the LTC workforce.
- Most countries expect shortages of LTC workers – even those where the supply is higher than the OECD average (e.g. Australia, Germany, Japan, Norway, The Netherlands and the United States).
- LTC workers' profile has remained unchanged since 2011. On average across countries, women represent more than 90% of the LTC workforce. The median age across countries is 45 years, which is one year and a half years older than the general workforce. Countries face two main age-related issues in the LTC workforce: attracting young workers is difficult and retaining workers aged 50 and over in the workforce is challenging.
- Home-based workers are lacking. While more than half of countries have started to move LTC out of residential facilities and into the community, personal care workers and institution-based workers still represent 70% and 56% of the total LTC workforce, respectively.
- Better policies are needed to attract new LTC workers. Only half of countries have implemented policies or reforms to enhance LTC worker recruitment since 2011. This is leading to challenges for employers seeking suitable applicants for LTC jobs.

- Where recruitment initiatives have occurred, countries have tried to improve the image of LTC or provide incentives to (re)-enter the sector. Some countries (e.g. Belgium, Portugal and the United Kingdom) have tried to improve the LTC image among young workers and students with Proud to Care and Care Ambassadors initiatives. Others (e.g. Cyprus, Israel and Romania) have provided financial support and perseverance grants for LTC education to train unemployed people or support people to come back into the sector (e.g. Japan). Finally, a smaller group (e.g. Germany, Norway, the United Kingdom) has targeted recruitment of men into the LTC workforce.
- On average, foreign-born workers represent over 20% of the OECD countries' LTC workforce. They are important contributors: they stay longer and work more hours than natives. However, most countries do not encourage their recruitment through channelled migration strategies. Only a handful of countries outside the European Union (EU) (Australia, Canada, Japan and Israel) have implemented managed migration channels to facilitate their entry and most initiatives are for nurses, not for personal care workers.

2.2. LTC workforce supply is not increasing enough to meet demand

This section explores recent trends and challenges associated with the recruitment of new LTC workers, who comprise nurses and personal care workers as defined in Annex 2.A. Identifying LTC workers to have a comprehensive picture of their working conditions is not straightforward. This chapter identifies them by cross-referencing industry codes and occupation codes (see Annex 2.A).

2.2.1. Population ageing is outpacing LTC workforce supply

Table 2.1 shows that the number of personal care workers increased in absolute terms between 2011 and 2016 in three-quarters of countries. Some countries saw opposing trends for personal care workers at home and in institutions. In Australia, Estonia, Hungary and the Slovak Republic, the number of personal carers at home decreased, while the number working in institutions increased. In Denmark and the United Kingdom, the opposite was true.

Similarly, the number of nurses working in LTC has increased in three-quarters of countries since 2011. For a number of countries, including Canada, Estonia, Germany, Israel, Japan, Korea, Luxembourg, Portugal, Switzerland and the United States, the nurse workforce increased for those working both at home and in institutions. These findings are consistent with an overall increase in supply of nurses observed among OECD countries that implemented efforts to increase nurses' training, retention rates and working conditions. On average, the overall number of nurses per 1 000 people in OECD countries doubled over the period 2000-15 (OECD, 2017[2]). Australia is the only country where the number of LTC nurses declined (both at home and in institutions) between 2011 and 2016.

Half the countries (Canada, Germany, Israel, Japan, Luxembourg, Portugal, Switzerland and the United States) were able to increase the numbers of both personal care workers and nurses.

Despite these overall increases in the number of LTC workers, the supply per 100 elderly people has not increased in most countries since 2011 (Figure 2.1). Data show that the LTC workforce has stagnated or declined even in most of the ten countries where its size was the largest in 2016. Several countries, including Israel (+1.2) Croatia (+0.8) Germany (+0.6), Luxembourg (+0.5), and Japan (+0.4), experienced an overall small increase in the number of LTC workers per 100 people aged 65+. There are on average five LTC workers per 100 people aged 65 and over across 28 OECD countries, including six LTC workers per 100 older people in the United States and Japan.

These trends show that the increase in LTC workforce supply was outpaced by population ageing in most countries, as the number of elderly people grew more rapidly than the number of LTC workers. This situation is concerning because a large proportion of the elderly population face LTC needs. On average, across 26 European countries half of adults aged over 65 reported that they faced limitations in their capacity to handle activities of daily living in 2015 (OECD, 2017[2]). Over the past decade the increase in the number of people aged 80+ has outpaced the change in the number of LTC workers in several countries (e.g. Estonia, the Slovak Republic, the Netherlands, Ireland, Spain, Hungary and Japan), and on average half of LTC recipients are over 80 years old in OECD19 countries (OECD, 2017[2]).

Table 2.1. The numbers of LTC workers grew in most OECD countries

Country	Personal carers at home	Personal carers in institutions	Nurses at home	Nurses in institutions	Personal carers (at home and in institutions)	Nurses (at home and in institutions)
Australia	-	+	-	-	+	-
Canada	+	+	+	+	+	+
Denmark	+	-	+	+	-	+
Estonia	-	+	+	+	-	+
France	n.a.	-	n.a.	-	n.a.	n.a.
Germany	+	+	+	+	+	+
Hungary	-	+	+	-	+	+
Ireland	+	+	n.a.	-	+	n.a.
Israel	+	+	+	+	+	+
Japan	+	+	+	+	+	+
Korea	+	+	+	+	+	+
Luxembourg	+	+	+	+	+	+
Netherlands *	-	-	+	-	-	+
New Zealand	-	n.a.	-	n.a.	n.a.	n.a.
Portugal	+	+	+	+	+	+
Slovak Republic	-	+	n.a.	-	+	n.a.
Switzerland	+	+	+	+	+	+
United Kingdom	+	-	n.a.	n.a.	+	n.a.
United States	+	+	+	+	+	+

Note: – represents a decrease, + an increase in number (headcount) between 2011 and 2016 (or nearest year); "n.a." represents "not applicable".
* Variations in the Netherlands may be due in part to a methodological break in 2012 as well as reforms (see Box 2.1).
Source: OECD Health Statistics 2018, https://doi.org/10.1787/health-data-en.

The situation is very concerning in some eastern and central European countries (Poland, Romania and the Slovak Republic), where the stock of LTC workers represents less than half the OECD average, and where no growth or even a small decrease has been seen in the LTC workforce. Several reasons contribute to explaining the limited supply of LTC workers in these countries. Families still represent the main source of LTC provision. Lacking or poor infrastructures in very rural areas contribute to reducing development of the LTC workforce supply (especially for home-based services) (Genet et al., 2013[3]). Many eastern European countries are also facing emigration of their LTC workforce: despite the high needs for LTC provision, many nurses are emigrating to participate in other countries' LTC workforces, where they are offered better wages and working conditions (OECD, 2016[4]). Finally, the financial crisis has negatively affected public spending directed towards LTC: it remains low in most of these countries (OECD, 2017[2]), and because LTC is a labour-intensive sector, low spending often means a low supply of workers.

Figure 2.1. The population aged 65+ grew at the same pace or faster than LTC workforce supply in most countries

Number of LTC workers per 100 individuals aged 65 and over, 2011 and 2016

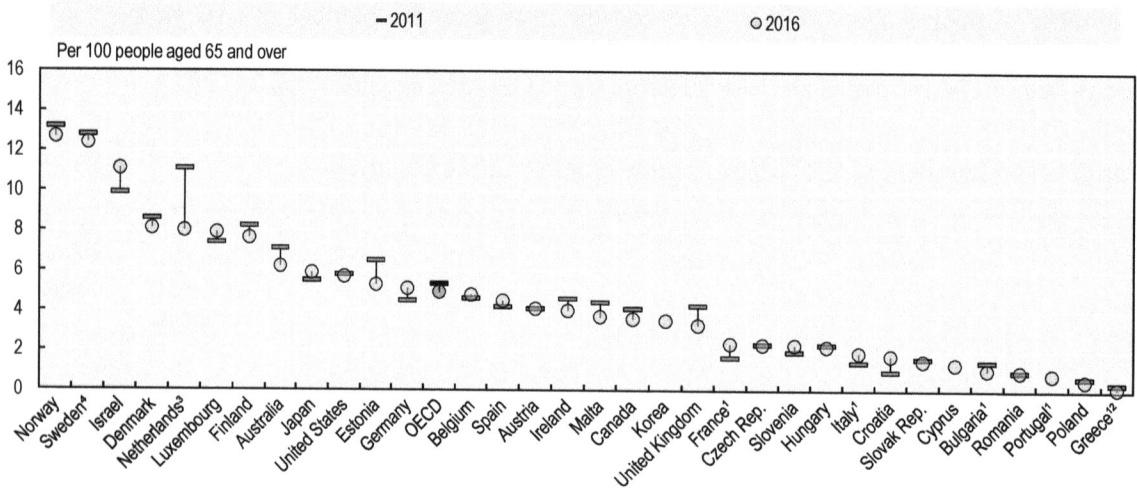

Note: The OECD data point is the unweighted average of the 28 OECD countries shown in the chart. EU-Labour Force Survey data are based on the International Standard Classification of Occupations (ISCO) 4-digit codes and the Nomenclature Statistique des Activités Economiques dans la Communauté Européenne (NACE) 2-digit codes.
1. Data are based on ISCO 3-digit and NACE 2-digit codes. 2. Data must be interpreted with caution as sample sizes are small. 3. The decrease in the Netherlands is due in part to a methodological break in 2012 but also to reforms in the sector (see Box 2.1). 4. Data refer only to the public sector.
Source: EU-Labour Force Survey and OECD Health Statistics 2018, https://doi.org/10.1787/health-data-en, with the exception of the Quarterly Labour Force Survey for the United Kingdom and the Annual Social and Economic Supplement of the Current Population Survey (ASEC-CPS) for the United States; Eurostat Database for population demographics. Data refer to 2011 and 2016 or nearest year.

Some southern European countries (Italy and Portugal) have low numbers of total available carers for elderly people. For instance, the Portuguese LTC system is under high pressure to change the way it operates, as a lack of funding contributes to long waiting lists and considerable out-of-pocket contributions. While more investment needs to be made to secure an effective LTC workforce, there is no sign of a long-term commitment either to raise workforce numbers in the face of future shortages or to improve skills.

It is important to note that a decrease or stagnation of the LTC workforce supply per 100 people aged 65 and over has also been observed in countries where the LTC workforce supply is sizeable (Belgium, Scandinavian countries and the Netherlands). Among these, the Netherlands has seen the greatest reduction in LTC workforce supply since 2011 (see Box 2.1 for an explanation). The decline in supply of LTC workers per 100 people aged 65 and over may be less of a concern in Sweden and Norway, where healthy life expectancy among elderly people is among the highest in OECD countries, and where the proportion of elderly people facing limitations in activities of daily living is far below the OECD average: 17.7% in Sweden and 22.9% in Norway vs. 68.3% for OECD (OECD, 2017[2]).

Low staffing ratios can raise concerns about the quality of care (de Bienassis, Llena Nozal and Klazinga, forthcoming[5]). To ensure an adequate level of care, some countries have requirements regarding staffing standards related to the number of workers needed and/or their competences. For instance, the United States requires that certified nursing homes have at least one registered nurse on duty for 8 consecutive hours 7 days a week (Harrington et al., 2012[6]). In Canada, staffing standards are set at the provincial level, of which three required the staffing of a registered nurse director of nursing and seven required a registered nurse to be on duty at all times (Harrington et al., 2012[6]). In France, the latest recommendations proposed to increase the staffing ratio in nursing homes by 20% by 2024, up from 62.8

full time equivalent staff per 100 residents in 2015 (an equivalent of 66 500 additional full time equivalent positions) (El Khomri, 2019[7]). In Germany, a scientifically based skill mix determination tool is being developed to establish adequate staffing levels and numbers in nursing homes. The tool will take into account (1) the mix of care interventions required per resident, (2) the required time per person per intervention, and (3) the assessed qualification level of the person providing the intervention. Preliminary results suggest that substantially more nursing assistants will be required to achieve optimal nursing home staffing levels, but only a small number of additional specialist nurses will be needed (Rothgang, Fünfstück and Kalwitzki, 2020[8]; de Bienassis, Llena Nozal and Klazinga, forthcoming[5]).

> **Box 2.1. The LTC workforce supply decreased in the Netherlands between 2011 and 2016**
>
> Two reasons may contribute to explaining why the LTC workforce has been decreasing in the Netherlands since 2011:
>
> - First, recent evidence shows that the LTC reform introduced in 2015 increased budgetary pressure on municipalities, which led to negotiation of lower tariffs (Maarse and Jeurissen, 2016[9]). Moreover, the reform led to closure of homes for elderly people and lay-offs of LTC staff hired through municipal contracts (mostly nurses with lower education levels). A challenge is to get these staff back into the LTC workforce, particularly because the image of LTC employers suffered greatly from these lay-offs. While the need for "hands on beds" is increasing, the government is expecting a shortage of workers mounting to around 130 000 professionals in the total care sector within the next four years.
> - Second, according to OECD Health Statistics, the number of LTC workers per 100 elderly people decreased from 11.1 to 8 between 2011 and 2016. A methodological break was reported in 2012, and the number of LTC workers per 100 elderly people decreased from 2011 to 2012. However, the methodology did not change after 2012 and the rate slowed from 10.6 to 8 LTC workers per 100 elderly people between 2012 and 2016.
>
> In addition, the Netherlands faces a structural shortage of workers in care (not only in LTC). The Ministry of Health reports that an extra 70 000 workers are needed to meet current demand, and that without further action the deficit will be between 100 000 and 120 000 people for the entire care sector by 2020.

2.2.2. Home-based workers are increasingly needed

Historically, most countries have provided LTC in institutions. A non-exhaustive list of institutions includes medical and health care facilities, rehabilitation facilities, specialised institutions for providing social services and social care establishments with accommodation.

However, over the past few decades, many countries have supported a "deinstitutionalisation" LTC strategy, promoting home-based care solutions in order to match elderly people's preferences for home-based ageing and contain LTC spending. In addition to enhancing home-based services, these countries have promoted use of community-based facilities as, for instance, hospices for terminally ill people, day care centres and homes for disabled people. Figure 2.2 shows that more than half of countries have started to move LTC out of residential facilities and into the community (OECD, 2017[2]).

Some countries have only recently embarked on the deinstitutionalisation of their LTC systems. This is the case in the Czech Republic, for example, which increased its efforts to develop home-based care later than many western European countries. Surprisingly, the home-based care workforce supply declined just after the introduction of the Act on Social Services (between 2008 and 2012). This can be explained by the cost of this policy for municipalities, which have to monitor and supervise the home-based care workforce supply (Kubalčíková and Havlíková, 2016[10]). Belgium has also historically provided care in institutions: availability of beds is one of the highest among OECD countries, and 74% of LTC workers are based in institutions. Two measures (Protocol 3 and the Flemish Home and Care Decree) have been implemented to ensure that home-based prices remain low: they are defined at the federal and community levels, and ceiling amounts per year have been introduced for nursing. Hungary engaged its deinstitutionalisation process in 2011, with the creation of a National Body for the Co-ordination of Deinstitutionalisation. The strategy aims to deinstitutionalise 10 000 people with disabilities, moving them from large residential institutions to community-based forms of housing.

Figure 2.2. More than half of countries have started to move LTC out of residential facilities and into the community

Trends in LTC beds in institutions, 2005-15 (or nearest year)

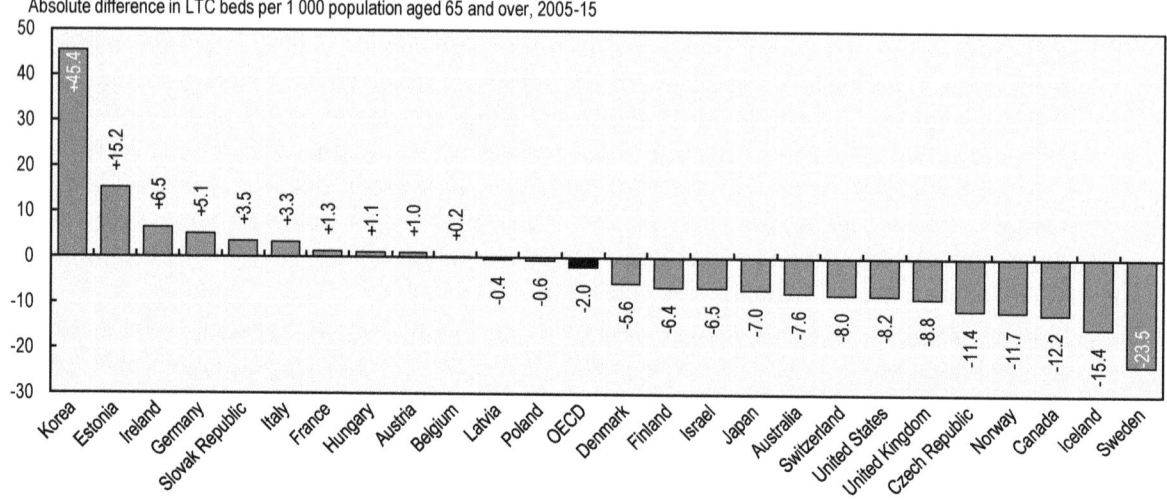

Note: The OECD25 data point is the unweighted average of the 25 countries shown in the chart.
Source: OECD Health Statistics 2017, https://doi.org/10.1787/health-data-en (data refer to 2005 and 2015 or nearest year).

A few countries, however, have followed the opposite trend and experienced large increases in institution beds over the past decade. Among these, Korea and Estonia experienced the largest increases (+45.4% and +15.2%, respectively). Despite a large supply of home-based workers, the LTC Insurance Programme in Korea favours institution-based care over home-based care. The average proportion of elderly people using home-based services has steadily decreased since 2009, and home-based support relies greatly on informal care provision (Sunwoo, 2017[11]), meaning that informal caregivers face large burden levels and health issues (Do et al., 2015[12]). In Estonia, nursing care services have been reorganised via two plans: the Nursing Care Master Plan 2015 and the Hospital Master Plan 2015 (Somanathan et al., 2017[13]). These led to the creation of "nursing care hospitals", which provide inpatient and outpatient LTC. In parallel, local municipalities provide several services (including domestic care and social transport services), while the state provides special care services for elderly people with severe disabilities (including, for instance, everyday life support services, community living services and 24-hour special care services). The Social Welfare Act of 2015 requires that municipalities offer at least 13 services, ranging from domestic to alarm-button services. However, the home-based workforce supply is currently too fragmented in Estonia to cover needs, and institution-based care and informal care meet most of the demand. Other countries have experienced small increases in the supply of beds. In France, for instance, four national plans since 2003 (Vieillissement Solidarité 2003-06, Solidarité Grand Age 2007-12, Plan Alzheimer 2008-12 and Plan Maladies Neurodégénératives 2014-19) led to expansion of the bed supply in institutions between 2005 and 2015 (Muller, 2017[14]; CNSA, 2017[15]).

Despite the deinstitutionalisation trends found in many countries, institution-based workers still represent the bulk of the workforce in most countries (see Figure 2.3). Institutions still cater for most disabled people and hence require more workers. Some countries, like Portugal, continue to heavily rely on residence-based care. Communities are not yet prepared to take care of complex cases, although pilots for home-based integrated care exist. Across 19 OECD countries, 56% of LTC workers are based in institutions. However, this share varies widely by country, reaching 88% in Canada and 81% in France, but below a quarter in Japan, Estonia and Israel. In most countries, both nurses and personal care workers are more likely to work in institutions.

Figure 2.3. Home-based workers and nurses often represent a small share of carers

Composition of the LTC workforce, selected countries, 2016 (or nearest year)

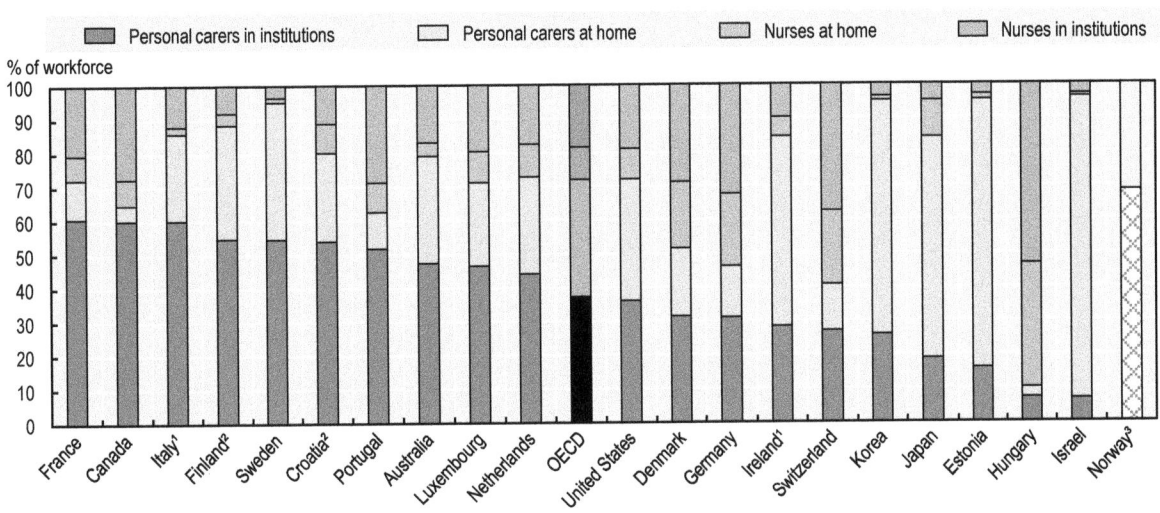

Note: The OECD data point is the unweighted average of the 19 OECD countries shown in the chart. EU-Labour Force Survey data are based on ISCO 4-digit and NACE 2-digit codes. Data are not displayed for European countries when the sample sizes for the LTC nurse workforce are too small and therefore not reliable.
1. Data are based on ISCO 3-digit and NACE 2-digit codes. 2. Data must be interpreted with caution as sample sizes are small. 3. Data for Norway do not have a breakdown by setting; 70% of LTC workers are personal carers.
Source: OECD Health Statistics 2018, https://doi.org/10.1787/health-data-en; EU-Labour Force Survey (data refer to 2016 or nearest year).

Because more than half of the countries are transferring public LTC spending away from residential care and towards home-based care (Table 2.2), it is expected that the situation will change in the future and that the proportion of home-based workers will increase. Indeed, LTC is very labour intensive, and most public LTC expenditure is on services provided by workers. The situation is likely to change rapidly in countries that have implemented large programmes to balance LTC spending. For instance, in the United States, the 50/50 balance between home-based and institution-based Medicaid spending was reached in 2013. The Balancing Incentive Program (BIP) led to investment of USD 2.4 billion over 2011-15 in 21 selected states that committed to increase state-level investments towards home-based services. To be eligible for the BIP, states had to spend less than 50% of their total Medicaid medical assistance expenditure on non-institutionally based long-term services and support for fiscal year 2009.

A few countries already have a larger home-based LTC workforce supply. In Japan and Israel, institution-based workers represent less than a quarter of the overall LTC workforce. Japan actively promotes community-based disability prevention and healthy ageing. Since 2011, the Japanese LTC Prevention Project has focused on three main objectives: to strengthen social connections of older people in their community, irrespective of their age and mental/physical conditions, and help their proactive efforts to organise exercise classes and other local gatherings; to use professionals with rehabilitation knowledge in their community to help older people live independent lives; and to develop a local community in which older people can live worthwhile lives and play a role, even if they are in serious need of LTC. The situation in Israel is explained by a lack of LTC nurses both at home and in institutions, and by the fact that the LTC system relies heavily on the work of home-based personal care workers, who represent almost 90% of the total LTC workforce.

Table 2.2. Public spending on LTC home-based LTC care increased

Absolute changes in LTC public spending allocated to inpatient and home-based care over the period 2011-16 (or nearest year)

Country	Inpatient-based	Home-based
Austria	-0.88%	0.55%
Belgium	-5.11%	5.80%
Canada	0.95%	-0.96%
Czech Republic	0.04%	-3.96%
Denmark	-1.11%	1.11%
Estonia	-2.91%	2.98%
Finland	-3.74%	3.74%
France	0.26%	-0.26%
Germany	-5.48%	4.91%
Greece	-2.85%	2.85%
Hungary	1.64%	-3.02%
Iceland	-0.89%	1.10%
Ireland	-1.76%	2.02%
Italy	1.05%	0.23%
Japan	-3.82%	1.62%
Korea	3.32%	-4.82%
Latvia	-8.82%	4.92%
Lithuania	-1.55%	1.70%
Netherlands	-4.38%	5.22%
Norway	-5.61%	5.61%
Poland	-3.35%	3.20%
Portugal	5.82%	-5.82%
Slovenia	-0.26%	0.04%
Spain	1.50%	-1.08%
Sweden	-1.99%	2.52%
Switzerland	-2.92%	2.92%

Note: Due to methodological breaks, Canada and Finland compare 2015 to 2017.
Source: OECD Health Statistics 2018, https://doi.org/10.1787/health-data-en.

The lower prevalence of nurses in the LTC workforce is found in most countries. On average in OECD countries, about 70% of LTC workers are personal care workers. In a few countries (Estonia, Israel, Korea and Sweden), 90% of LTC workers are personal care workers.

The only exceptions are Germany, Hungary and Switzerland, where the supply of nurses is greater than the supply of personal care workers. In Switzerland, personal care workers represent 41% of the LTC workforce. Switzerland relies heavily on immigration, and more specifically on foreign-born nurses. In Hungary, social help for elderly people with low needs can be provided by social carers without relevant education in the framework of volunteering or public sector employment, but professional education is required to provide personal care for elderly people with more intensive needs. Consequently, nurses provide most LTC. Fully qualified nurses have been a key component of the German LTC workforce since the early 2000s. However, this situation may change in the future and nurses may be lacking, as Germany faces two main challenges associated with the difficulty of attracting highly qualified nurses into the LTC workforce and the ageing of the reservoir of nurses (fully qualified geriatric nurses).

2.2.3. Shortages of LTC workers are foreseen

Several factors contribute to fuelling demand for LTC services in most countries. First, the ageing of the postwar "baby-boomer" generation is likely to increase frailty and disability trends, raising new needs for LTC services (Lin et al., 2012[16]; Lynn, 2013[17]). In particular, preferences of elderly people towards more independent living have been changing. Second, research has documented the increase in burden of care issues observed among informal care providers, whose workload has increased dramatically over recent decades (Kikuzawa, 2015[18]), and observed that the use of institution-based care solutions can contribute to reducing that burden (Rapp, Apouey and Senik, 2018[19]). Third, several factors contribute to reducing availability of informal caregivers: birth rates have been declining over the past few decades; more mobility is observed across society; there are more nuclear families; and the number of working women has been growing (OECD, 2017[2]).

Consequently, shortages of LTC workers are expected and countries urgently need to recruit to the workforce. For instance, studies show the number of LTC workers will decrease in Germany and Poland and stagnate in the Netherlands, while demand for LTC services will increase in the coming decades (Geerts, 2011[20]). In Japan, there are also concerns that the increasing demand for formal LTC providers may lead to shortages. Despite an increase in its supply of LTC workers per 100 people aged 65 and over, the Japanese government forecasts that the LTC workforce needs to increase by 12% (250 000 new workers) to meet growing LTC demand by 2020. Needs are increasing dramatically, as people aged 65 and over will represent 27% of Japan's overall population by 2050. In the United States, the Institute of Medicine reports widespread consensus that there were insufficient numbers of licensed direct care staff to deliver the LTC required by the population (Institute of Medicine, 2008[21]) and recent evidence underlines the existence of shortage issues within the LTC workforce (Frogner and Spetz, 2015[22]) (Osterman, 2017[23]). In Australia, predictions shows that the LTC workforce will need to increase to 980 000 workers by 2050 in order to prevent shortages, a nearly threefold increase from 366 000 workers in 2016 (Mavromaras et al., 2017[24]). In France, it is estimated that over 150 000 full-time equivalent workers will be needed by 2030 (Libault, 2019[25]). A more recent report in France estimated that about 92 300 full-time equivalent positions would be needed by 2024, among others because population ageing would require the creation of 20 700 positions and improved working conditions (via the increase by 20% of the ratio of LTC workers by person with a loss of autonomy) would require another 66 500 FTE positions. Another scenario taking into account current unfilled positions, turnover and retirement showed that over 350 000 people would need to be trained by 2024 in France to be able to address the LTC needs while ensuring decent working conditions (El Khomri, 2019[7]). In Ireland, while the public sector does not report significant shortages, they exist in the private LTC sector.

The importance of future needs varies across types of worker. In Norway, a large proportion of health care workers with secondary school education are more than 50 years old and will retire in 10-15 years (Stølen and Texmon, 2010[26]). While the supply of auxiliary nurses may stay constant, that of occupational therapists may decrease in the future. For health and social care personnel educated at the tertiary undergraduate level, a combination of growth in demand and modest growth in supply will cause rising shortages of nurses, physiotherapists and health visitors in the decades to come. For social workers, a strong increase in educational capacity during the 1990s causes projections to show growing excess supply. In the United States, demand for occupational therapists is already strong (especially for those specialising in geriatrics), and is expected to outpace supply for all 50 states in the coming decades (Lin, Zhang and Dixon, 2015[27]).

Increasing shortages of LTC workers may have a severe impact on care quality (Harrington et al., 2012[28]) and result in unmet care needs. In the United States, demand for LTC occupations has become one of the ten fastest growing over the past 20 years; by 2024, the LTC demand growth rate is predicted to reach 30% (Bureau of Labor Statistics and U.S. Department of Labor, 2015[29]). Because of shortages of services, it is estimated that over 2 million older US citizens based in the community experienced an adverse consequence (such as soiled clothes) at least once due to an unmet self-care need, and that over 3 million people suffer from the adverse consequences of unmet needs for assistance with mobility-related activities, representing one-third of people requiring LTC care in settings other than nursing homes (Allen, Piette and Mor, 2014[30]). For community residents with a paid caregiver, this figure rises to 60% (Freedman and Spillman, 2014[31]). In Canada (Alberta), findings suggest that hospital admission rates are higher in publicly funded assisted living facilities that have no licensed practical nurse or registered nurse on site, or one on site less than 24/7 (Hogan et al., 2014[32]). This situation leads frail elderly people to use more expensive care solutions, as a direct consequence of the lack of proper LTC services. Moreover, a higher number of care hours provided by nurse assistants per resident per day is associated with better quality of care in institutions in Ontario (Boscart et al., 2018[33]).

2.3. LTC workers' profiles are unchanged

2.3.1. Most LTC workers are middle-aged women

Prior work underlined that the LTC workforce was ageing (Colombo et al., 2011[1]). In Australia, up to 70% of the LTC workforce are aged 45+; in Japan, 42% are aged 50+ (Scheil-Adlung, 2015[34]). Figure 2.4 confirms that the median age across OECD countries is 45, which is one year and a half older than the median age in the overall workforce. Data also show that the median age has remained fairly stable in most OECD countries since 2011. Young workers comprise a relatively small share of the LTC workforce. Those under 26 represent only 13% of the LTC workforce in EU countries.

Figure 2.4. The median age of LTC workers is 45 years old across OECD countries

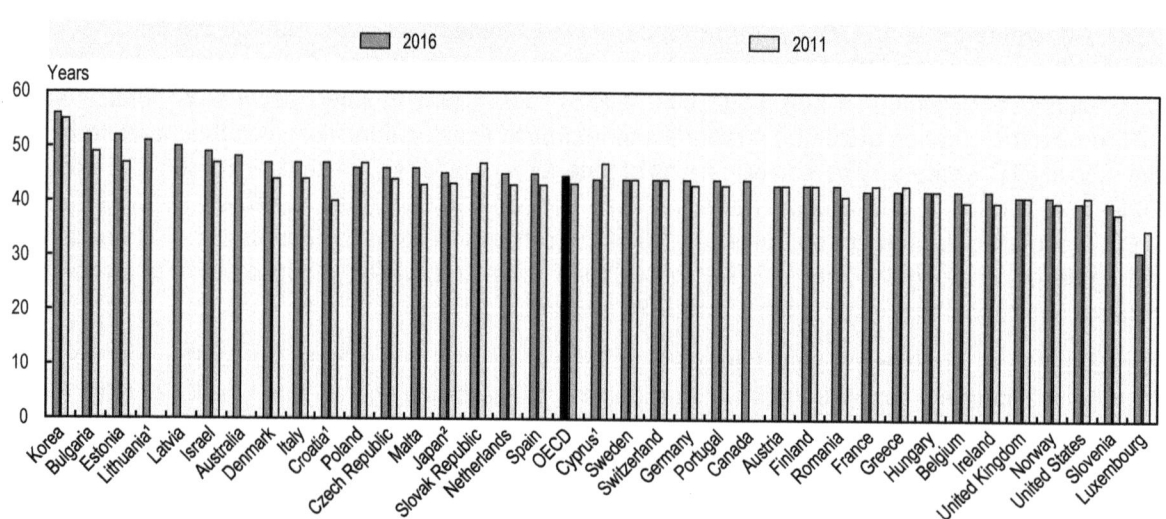

Note: The OECD data point is the unweighted average of the 30 OECD countries shown in the chart. For European countries, LTC workforce supply covers nurses and personal workers who do not work in hospital and education.
1. Data must be interpreted with caution as sample sizes are small. 2. Data refer to the average.
Source: EU-Labour Force Survey; ASEC-CPS for the United States; National Health Insurance System for Korea; Census 2016 for Canada; Labour Force Survey for Israel, Survey on Long-term Care Workers 2016 for Japan; OECD estimate based on national source for Australia. Data refer to 2011 and 2016 or nearest year.

The two main age-related issues in the LTC workforce are that attracting young workers is difficult and retaining workers aged 50+ is challenging. Indeed, young female workers tend to be attracted by sectors that have a better image than LTC, such as childcare or hospital care. Moreover, the oldest workers are likely to experience health issues (such as back problems) and can face increasing difficulties with carrying out LTC tasks like transporting and moving elderly people; this reduces the probability of staying into the workforce after a certain age. Micro-econometric analyses confirm the difficulty of attracting young and old workers into the LTC workforce. Indeed, Box 2.2 shows that middle-aged LTC workers are those who work the longest in the United States (working hours and tenure) and in the United Kingdom (working hours).

Box 2.2. Engagement in the LTC workforce varies across the life cycle

Micro-econometric analyses suggest the presence of a non-linear association between age and LTC workforce participation; they confirm that middle-aged workers produce the highest volume of care and have greater retention rates (Table 2.3). Results are estimated using regressions that included variables on age, age-squared, education categories (low vs. medium, low vs. high), foreign-born status (yes vs. no), number of children (0 vs. 1, 0 vs. 2, 0 vs. 3 and 0 vs. 4+), gender, ethnicity (white vs. other) and year dummies. In the model exploring the correlation between age and hours worked per week, the dependent variable is log-transformed. The two other models are linear probability models.

- In the United Kingdom, working time per week is highest when LTC workers reach 34 years of age, and the probability of working full time reaches its maximum value at 35. However, older people are more likely to have longer tenure: having at least two consecutive years of tenure increases as age increases.
- In the United States, the number of hours provided by LTC workers is highest at 46 years of age, and the probability of being employed full time is at the maximum at 43. The probability of staying at least two consecutive years in the LTC workforce is highest when workers are 51 years old.

Table 2.3. Age at which LTC work participation is highest

Results from multivariate analyses – estimations from samples of LTC workers

	Age at which most hours worked per week	Age with highest probability of full-time work	Age with highest likelihood of 1+ year tenure
United Kingdom	34	35	n.s.
United States	46	43	51

Note: n.s. = non-significant (10% level threshold). In the United States, tenure regressions estimate the probability of staying two consecutive years in the LTC workforce, while in the United Kingdom, tenure regressions estimate the probability of staying two consecutive years with the same employer. All regressions for the United Kingdom control for a dichotomous variable describing whether the worker lives in Great Britain or in Northern Ireland. All regressions for the United States control for state-level fixed effects.
Source: Pooled cross-sections of UK Labour Force Survey (UK-LFS) (2012 to 2016) and ASEC-CPS (2012 to 2016).

Women represent more than 90% of the LTC workforce (Figure 2.5). The overwhelming participation of women in the LTC workforce was observed in 2011 (Colombo et al., 2011[1]). LTC jobs are traditionally considered to be feminine and, while this perception may be changing slowly, stigma is still attached to men performing them. This large share of women among LTC workers contrasts with the share of women in more skilled health occupations such as physicians, where under half are female across OECD countries.

Figure 2.5. Women represent the overwhelming majority of LTC workers in all countries

Share of women in the LTC workforce, 2016 (or nearest year)

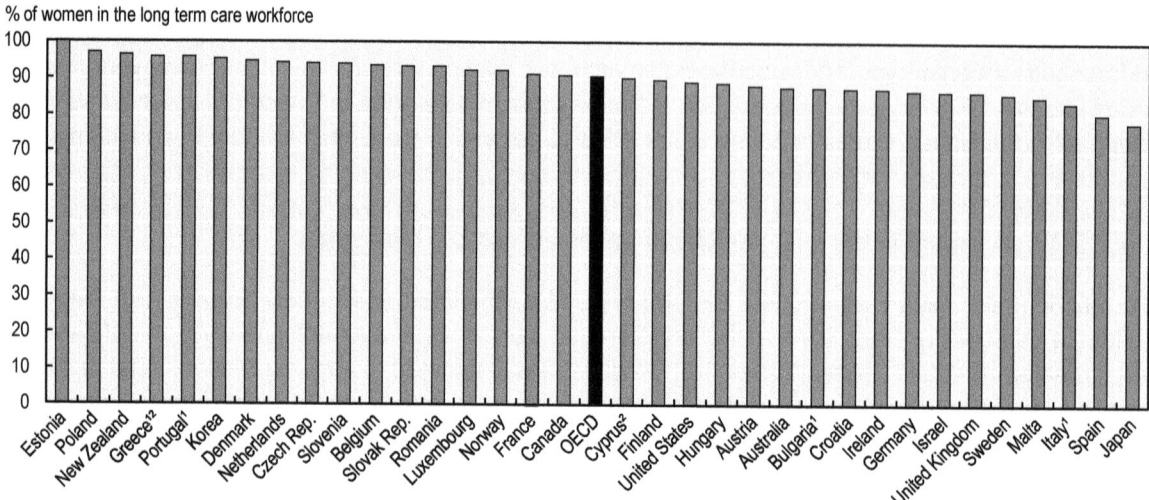

Note: The OECD data point is the unweighted average of the 29 OECD countries shown in the chart. EU-Labour Force Survey data are based on ISCO 4-digit and NACE 2-digit codes.
1. LTC workforce supply data are based on ISCO 3-digit and NACE 2-digit codes. 2. Data must be interpreted with caution as sample sizes are small.
Source: EU-Labour Force Survey; OECD Health Statistics 2018, https://doi.org/10.1787/health-data-en; Survey on Long-term Care Workers 2016 for Japan; OECD estimates based on national sources for Australia and New Zealand. Data refer to 2016 or nearest year.

2.3.2. Foreign-born workers represent an important proportion of LTC workers in some countries

On average, the share of foreign-born workers in LTC represents twice the overall share of foreign-born in the total population. The share in the LTC workforce is highest in Israel (71%), Ireland (48%), Canada (34%), Switzerland (31%) and Australia (29%) (Figure 2.6). In these countries, foreign-born people represent over 20% of the population. However, countries where the foreign-born population is high do not necessarily have the largest share of foreign-born workers in LTC.

The importance of foreign-born workers in the LTC workforce is more limited in the Netherlands and some Nordic countries (Finland, Denmark and Norway) compared to continental and southern European countries and the United Kingdom. These data are consistent with earlier evidence (Da Roit and van Bochove, 2015[35]).

While cross-country variation is often related to the overall share of foreign-born people in the population, foreign-born workers tend to be over-represented in the LTC sector in OECD countries: over 20% of carers in the LTC sector are foreign-born across OECD countries, a share relatively higher than across workers all sectors. This share is especially large in some countries such as Israel, Canada and Ireland. This may be the result of specific migration policies (as in Israel) or of a lack of opportunities in other sectors. It can also reflect the degree of institutionalisation of the LTC system (such as in Belgium). At the same time, these statistics often fail to include live-in home care work, where foreign-born workers might be over-represented in some countries (such as Italy and Spain).

Figure 2.6. Over 20% of LTC workers are foreign-born in OECD countries

Share of foreign-born among the LTC workforce, 2015 (or nearest year)

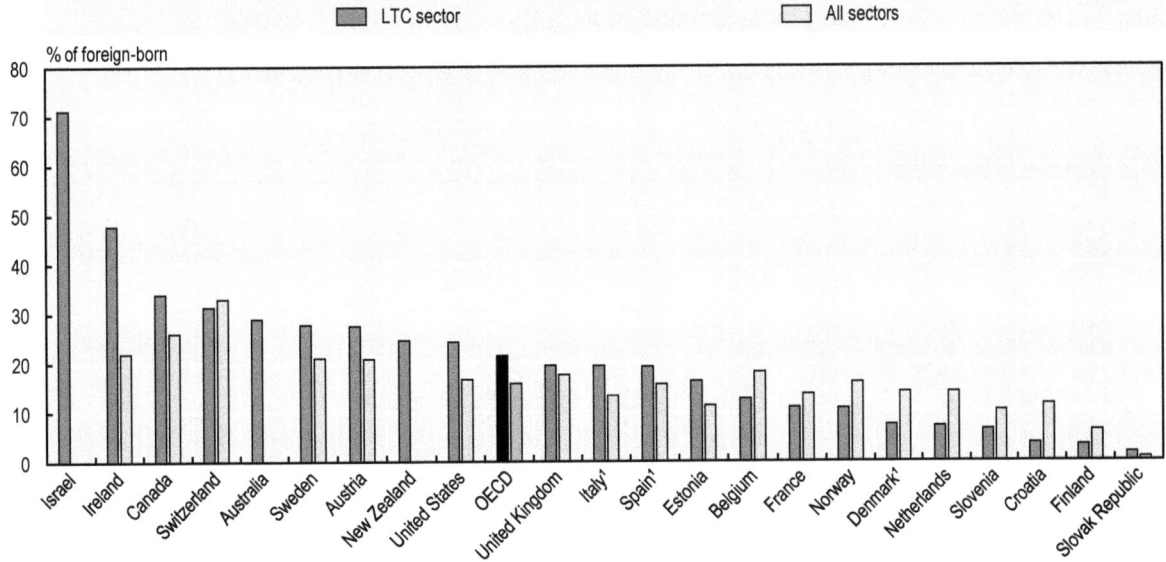

Note: The OECD data point is the unweighted average of the 21 OECD countries shown in the chart for which data are available about the LTC sector and across all sectors. EU-Labour Force Survey data are based on ISCO 4-digit and NACE 2-digit codes.
1. Data are based on ISCO 3-digit and NACE 2-digit codes. 2. Data must be interpreted with caution as sample sizes are small.
Source: EU-Labour Force Survey; ASEC-CPS for the United States; Census 2016 for Canada; LFS for Israel; OECD estimates based on national sources for Australia and New Zealand. Data refer to 2015 or nearest year.

The size of the foreign-born workforce varies little across LTC professions. In Belgium and in the United States, the share of foreign-born workers is slightly larger among personal care workers than among nurses; in other countries, proportions are about the same for both (they represent over 20% in Ireland, and Austria). In Germany, currently around 11% of nurses are foreign-born, a share that has risen from 7% in 2013.

In most European countries, the share of foreign-born workers is greater among institution-based providers than among home-based care providers. In the United States, more foreign-born workers are in home-based care than in institutions; similarly, in Australia, 32% of institution-based workers are migrants, while the share is 23% among home-based workers (Mavromaras et al., 2017[24]). At the same time, in several countries in southern Europe and in the Netherlands there is a grey market for live-in home care workers with a high incidence of foreign-born workers (Da Roit and van Bochove, 2015[35]).

Foreign-born LTC workers are often young and usually highly skilled (nurses in their home country). They have often migrated because of the geographical proximity, language, culture and wealth of the host country, and usually come to the host country to work at a lower level than the one for which they are qualified (Colombo et al., 2011[1]). The overqualification of foreign-born workers has been documented in recent work for countries like Canada, Spain, the United Kingdom and the United States (The Global Ageing Network Leading Age LTSS Center@UMass, 2018[36]). In most European countries, the share of migrants reporting that they are overqualified for the work they do is greater in the LTC sector than any other (see Figure 2.7).

LTC workers follow the common migration routes between lower- and higher-income countries (Luppi et al., 2014[37]). Several countries are primarily sources of outflows: the Philippines, India, Mexico, Romania, Poland, Bulgaria, Nigeria, Kenya and Liberia. Among these, the Philippines, Mexico, Romania, Poland and Bulgaria were in the top 20 countries of origin of new immigrants to OECD countries in 2015

(OECD, 2017[38]), and a proportion of these flows were driven by demand for LTC workers. Figure 2.8 shows the distribution of workers across continents.

Figure 2.7. Migrants report being overqualified more frequently in the LTC sector

Proportion of overqualified workers among the migrants in LTC and women across sectors, 2013

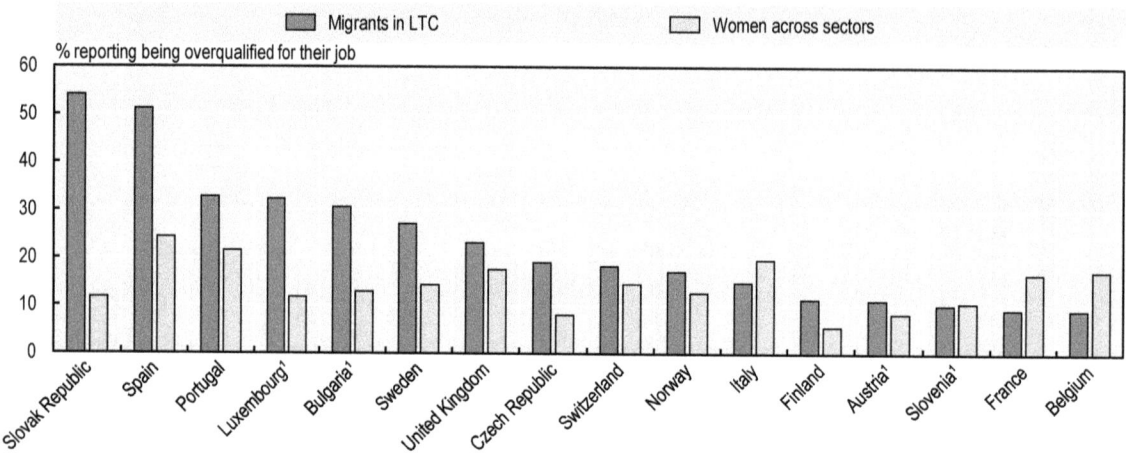

Note: EU-Labour Force Survey data were calculated based on ISCO 3-digit and NACE 2-digit codes.
1. Data on migrants must be interpreted with caution as sample sizes are small.
Source: Ad hoc module EU-Labour Force Survey for data on migrants; OECD Statistics 2019 for data on the female general population (data refer to 2013).

Figure 2.8. Foreign-born workers' regions of origin vary widely

Composition of the foreign-born LTC workforce, by world region of birth, 2015 (or nearest year)

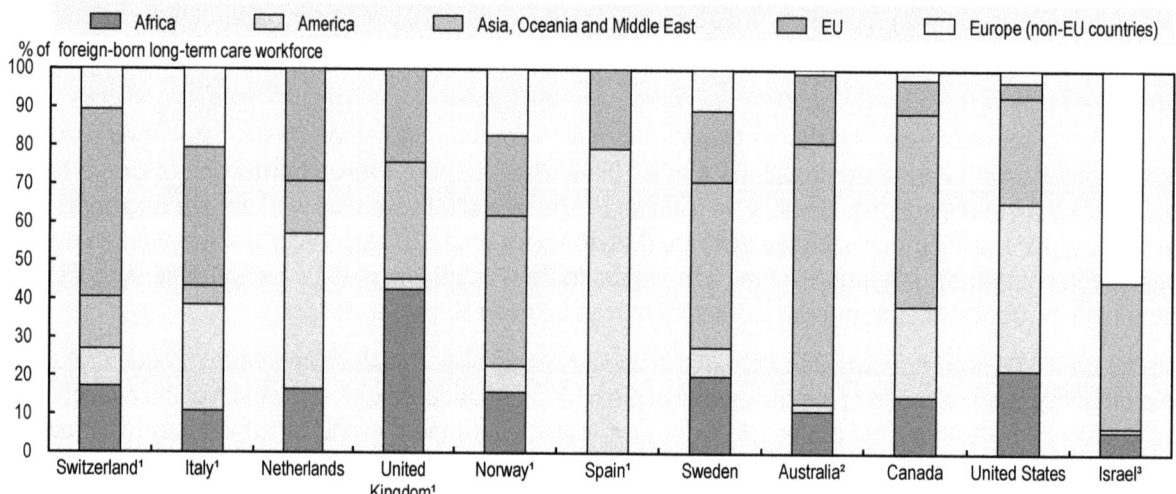

Note: Data were calculated based on ISCO 3-digit and NACE 2-digit codes. Countries of birth were grouped by localisation and, for European countries, membership of the EU: Africa, America, EU, Europe (non-EU) and lastly Asia, Oceania and Middle East.
1. Data must be interpreted with caution as sample sizes are small. 2. Australia's data cover only nurses in residential health care. 3. The white category for Israel refers to European countries (EU and non-EU countries) and America and Oceania are grouped together (in light grey), as Asia and Middle East (in light blue).
Source: EU-Labour Force Survey; ASEC-CPS for the United States; Census 2016 for Canada; Labour Force Survey for Israel. Data refer to 2015 or nearest year.

Micro-econometric analyses suggest that foreign-born workers are important LTC workforce contributors. In both the United States and the United Kingdom, they work more hours and tend to have higher retention rates than natives (Box 2.3).

> ### Box 2.3. Foreign-born workers tend to work more than natives
>
> Micro-econometric analyses in the United States and the United Kingdom suggest that foreign-born carers work generally more than natives. Results were estimated using regressions that include variables on age, age-squared, education categories (low vs. medium, low vs. high), foreign-born status (yes vs. no), number of children (0 vs. 1, 0 vs. 2, 0 vs. 3 and 0 vs. 4+), gender, ethnicity (white vs. other), and year dummies. In the model exploring the correlation between age and hours worked per week, the dependent variable was log-transformed. The two other models were linear probability models.
>
> On average, foreign-born care providers work more hours than natives: 14.7% more in the United States and 15.2% more in the United Kingdom (Table 2.4). They have higher chances of working full time than native workers: 4.6 percentage points higher in the United States, and 13.4 percentage points higher in the United Kingdom. In the United States, the probability of having more than one year of tenure is 2.3 percentage points higher among foreign-born workers than among natives.
>
> #### Table 2.4. Foreign-born workers are more likely to work more hours and stay longer in the LTC sector
>
> Results from multivariate analyses, estimations from samples of LTC workers
>
> | | United States | United Kingdom |
> |---|---|---|
> | Hours of care provided by week (logged) | 0.147*** (0.027) | 0.152*** (0.041) |
> | Probability of working full time | 0.046*** (0.011) | 0.134*** (0.038) |
> | Probability of staying at least two consecutive years | 0.023** (0.010) | 0.005 (0.033) |
>
> Note: * $p<0.10$, ** $p<0.05$, *** $p<0.01$. Robust standard errors are in parentheses. In the United States, regressions estimate the probability of staying two consecutive years in the LTC workforce, while in the United Kingdom, regressions estimate the probability of staying two consecutive years with the same employer. All regressions for the United Kingdom control for a dichotomous variable describing whether the worker lives in Great Britain or in Northern Ireland. All regressions for the United States control for state-level fixed effects.
> Source: Pooled cross-sections of UK-LFS (2012 to 2016) and ASEC-CPS (2012 to 2016).

Immigrant workers are more likely to accept difficult working conditions than native workers. Research (Borjas, 2017[39]) has shown lower wage sensitivity among immigrant LTC workers, especially among undocumented immigrants.

2.4. Policies have been implemented to attract more people into LTC careers

2.4.1. Finding workers with adequate skills is challenging

Countries are struggling to find skilled and motivated LTC workers (Figure 2.9). Indeed, the reservoir of suitable workers is small, and the attractiveness of the LTC sector is low.

Figure 2.9. In most surveyed countries, the policy challenge associated with recruitment of new LTC workers is high

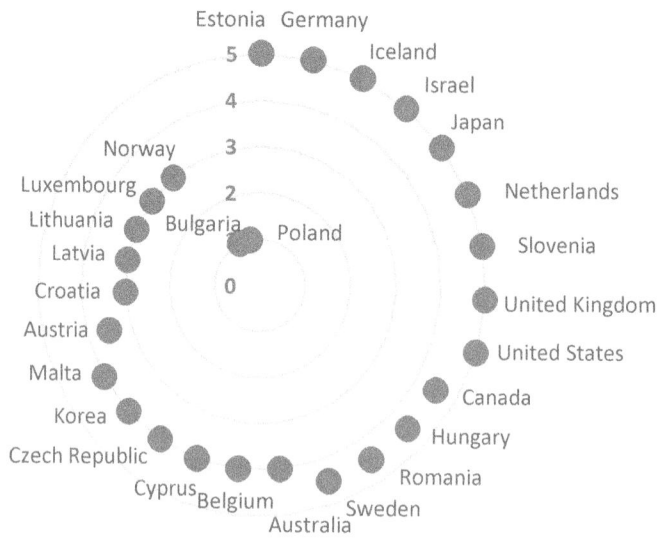

Note: Countries answered the following question: "On a scale between 1 (low-level) and 5 (high-level), what is the challenge faced to recruit new LTC workers in your country?".
Source: OECD LTC workforce survey (2018) – see Annex 2.A for a description.

Countries experience two main issues with finding new LTC workers. First, it is difficult to find candidates interested in applying for LTC job openings. In Australia, for instance, 37% of vacancies for personal carers were not filled because nobody applied for them (Australian Government, 2017[40]). Second, employers do not always find suitable profiles among the few applicants. In the reduced pool of candidates applying for a job in LTC, some cannot be recruited because they lack basic skills, qualifications and experience. In the Netherlands, municipalities have noted that they face issues recruiting workers with sufficient competencies. In Australia, these issues are mentioned in 85% of unfilled vacancies for personal care worker jobs (Australian Government, 2017[40]). In France, 41.1% of institutions for disabled elders (EHPADs) and 33.3% of long-stay facilities declared that they faced recruitment issues in 2015. In addition, 63% of institutions reported having LTC job vacancies for more than six months (Muller, 2017[14]) (Bazin and Muller, 2018[41]). In the United States, where the recruitment challenge is high, 10% of openings for nurse practitioners and physician assistants were focused on care for older people and/or people with disabilities (Himmerick et al., 2017[42]).

To find new sources of workers, countries have focused on four main policies. Several countries have targeted recruitment of workers from the traditional pool (students of health or social care or former LTC workers). Some countries have tried to improve the image of the sector, especially to attract more students of nursing or social care. Others have tried to recruit outside the traditional pool by targeting men, unemployed people or those looking for a career change. Finally, increasing the recruitment of foreign-born workers is another strategy (Colombo and Muir, 2015[43]; Fujisawa and Colombo, 2009[44]). However, only half of countries have implemented policies or reforms in any of these directions since 2011[1] (Table 2.5).

Table 2.5. Many countries implemented recruitment measures targeting underrepresented profiles of workers

Measure	Countries implementing the measure
Recruiting from the traditional pool (making sure people return to the sector), with "Get back to work" initiatives	Australia, Estonia, Germany, Japan, Netherlands, Norway, Romania, United Kingdom
Improving image of LTC jobs with Proud to Care and Care Ambassadors initiatives	Australia, Belgium, Netherlands, Portugal, United Kingdom
Providing financial support and perseverance grants for LTC education to train unemployed people or caregivers willing to get licences or certification	Cyprus, Germany, Israel, Japan, Netherlands, Romania, United States
Targeting the recruitment of men into the LTC workforce	Germany, Norway, United Kingdom, Hungary

Source: OECD LTC workforce survey 2018.

2.4.2. Some countries are targeting recruitment from the traditional pool

Since 2011, some countries have been implementing measures to increase students' exposure to LTC practice. Strategies include offering placement opportunities to nurse students and personal care workers during their studies. In Germany, successful LTC employers report that they are able retain nurse students during their time in placements by providing professional mentoring and encouraging their academic progress. Such companies create a strong link with vocational training institutes to attract and retain students. The US Bureau of Health Workforce initiated the Geriatric Workforce Enhancement Program in 2015, providing funding to 44 communities in 29 states to develop new curricula and geriatric care experience and involving collaborations between various professions and partners (Spetz and Dudley, 2019[45]). Similarly, in its Aged Care Workforce Strategy 2018, Australia is exploring the potential for the introduction of a retention strategy to offer LTC placements to nurse students.

In addition to raising students' interest in LTC careers, these measures also have the advantage of providing them with basic experience, which may ease their entry into the job market. Indeed, young graduates can sometimes face issues finding jobs in the LTC sector because employers may require some minimum experience. In the United States, for example, half of the job openings for nurse practitioners and physician assistants for elderly people required at least one year of experience, reducing opportunities for new graduates (Himmerick et al., 2017[42]).

A second set of measures aims to recruit workers from the traditional pool who have left the LTC workforce. Although not specifically focused on LTC, Estonia implemented the Nurse Back to Health Care Programme for nurses working in other fields to return to health care. Germany launched Concerted Action on Nursing in 2018, involving employers and job centres, which seeks to promote retraining into the profession using full-time funding for professional training courses. Low wages and benefits often represent a barrier to recruitment of these workers. For instance, in the United Kingdom, urban LTC agencies often face issues attracting workers who cannot afford housing costs in urban locations, and therefore face significant work-travelling distances (Moriarty, Manthorpe and Harris, 2018[46]). While some employers provide access to short-term accommodation for newly appointed employees, long-term housing solutions are often needed to facilitate the recruitment of new LTC workers. Wage issues are further discussed in Chapter 4.

2.4.3. Work is under way to improve the image of LTC work

LTC jobs suffer from a lack of status and recognition. The poor image of LTC is an important barrier to recruitment, especially for young people who tend to stigmatise LTC professions as low- or unskilled, and men who may traditionally regard LTC jobs as "women's work". Several countries have implemented advertisement campaigns to change the mindset on LTC by presenting a positive side of ageing and promoting the good aspects of LTC careers. Image campaigns can also be used to promote "values-based recruitment": they underline important values needed to work in LTC, such as empathy, and highlight workers' capacity to make a difference on small things. They show a more positive and joyful side of LTC and emphasise its key contribution to the society. In France, the Caisse nationale de solidarité pour l'autonomie (CNSA) launched a TV campaign in 2018, showing the positive aspects of LTC provision in a short cartoon, which involved male characters as care providers. While their true impact on the public is difficult to assess (Colombo et al., 2011[1]), image campaigns are not necessarily expensive. Specifically, social media represents interesting ways of reaching a broader audience at low cost.

Objectives of such campaigns are not only to encourage students to choose LTC as a profession but also to encourage job changers to stay in LTC. Australia is working to introduce a social change campaign to reframe caring and promote the workforce. Similarly, in Belgium (Flanders), two campaigns called Normale Helden and Proud to Care started in 2018 to improve the image of the LTC sector among young workers. In the United Kingdom, additional approaches include the development of outward-facing activities to improve the public understanding of LTC work (such as the Proud to Care initiative) and the improvement of information among those who provide social care career advices (teachers, staff in job centres etc.), with initiatives such as the Care Ambassadors, who visit schools and job centres to talk about their jobs. In the Czech Republic, the Ministry of Labour and Social Affairs regularly patronises events aimed at rewarding workers in social services, such as the Caregiver of the Year Award.

Some countries promote local/regional initiatives. In the Netherlands, regional agencies have implemented various campaigns (including Ambassadors, We have Something for You, Care Xperience and Open Days) to promote a better image of LTC and attract students by providing short lectures and training sessions, focusing on a regional labour market policy. Regional employers' organisations also co-operate with educators and care providers. In Portugal, a few local programmes – with the support of municipalities – have been established to promote a positive image of the LTC workforce.

2.4.4. Initiatives have been created to retrain unemployed people

One of the main avenues used to increase recruitment in LTC has been to target unemployed people and widen the pool of new applicants. These initiatives can require co-ordination of action by several stakeholders: governments providing funding for training, vocational schools organising training, job centres and employers. Agreements between employers, schools and job centres can also facilitate sharing of existing networks, databases and resources to target potential candidates for these programmes. For instance, a council-run Learning to be Job Ready pilot project aimed to attract unemployed people back into work in the north-east of England, targeting those who might be interested by using data on prior course attendance at local colleges and offering a six-month paid placement and four weeks of training (Bennett, 2011[47]).

Since 2011, a few countries have implemented strategies to offer unemployed people job opportunities in LTC. Examples include the Job Winner (Norway) and We have Something for You (Netherlands) campaigns. As LTC is mostly a low-skilled sector, these have been opened to a large pool of applicants, including former LTC staff and unemployed people without a care background. Japan has introduced basic LTC training courses targeting middle-aged and older workers to prepare themselves to return to work after a long break, and provides support for beginners to take LTC training courses. This led to an increase of 320 000 in the number of LTC workers between 2011 and 2015 and contributed to the acceleration of growth in the number of new workers in the LTC market. In Cyprus, since 2014, there has been a co-ordinated attempt to provide better training programmes to attract unemployed people into LTC. This initiative is co-ordinated by two public entities: the Ministry of Labour, Welfare and Social Insurance (in charge of LTC staff competencies qualification) and the Human Resource Development Authority. In Hungary, similar schemes were launched to provide education, training and employment in LTC to unemployed Roma women.

2.4.5. Policies to attract men into LTC careers could increase worker supply

The objective to widen participation in the LTC workforce could also be reached through action targeting the recruitment of men. Bringing more men into the LTC workforce represents a promising policy option to improve supply: empirical analyses suggest that once recruited into the LTC workforce, they have higher engagement than women (see Box 2.4).

Only a few countries (Norway, the United Kingdom and Germany) reported that they have implemented specific programmes to target the recruitment of men since 2011. The Norwegian Men in Health Recruitment Programme was instigated to recruit (unemployed) men aged 26-55 years to the health and care sector. It entails eight weeks of guided training as health recruits in a regional health institution or health care service. The Programme has been very effective in the Norwegian context to motivate men for a job in LTC. In the United Kingdom, Skills for Care commissioned the Men into Care Programme to attract more men into the LTC workforce. One of the main goals of Germany's Concerted Action on Nursing is to make nursing work more attractive to both women and men.

Box 2.4. Compared to women, men are more likely to work longer hours

Micro-econometric analyses in the United States and the United Kingdom suggest that when they participate in the LTC workforce, men tend to work a greater number of hours than women (Table 2.6). Results were estimated using regressions that included variables on age, age-squared, education categories (low vs. medium, low vs. high), foreign-born status (yes vs. no), number of children (0 vs. 1, 0 vs. 2, 0 vs. 3 and 0 vs. 4+), gender, ethnicity (white vs. other), and year dummies. In the model exploring the correlation between age and hours worked per week, the dependent variable was log-transformed. The two other models were linear probability models.

Men work on average 14.6% more hours than women in the United States and 15.2% more in the United Kingdom. Moreover, men have a higher probability of working full time than women: 18 percentage points higher in the United Kingdom and 8 percentage points higher in the United States. These results suggest that men may represent a promising source of potential LTC workers.

Table 2.6. Men tend to work more than women once in the LTC workforce

Results from multivariate analyses, estimations from samples of LTC workers

	United States	United Kingdom
Hours of care provided per week (men compared to women)	0.146*** (0.038)	0.152*** (0.027)
Probability of working full time (men compared to women)	0.080*** (0.0143)	0.180*** (0.0277)
Probability of staying 2 consecutive years (men compared to women)	0.000 (0.014)	0.008 (0.026)

Note: * $p<0.10$, ** $p<0.05$, *** $p<0.01$. Robust standard errors are in parenthesis. In the United States, regressions estimate the probability of staying two consecutive years in the LTC workforce, while in the United Kingdom, regressions estimate the probability of staying two consecutive years with the same employer. All regressions for the United Kingdom control for a dichotomous variable describing whether the worker lives in Great Britain or in Northern Ireland. All regressions for the United States control for state-level fixed effects.
Source: Pooled cross-sections of UK-LFS (2012 to 2016) and ASEC-CPS (2012 to 2016).

2.4.6. Encouraging the hiring of foreign-born workers

2.4.6.1. Recruiting foreign-born workers via labour migration channels is rare

While LTC has started to appear in debates over migration policy in many OECD countries, introducing or expanding labour migration channels to attract more foreign workers from abroad is not a strategy pursued in most countries. Recruitment from abroad is a potential response to cover the unmet needs of OECD countries' ageing populations, but the presence of foreign workers in this sector is uneven across OECD countries, and most countries do not have specific labour migration channels into LTC. Most recruitment of foreign-born LTC workers draws on the pool of people who have arrived through non-economic migration channels, such as family reunification, student visas, general migration channels for low-skilled workers and international protection (Fujisawa and Colombo, 2009[44]; Cangiano, 2014[48]). For instance, a study among Filipino health care aides in Canada (Winnipeg) showed that they often are recruited locally through informal networks within migrant communities (Novek, 2013[49]). In the United Kingdom, recruitment of foreign-born carers for older adults is mainly explained by the difficulty of hiring native-born workers, and often relies on use of regional/local advertising, informal networks and recruitment agencies (Cangiano and Walsh, 2014[50]).

Registered nurses are generally eligible for labour migration programmes. A number of countries have general programmes for nurses, who might come into LTC or other sectors. For instance, Australia includes registered nurses in its skilled migration programme, which includes a list of occupations for which either the short-term or medium/long-term demand cannot be met by the local market. In Germany, where nurses are eligible for recruitment, a discussion is under way about how to attract more foreign workers, and a dedicated working group is preparing an action plan under the Concerted Action. The Federal Employment Agency has tried to attract workers from other EU countries, in particular southern European countries, which is facilitated as these workers are not subject to labour migration regimes but enjoy free movement. In addition, a programme called Triple Win has been introduced with Serbia, Bosnia, the Philippines and Tunisia, together with Deutsche Gesellschaft für Internationale Zusammenarbeit (GIZ), for the placement of nurses, leading to 1 000 nurse placements since 2017. Another programme includes training and recruitment of foreign nurses in Vietnam, through which nurses complete their Vietnamese degree and take a full year of German language courses provided by Goethe Institute in Vietnam before coming to Germany. They complete a shorter training course of up to two years on arrival, which includes theoretical and practical aspects and additional language courses. After getting the German degree, they need to work in the care sector for three years to obtain a permanent residence permit. The programme has been successful and the nurse trainees have remained with the participating firms. At the same time, it remains limited in size, with only 150 nurses trained so far since 2013.

Recruitment from abroad of LTC workers who are *not* nurses may not be possible in countries where qualification requirements are in place for labour migrants, or where their salary is below the threshold. Where such recruitment is allowed, it is mostly under general procedures, although a few countries have specific measures. In several European countries (France, Spain, Portugal, Italy and Finland), recruitment from abroad for LTC is exempt from a labour market test if it appears on the list of occupations for which there are labour market shortages. Specific measures for LTC exist in Canada, through caregiver schemes (the cancelled Live-in Care Programme and its replacement pilot programmes), and in Israel through the LTC sector visa. The Canadian programme has been in place in one form or another since 1992 and requires workers to stay in LTC employment for a specific period of time to apply for permanent residence. In 2019, Canada launched the Home Support Worker Pilot, which provides caregivers the ability to change jobs and bring their family members, unlike the previous programme. The Israeli care worker permit is a temporary programme with a maximum stay, is uncapped and has led to a steady increase of foreign LTC workers (up to 70% from 10% of workers in 1990). In 2018, 54 000 temporary foreign workers were legally employed in live-in care in Israel.

2.4.6.2. Dealing with workplace discrimination

Several issues are associated with the recruitment of foreign personal care workers. Some are specific to labour migration channels. When individuals or families are the employer (or sponsor), international recruitment, even when allowed, may be problematic. It can difficult to match supply to demand and choose workers with sufficient skills. There is also the issue of the visa and work permit processing time, which does not always meet the urgency of the demand (home care needs often arise after a fall or an emergency). More generally, some people may be reluctant to receive LTC provided by a foreign-born personal care worker, whether resident or recruited from abroad. In particular, ethnic or religious discrimination might be an issue for older people in some countries.

Given that migrants will probably play a bigger role in the future of the LTC workforce, several actions should be implemented to ensure that beneficiaries accept immigrant care suppliers who are entitled to work in the sector. Potential strategies could consist of implementing training and coaching programmes to improve immigrant personal care workers' communication skills, to educate clients and co-workers in a zero-tolerance policy towards racism and to develop training on the local cultural environment and care delivery.

In some cases, agency mediation can represent a solution. However, it can also bring additional risks. Agencies should be in charge of guaranteeing that workers satisfy training and certification requirements. While they have the capacity to identify new candidates and facilitate their access to training and education, they are often unregulated, which may raise concerns (The Global Ageing Network Leading Age LTSS Center@UMass, 2018[36]). Agency fees can be high, and the recruitment process is not always transparent, especially when agencies do not involve LTC providers in the selection process. Concerns are high for personal care workers and home-based workers.

Another issue relates to the fact that immigrant personal care workers are at higher risk of illegal employment. It is likely that foreign-born workers are over-represented in the grey market. A large proportion are likely to face difficult labour conditions. In countries where LTC subsidies are provided through cash benefits, they may face lower salaries and benefits, lower job stability and very difficult working conditions (such as unpaid extra hours). For instance, this is the case in Italy, where cash purchases of LTC services are common and seem to have fuelled the use of services from low-paid immigrant women (OECD, 2014[51]). Therefore, policies should enhance protection of workers who rely on their sponsor for visas or social benefits, increase awareness about foreign-born workers' legal rights and be proactive in the defence of these rights (for instance, by sending warning letters when encountering an issue).

Improving education and training access for foreign-born workers is central. While not specifically targeting LTC workers, some countries (Japan, Canada) have implemented initiatives to encourage foreign-born workers to get training and certification. The Japanese government introduced economic partnership agreements, through which candidates for certified care workers from three countries can get a visa for a total duration of stay of four years. Their period of stay can be extended for a year under certain conditions and, if they pass the national caregiver examination, it can be renewed without restriction. In Canada, the Prior Learning Assessment and Recognition Process improves immigrants' employability and facilitates their entry into post-secondary education institutions. It allows recognition of the international credentials of immigrants willing to work in health occupations. The programme involves post-secondary education institutions, provincial governments, professional self-regulating bodies and employers.

2.5. Conclusion

This chapter shows that, despite the large increase in LTC service demand, the size, structure and characteristics of the LTC workforce have not changed much since the publication of *Help Wanted? Providing and Paying for Long-Term Care* in 2011 (Colombo et al., 2011[1]). Indeed, the LTC sector is mainly composed of middle-aged women, who mostly work as personal care providers in institutions. Data also reveal the urgency of increasing the size of the LTC workforce in many OECD countries. In 2011, the OECD estimated that the size of the LTC workforce would have to double in order to meet the increase in demand (Colombo et al., 2011[1]). Recent data show that there is still a long way to go to meet this objective. The situation is not uniform across OECD countries, however. International comparisons reveal that Nordic countries (Sweden, Denmark, Norway and Finland) and Japan have successfully enhanced the number of LTC workers over the past ten years. Other countries urgently need to implement reforms to attract new workers into the LTC sector and match growing demand to supply.

Better policies are needed to improve recruitment in the LTC sector. The evidence shows that only a few countries have implemented policies to increase recruitment in LTC. Attracting and training new domestic (currently employed) workers, targeting undersupply by attracting young workers and men to the sector and developing image campaigns are the most prevalent measures. They have a strong potential in terms of effectiveness and magnitude.

This chapter also underlines some forthcoming challenges for organisation of LTC workforce supply. Most countries are implementing a deinstitutionalisation of the LTC workforce by increasing spending on home-based care and reducing spending on institution-based care. While these policies answer elderly people's desire to remain at home as long as possible, their implementation raises new challenges for the LTC market. Specifically, countries need to increase the supply of home-based workers, but must also make sure that nursing homes are prepared to face the associated change in the profile of their residents (who will be more disabled).

References

Allen, S., E. Piette and V. Mor (2014), "The adverse consequences of unmet need among older persons living in the community: dual-eligible versus Medicare-only beneficiaries", *The Journals of Gerontology: Series B*, Vol. Vol. 69/Suppl 1, pp. S51-S58, http://dx.doi.org/10.1093/geronb/gbu124. [30]

Australian Government (2017), *The Labour Market for Personal Care Corkers, in Aged and Disability Care - Australia 2017*, Australian Government Department of Jobs and Small Business, Canberra, https://www.employment.gov.au/newsroom/demand-personal-care-workers-growing. [40]

Bazin, M. and M. Muller (2018), "Le personnel et les difficultés de recrutement dans les Ehpad", *DREES Études et Résultats*, Vol. 1067, https://drees.solidarites-sante.gouv.fr/etudes-et-statistiques/publications/etudes-et-resultats/article/le-personnel-et-les-difficultes-de-recrutement-dans-les-ehpad. [41]

Bennett, A. (2011), "Learning to be job ready: strategies for greater social inclusion in public sector employment", *Journal of Business Ethics*, Vol. 104/3, pp. 347-359, http://dx.doi.org/10.1007/s10551-011-0913-y. [47]

Borjas, G. (2017), "The labor supply of undocumented immigrants", *Labour Economics*, Vol. 46, pp. 1-13, http://dx.doi.org/10.1016/j.labeco.2017.02.004. [39]

Boscart, V. et al. (2018), "The associations between staffing hours and quality of care indicators in long-term care", *BMC Health Services Research*, Vol. 18/1, http://dx.doi.org/10.1186/s12913-018-3552-5. [33]

Bureau of Labor Statistics and U.S. Department of Labor (2015), *Occupational Outlook Handbook: Registered Nurses*, Bureau of Labor Statistics, Washington DC, https://www.bls.gov/ooh/healthcare/registered-nurses.htm. [29]

Cangiano, A. (2014), "Elder care and migrant labor in Europe: a demographic outlook", *Population Development Review*, Vol. 40/1, pp. 1-3-1-1-5-4, https://doi.org/10.1111/j.1728-4457.2014.00653.x. [48]

Cangiano, A. and K. Walsh (2014), "Recruitment processes and immigration regulations: the disjointed pathways to employing migrant carers in ageing societies", *Work, Employment and Society*, Vol. 28/3, pp. 372-389, http://dx.doi.org/10.1177/0950017013491453. [50]

CNSA (2017), *La situation des EHPAD en 2016*, Caisse nationale de solidarité pour l'autonomie, Paris, https://www.cnsa.fr/documentation/cnsa_portrait_ehpad_2017_vf.pdf. [15]

Colombo, F. et al. (2011), *Help Wanted? Providing and Paying for Long-Term Care*, OECD Health Policy Studies, OECD Publishing, Paris, http://dx.doi.org/10.1787/9789264097759-en. [1]

Colombo, F. and T. Muir (2015), "Developing a skilled long-term care workforce", in Cristiano Gori, Jose-Luis Fernandez, A. (ed.), *Long-Term Care Reforms in OECD Countries*, Policy Press, London, http://dx.doi.org/DOI:10.1332/policypress/9781447305057.003.0009. [43]

Da Roit, B. and M. van Bochove (2015), "Migrant care work going Dutch? The emergence of a live-in migrant care market and the restructuring", *Social Policy and Administration*. [35]

de Bienassis, K., A. Llena Nozal and N. Klazinga (forthcoming), "The Economics of Patient Safety Part III: Long-Term Care", *OECD Health Working Papers*, OECD Publishing, Paris. [5]

Do, Y. et al. (2015), "Informal care and caregiver's health", *Health Economics (United Kingdom)*, Vol. 24/2, pp. 224-237, http://dx.doi.org/10.1002/hec.3012. [12]

El Khomri, M. (2019), *Plan national en faveur de l'attractivité des métiers du grand-âge 2020-2024*, Ministère des Solidarités et de la Santé, Paris, https://solidarites-sante.gouv.fr/IMG/pdf/rapport_el_khomri_-_plan_metiers_du_grand_age.pdf. [7]

Freedman, V. and B. Spillman (2014), "Disability and care needs among older Americans", *Milbank Quarterly*, Vol. 92/3, pp. 509-41, http://dx.doi.org/10.1111/1468-0009.12076. [31]

Frogner, B. and J. Spetz (2015), *Entry and Exit of Workers in Long-Term Care*, USCF Health Workforce Research Center on Long-Term Care Frogner, San Francisco, CA, https://healthworkforce.ucsf.edu/sites/healthworkforce.ucsf.edu/files/Report-Entry_and_Exit_of_Workers_in_Long-Term_Care.pdf. [22]

Fujisawa, R. and F. Colombo (2009), "The Long-Term Care Workforce: Overview and Strategies to Adapt Supply to a Growing Demand", *OECD Health Working Papers*, No. 44, OECD Publishing, Paris, https://dx.doi.org/10.1787/225350638472. [44]

Geerts, J. (2011), *The Long-Term Care Workforce: Description And Perspectives*, Centre for European Policy Studies, Brussels, http://www.ancien-longtermcare.eu/sites/default/files/ENEPRIRR93_ANCIENWP3_0.pdf. [20]

Genet, N. et al. (2013), "Home Care Across Europe: Case Studies.", *WHO Regional Office for Europe, Copenhagen*, https://www.nivel.nl/sites/default/files/bestanden/Home-care-across-Europe-case-studies.pdf. [3]

Harrington, C. et al. (2012), "Nursing home staffing standards and staffing levels in six countries", *Journal of Nursing Scholarship*, Vol. 44, pp. 88-98, http://dx.doi.org/10.1111/j.1547-5069.2011.01430.x. [28]

Harrington, C. et al. (2012), "Nursing Home Staffing Standards and Staffing Levels in Six Countries", *Journal of Nursing Scholarship*, Vol. 44/1, pp. 88-98, http://dx.doi.org/10.1111/j.1547-5069.2011.01430.x. [6]

Himmerick, K. et al. (2017), *Employer Demand for Physician Assistants and Nurse Practitioners to Care for Older People and People with Disabilities*, UCSF Health Workforce Research Center on Long-Term Care, San Francisco, CA. [42]

Hogan, D. et al. (2014), "High rates of hospital admission among older residents in assisted living facilities: Opportunities for intervention and impact on acute care", *Open Medicine*, Vol. 8/1, pp. e33-45. [32]

Institute of Medicine (2008), *Retooling for an Aging America: Building the Health Care Workforce*, https://doi.org/10.17226/12089. [21]

Kikuzawa, S. (2015), "Elder care, multiple role involvement, and well-being among middle-aged men and women in Japan", *Journal of Cross-Cultural Gerontology*, Vol. 30/4, pp. 423-438, http://dx.doi.org/10.1007/s10823-015-9273-x. [18]

Kubalčíková, K. and J. Havlíková (2016), "Current developments in social care services for older adults in the Czech Republic: trends towards deinstitutionalization and marketization", *Journal of Social Service Research*, Vol. 42/2, pp. 180-198, http://dx.doi.org/10.1080/01488376.2015.1129014. [10]

Libault, D. (2019), *Concertation: Grand âge et autonomie*, Ministère des Solidarités et de la Santé, Paris, https://solidarites-sante.gouv.fr/IMG/pdf/rapport_grand_age_autonomie.pdf. [25]

Lin, S. et al. (2012), "Trends in US older adult disability: exploring age, period, and cohort effects", *American Journal of Public Health*, Vol. 102/11, pp. 2157-2163, http://dx.doi.org/10.2105/AJPH.2011.300602. [16]

Lin, V., X. Zhang and P. Dixon (2015), "Occupational therapy workforce in the United States: forecasting nationwide shortages", *PM&R: the Journal of Injury, Function, and Rehabilitation*, Vol. 7/9, pp. 946-54, http://dx.doi.org/10.1016/j.pmrj.2015.02.012. [27]

Luppi, M. et al. (2014), *Report on the Legal-sociological Analysis of Discrepancies and Dilemmas in Care Workers' Rights*, Centre for Social Policy and Intervention Studies, Utrecht, https://www.uu.nl/en/research/beucitizen-european-citizenship-research/publications. [37]

Lynn, J. (2013), "Reliable and sustainable comprehensive care for frail elderly people.", *JAMA*, Vol. 310/18, pp. 1935-1936, http://dx.doi.org/10.1001/jama.2013.281923. [17]

Maarse, J. and P. Jeurissen (2016), "The policy and politics of the 2015 long-term care reform in the Netherlands", *Health Policy*, Vol. 120/3, pp. 241-245, http://dx.doi.org/10.1016/j.healthpol.2016.01.014. [9]

Mavromaras, K. et al. (2017), *The Aged Care Workforce, 2016*, Department of Health, Canberra, https://agedcare.health.gov.au/sites/g/files/net1426/f/documents/03_2017/nacwcs_final_report_290317.pdf. [24]

Moriarty, J., J. Manthorpe and J. Harris (2018), *Recruitment and Retention in Adult Social Care Services*, Policy Institute at King's College London, London, https://www.kcl.ac.uk/scwru/pubs/2018/reports/recruitment-and-retention-report.pdf. [46]

Muller, M. (2017), *L'accueil des personnes âgées en établissement : entre progression et diversification de l'offre*, DREES, Paris. [14]

Novek, S. (2013), "Filipino health care aides and the nursing home labour market in Winnipeg", *Canadian Journal on Aging*, Vol. 32/4, pp. 405-416, http://dx.doi.org/10.1017/S071498081300038X. [49]

OECD (2017), *Health at a Glance 2017: OECD Indicators*, OECD Publishing, Paris, http://dx.doi.org/10.1787/health_glance-2017-en. [2]

OECD (2017), *International Migration Outlook 2017*, OECD Publishing, Paris, http://dx.doi.org/10.1787/migr_outlook-2017-en. [38]

OECD (2016), *Health Workforce Policies in OECD Countries: Right Jobs, Right Skills, Right Places*, OECD Health Policy Studies, OECD Publishing, Paris, https://dx.doi.org/10.1787/9789264239517-en. [4]

OECD (2014), *Jobs for Immigrants (Vol. 4): Labour Market Integration in Italy*, OECD Publishing, Paris, https://dx.doi.org/10.1787/9789264214712-en. [51]

Osterman, P. (2017), *Who Will Care for Us? Long-term Care and the Long-term Workforce*, Russell Sage Foundation, New York, http://www.jstor.org/stable/10.7758/9781610448673. [23]

Rapp, T., B. Apouey and C. Senik (2018), "The impact of institution use on the wellbeing of Alzheimer's disease patients and their caregivers", *Social Science and Medicine*, Vol. 207/1-10, http://dx.doi.org/10.1016/j.socscimed.2018.04.014. [19]

Rothgang, H., M. Fünfstück and T. Kalwitzki (2020), "Personalbemessung in der Langzeitpflege", in *Pflege-Report 2019*, Springer Berlin Heidelberg, http://dx.doi.org/10.1007/978-3-662-58935-9_11. [8]

Scheil-Adlung, X. (2015), *Extension of Social Security Long-term care protection for older persons: A review of coverage deficits in 46 countries*, http://www.ilo.org/publns. [34]

Somanathan, A. et al. (2017), *Reducing the Burden of Care in Estonia*, Word Bank Group, Washington DC, http://www.share-estonia.ee/fileadmin/pdffailid/estonia_ltc_report_final.pdf. [13]

Spetz, J. and N. Dudley (2019), "Consensus-Based Recommendations for an Adequate Workforce to Care for People with Serious Illness", *Journal of the American Geriatrics Society*, Vol. 67/S2, pp. S392-S399, http://dx.doi.org/10.1111/jgs.15938. [45]

Stølen, N. and I. Texmon (2010), *Projections of the Norwegian Labour Market for Employees in the Health and Social Sector towards 2030*, Statistics Norway, Oslo. [26]

Sunwoo, D. (2017), *Public Long-Term Care Insurance Program for the Elderly (LTCI)-Performance Evaluation and Policy Implications*, Korea Institute for Health and Social Affairs, Sejong City, http://www.kihasa.re.kr. [11]

The Global Ageing Network Leading Age LTSS Center@UMass (2018), *Filling the Care Gap Integrating Foreign-Born Nurses and Personal Care Assistants into the Field of Long-Term Services and Supports*, The Global Ageing Network, Washington DC, https://leadingage.org/sites/default/files/LA_SodexoReport2018_Digital_r2.pdf. [36]

Annex 2.A. Definitions and data sources

Definitions

This chapter uses OECD's definitions of long-term care (LTC), of the LTC workforce and of LTC settings. The following subsections provide comprehensive descriptions of these definitions, as provided by the OECD Health Statistics 2018.[2]

LTC definition: Health and social care provided for Activities of Daily Living (ADL) and Instrumental Activities of Daily Living (IADL)

LTC is a highly labour-intensive sector, which consists of a range of medical, personal care and assistance services that are provided with the primary goal of alleviating pain and reducing or managing the deterioration in health status for people with a degree of long-term dependency, assisting them with their personal care (through help for ADL, such as eating, washing and dressing) and assisting them to live independently (through help for IADL, such as cooking, shopping and managing finances). As a result, the LTC workforce is its most precious resource.

LTC workforce definition: Nurses and personal care workers

LTC workers are individuals who provide care to LTC recipients at home or in LTC institutions (other than hospitals). Following the OECD definition, formal LTC workers comprise two main professional categories: nurses and personal care workers. The other professional categories are not included in the LTC workforce definition. For instance, the OECD definition does not consider that doctors who work in institutions are LTC workers. LTC workers can come from the health or the social care branch. Their services can be publicly or privately financed.

Nurses include people who have completed their studies/education in nursing and who are licensed to practise (including both professional nurses and associate/practical/vocational nurses); salaried and self-employed nurses delivering services at home or in LTC institutions (other than hospitals); foreign nurses licensed to practise and actively practising in the country; and nurses providing LTC to care recipients affected by dementia and/or Alzheimer's disease.

The following categories of nurses are excluded from the OECD definition (and therefore not covered by the analysis of this chapter): students who have not yet graduated; nursing aides/assistants and care workers who do not have any recognised qualification/certification as licensed nurses; nurses working in administration, research and other posts that exclude direct contact with care recipients; unemployed nurses and retired nurses; nurses working abroad; nurses providing social services; and psychiatric nurses.

Personal care workers include formal workers providing LTC services at home or in institutions (other than hospitals) and who are not qualified or certified as nurses. Personal care workers are defined as people providing routine personal care, such as bathing, dressing or grooming, to elderly, convalescent or disabled people in their own homes or in institutions. They include nursing aides/assistants and care workers providing LTC services, who do not have any recognised qualification/certification in nursing; family members, neighbours or friends employed (i.e. under a formal contractual obligation and/or declared to social security systems as caregiver) by the care recipient or a person/agency representing the care recipient, and/or by public care services and private care service companies, to provide the care services to the person in need.

The following categories of workers are excluded from the OECD definition (and therefore not covered by the analysis of this chapter): informal caregivers, defined as family, friends or neighbours, receiving income support or other cash payments from the care recipient as part of cash programmes and/or consumer-choice programmes, but who are not formally employed, or paid for, by the care recipient (or the person/agency representing the care recipient, including providers/organisations, such as public social care services and private care service companies); unemployed and retired caregivers; caregivers working abroad; caregivers in assessment teams employed to evaluate care needs and other people employed in administrative positions; and social workers/community workers.

LTC settings definition: Home-based and institution-based LTC

Nurses and personal care workers can be either home-based or institution-based. LTC at home is provided to people with functional restrictions who mainly reside in their own homes. It also applies to the use of institutions on a temporary basis to support continued living at home – such as in the case of community care and day care centres and respite care. Home-based LTC also includes specially designed or adapted living arrangements (for instance, sheltered housing) for people who require help on a regular basis while guaranteeing a high degree of autonomy and self-control, and supportive living arrangements. LTC at home is provided to people with functional restrictions who mainly reside in their own homes.

In the OECD definition, LTC institutions refer to nursing and residential care facilities, which provide accommodation and LTC as a package. They refer to specially designed institutions or hospital-like settings where the predominant service component is LTC and the services are provided for people with moderate to severe functional restrictions. LTC institutions include nursing and residential care facilities dedicated to long-term nursing care. LTC facilities comprise establishments primarily engaged in providing residential LTC that combines nursing, supervisory or other types of care, as required by the residents. In these establishments, a significant part of the production process and the care provided is a mix of health and social services, with the health services largely at the level of nursing care, in combination with personal care services. The medical components of care are, however, much less intensive than those provided in hospitals.

According to the OECD definition, institution-based LTC excludes institutions used on a temporary basis to support continued living at home – such as community care, day care centres and respite care. It also excludes LTC services provided in specially designed or adapted living arrangements for people who require help on a regular basis while guaranteeing a high degree of autonomy and self-control (defined as home, and included in the home-based setting). Finally, the definition excludes LTC services provided in hospitals.

Data sources to compare the LTC workforce internationally

Data sources

Given the specificity of the above definition, identifying LTC workers in the LFS is very challenging, which explains why few reports provide international comparisons. Two prior publications offered insights, but faced several data limitations. In *Help Wanted? Providing and Paying for Long-Term Care*, Colombo et. al. (2011[1]) used data collected from a pilot study regrouping several countries, but only focused on five main characteristics: gender, occupation, care setting, country of birth and education. In another report from the ENEPRI European project ANCIEN provided additional information, but only for four countries (Germany, the Netherlands, Spain, and Poland), and were not able to accurately identify LTC workers.

One of the main contributions of this chapter is to provide international comparisons relying on accurate and reliable data. The first source was the OECD Health Statistics Database, which provides data for some relatively basic socio-demographic characteristics of LTC workers. The second main source is labour force surveys (LFSs), because these provide more information on detailed characteristics of the LTC labour force. LFSs are conducted by national statistics institutions (and harmonised by Eurostat for Europe) every year. They supply data on professions, working conditions, unemployment situations, education and socio-demographic characteristics. Further, an ad hoc module each year focuses on a particular topic. The ad hoc module of the LFS on accidents at work and other work-related health problems, for example, is repeated every seven years. Specifically, this chapter uses two main data sources: the March supplements of the Annual Social and Economic Supplement of the Current Population Survey (ASEC-CPS) for the United States and the European Union Labour Force Survey (EU-LFS), which includes Austria, Belgium, Bulgaria, Croatia, Cyprus, the Czech Republic, Denmark, Estonia, Finland, France, Germany, Greece, Hungary, Ireland, Italy, Latvia, Lithuania, Luxembourg, Malta, the Netherlands, Poland, Portugal, Romania, the Slovak Republic, Slovenia, Spain, Sweden and the United Kingdom. Data on earnings came from the Structure of Earnings Survey (SES) for European countries and ASEC-CPS for the United States. As for the EU-LFS, SES are conducted by national statistics institutions and harmonised by Eurostat, but it is run every four years.

For countries not included in these surveys (Australia, Canada, Israel, Japan, Korea and New Zealand), data requests were sent directly to government agencies. Australia's data were based on the Australia Aged Care Workforce 2016 report, published by the Department of Health of the Australian Government. For Canada, the source was the Census survey of 2016. Israel's data were based on their national LFS. For Japan, the source was the survey on Long-term Care Workers Financial Year 2016. Korea's data were from the National Health Insurance Survey (NHIS)'s database for the registry of LTC providers, using the Long Term Care Provider Report for Registration. New Zealand's data were based on the New Zealand Aged Care Workforce, 2016 report, published by the New Zealand Work Research Institute.

These data sources provide comprehensive geographical coverage of high-income countries, as well as a wealth of information on labour and socio-demographic characteristics. In addition, several countries provide micro-level data: the Korean Labour and Income Study, the UK labour force survey (UK-LFS), the ASEC-CPS and the German Socio-economic Panel. However, an accurate and reliable identification of LTC workers in micro-level detail was only possible in the United States, Germany and the United Kingdom surveys. In France, the French survey of long-term care institutions (EHPA: Établissement d'hébergement pour personnes âgées) provided complementary information on the characteristics of the LTC workers.

Methodology to identify LTC workers

This chapter identifies LTC workers by cross-referencing industry codes and occupation codes. While this methodology can be used for international comparisons, caution is needed when interpreting cross-country variations. The tasks undertaken by workers under similar occupation codes may vary from one country to another (this limitation motivated the LTC workforce survey described in Annex 3.A in Chapter 3, which allows more accurate mapping of LTC workers' functions and tasks).

For most European countries, this chapter uses semi-aggregated data obtained from specific extractions sent to Eurostat. The industry code of the EU-LFS is based on the Nomenclature Statistique des Activités Economiques dans la Communauté Européenne (NACE), the industry standard classification system used in the EU. The 2006-07 revision facilitated disentangling of hospital and non-hospital activities. The occupation codes of the EU-LFS are based on the International Standard Classification of Occupations (ISCO), the International Labour Organization classification for organising information on jobs. Note that a revision of ISCO codes in 2011 produced an important methodological break, which prevents any interpretation of time series prior to 2011.

This chapter uses NACE 2-digit and ISCO 4-digit codes, which enables identification of LTC workers with great accuracy. Note that NACE 2-digit and ISCO 3-digit codes were used in some figures when country information on ISCO 4-digits was not available. Annex Table 2.A.1 shows the ISCO codes used to identify nurses (2 221 for professional nurses and 3 221 for associate professional nurses) and personal care workers (5 322 for home-based personal care workers and 5 321 for personal care assistants). The use of NACE 2-digit codes is helpful to exclude hospital-based workers from the population of interest, while ISCO 4-digit codes enable exclusion of workers who are not in the scope of interest (for instance, midwifes, medical imaging assistants or dental assistants) from the definition. NACE code 88 (social work activities without accommodation) identifies home-based care and NACE code 87 (residential care activities) identifies institution care.

Annex Table 2.A.1. Industry and occupation codes for European countries

European countries			
Industry code (NACE)		Occupation code (ISCO)	
At home	Institutions	Nurses	Personal carers
88 Social work activities without accommodation	87 Residential care activities	2221 / 2230 (before 2011) Professional nurses 3221 / 3231 (before 2011) Associate professional nurses	5322 / 5132 (before 2011) Home-based personal care workers 5321 / 5133 (before 2011) Health care assistants

The size of the sample used to compute the semi-aggregated data was small for some countries or some specific characteristics. When small samples questioned the robustness of results, ISCO 3-digit codes were selected, resulting in the inclusion of midwives practising at home. This may have led to a small overestimation of the LTC workforce.

For European countries, NACE codes Q87 and Q88 are used. NACE Q87 describes residential care activities, which include residential nursing care activities; residential care activities for mental retardation, mental health and substance abuse; residential care activities for elderly and disabled people; and other residential care activities. NACE Q88 describes social work activities without accommodation, which include social work activities without accommodation for elderly and disabled people; other social work activities without accommodation; child day care activities; and other social work activities without accommodation. The interaction of ISCO occupation codes with NACE industry codes 87 (residential care activities) and 88 (social work activities without accommodation) is assumed to have led to selection of the subcategories highlighted in bold in Annex Table 2.A.2.

Annex Table 2.A.2. Result of cross-checking for European countries

2221 (Professional nurses)	3221 (associate professional nurses)	5321 (health care assistants)	5322 (home-based personal care workers)
Anaesthetist, nurse	Nurse, assistant	Aide, nursing: clinic	Aide, home care
Consultant, nurse: clinical	Nurse, associate professional	Aide, nursing: hospital	Aide, nursing: home
Educator, nurse	Nurse, enrolled	Aide, psychiatric	Assistant, birth: home
Nurse, anaesthetics	Nurse, practical	Assistant, birth: clinic or hospital	Assistant, day care: aged or disabled people
Nurse, charge	Sister, nursing: associate professional	Assistant, midwifery: clinic or hospital	Assistant, homecare: aged or disabled people
Nurse, professional: obstetrics		Assistant, patient care	Assistant, residential care: aged or disabled people
Nurse, professional: occupational health		Attendant, birth: clinic or hospital	Assistant, respite care
Nurse, professional: paediatric		Attendant, hospital	Attendant, birth: home birth
Nurse, professional: psychiatric		Attendant, midwifery: clinic or hospital	Attendant, midwifery: home birth
Nurse, public health		Attendant, nursing: except home	Attendant, nursing: home
Nurse, registered		Ayah, hospital	Carer, home: aged or disabled people
Nurse, specialist			Carer, respite
Practitioner, clinical nurse			Companion, aged care
Practitioner, nurse			Companion, disabled people
Sister, nursing: professional			Helper, aged care
Sister, operating theatre			Helper, companion
			Helper, home: caring for aged or infirm people
			Provider, personal care
			Worker, home care
			Worker, home support
			Worker, personal care: home
			Worker, respite care

For the United States, the ASEC-CPS data provide sufficient observations and detail to identify LTC workforce characteristics. The industry code uses the North American Industry Classification System (NAICS), while the occupation code is derived from the Standard Occupational Classification (SOC).

As described in Annex Table 2.A.3, NAICS codes 8170 (home health care services) and 9290 (private households health services) identify workers in home-based settings. NAICS codes 8270 (nursing care facilities), and 8290 (residential care facilities without nursing) identify institution-based care. Moreover, SOC codes 3130 (registered nurses) and 3258 (nurse practitioners) identify nurses, and SOC codes 3600 (nursing, psychiatric and home health aides) and 4610 (personal and home care aides) identify personal care workers.

Note that since a change in the nomenclature in 2010, registered nurses since 2011 have included midwifes, leading to an overestimation of the LTC workforce size. However, the importance the overestimation remains small, since the sample is restricted to nursing care facilities and home health care services. Moreover, the proportion of nurses in the US LTC workforce is small (20%).

Annex Table 2.A.3. Industry code and occupation code for the United States

Industry code (NAICS)		Occupation code (SOC)	
At home	Institutions	Nurses	Personal carers
8170 Home health care services 9290 Private household health services	8270 Nursing care facilities 8290 Residential care facility without nursing	3130 Registered nurses 3255 Registered nurses 3258 Nurse practitioners 3500 Licensed practical and licensed vocational nurses	3600 Nursing, psychiatric and home health aides 4610 Personal and home care aides

LTC workforce questionnaire and pilot study

In many OECD countries, the LTC workforce cannot be as clearly identified as the health workforce can. It rather consists of a mix of professions with different levels of training and skills, and different functions. Countries have a wide variety of professions performing different tasks in both social and health care. Social care ranges from improving elderly people's physical and cognitive state to ensuring better quality of life for vulnerable elderly people and those with chronic illnesses. The roles and skills of professions also vary between countries, even for professions with similar names, making it even more difficult to define LTC workers by job title.

To overcome that methodological issue, this chapter uses data from an LTC workforce questionnaire and a pilot study. Twenty-six OECD countries participated in the questionnaire: Australia, Austria, Belgium, Bulgaria, Cyprus, the Czech Republic, Denmark, Estonia, Germany, Hungary, Iceland, Israel, Japan, Korea, Latvia, Lithuania, Luxembourg, Malta, the Netherlands, Norway, Poland, Romania, Slovenia, Sweden, the United Kingdom and the United States. This survey focused on several themes: the different tasks provided by LTC workers, the professions that carry out LTC tasks, opportunities for tasks delegation between professionals, opportunities for career progression and raising status, the specificity of standards and regulations for LTC workers and the initial training and qualification levels in these professions.

The OECD LTC workforce questionnaire was supplemented by findings from a pilot study involving semi-structured interviews and fact-finding missions to five countries: France, Norway, the Netherlands, Germany and Portugal. Data collected from these interviews with key stakeholders reveal issues that quantitative data cannot always show. These countries were selected based on their ability to provide the relevant information, but also because of their specificity. LTC workforce development in Norway and the Netherlands is among the most advanced across OECD countries. Germany and the Netherlands have an LTC insurance system. France and the Netherlands implemented important dependency reforms in 2015 targeting several aspects of elderly care provision. Portugal is one of the European countries where the size of the LTC workforce is the smallest, but where its growth rate is high. In addition, semi-structured interviews were performed during teleconferences with experts from the United States and Australia. All evidence was collected between January 2018 and December 2018.

Notes

[1] This does not include measures improving pay and working conditions, which can also increase LTC workforce supply through retention.

[2] All definitions, sources and methods per country are available in the database online in OECD.Stat at http://stats.oecd.org//Index.aspx?QueryId=30140.

3 Tasks, qualifications and training of long-term care workers: reducing the skills gap

This chapter presents new analysis of the tasks and functions of long-term care (LTC) workers, providing a comparative overview of what workers do and how this varies across OECD countries. The tasks and knowledge required are compared with their training and education requirements to assess skills gaps. The chapter concludes by discussing policies to improve training and skills: both initial training and life-long learning.

3.1. A better skills match is needed

In many OECD countries, the LTC workforce cannot be identified clearly as part of the health workforce. LTC ranges from improving elderly people's physical and cognitive state to ensuring a better quality of life for vulnerable elderly people and those with chronic illnesses. The LTC workforce consists of a mix of professionals with different levels of training and skills, and different functions/tasks in both social and health care. Exploring the specific role of LTC workers and having a clear vision of their competencies and skills in each country is important when trying to understand the challenges faced by the LTC workforce, to learn from each country's experience and to design policies that meet the LTC needs of ageing populations now and in the future.

The three objectives of this chapter are: to provide a global and comprehensive view of LTC workers' tasks and functions in OECD countries, to explore current skills needs and training rules in the LTC workforce and to explore policy options to improve training participation and to address these needs. It tries to provide answers to several questions that need clarification: What are the specific tasks carried out by LTC workers? Do LTC workers have enough skills to perform these tasks? Do they have access to and participate in geriatric care training? What policies have been implemented to reduce potential gaps in workers' skills?

The remainder of the chapter is organised as follows. Section 3.2 maps LTC workers' tasks and functions, Section 3.3 explores training rules in the LTC workforce, Section 3.4 explores training policies to address the shortfall in skills and Section 3.5 provides a brief conclusion.

Key findings

- LTC jobs are more complex than often portrayed. In more than two-thirds of countries, personal care workers' tasks go well beyond activity of daily living provision. In more than three-quarter of countries, nurses working in the LTC sector perform case management tasks.
- Educational and training requirements for personal care workers are low. In most countries, almost anyone can become a personal care worker. Less than half of the surveyed countries require that personal care workers hold a minimum education level. Among those that do, the requirement varies from vocational training (Hungary, Latvia, Luxembourg, the Netherlands) to a high school certificate (Belgium and Sweden) or a technical qualification after high school (Canada (Ontario), Malta and Estonia after 2020). Very few countries (Canada, Denmark, Germany and Korea) have developed a career structure for LTC workers. This can be problematic when workers are asked to perform tasks beyond basic care, such as medication administration.
- Nurses usually have high education but do not necessarily participate in specialised geriatric care training. Nurses are required to hold a bachelor's degree in half of OECD countries, but only a few (Iceland, Israel, Estonia, Poland, and Sweden) include geriatric care training in the general curriculum, or require nurses to follow such training when working in the LTC sector. In more than half of the surveyed countries, there is no national curriculum for LTC nurses, and geriatric care training remains optional (participation rates can be low). Therefore, nurses in LTC may lack important knowledge in health care for specific conditions of elderly people, such as dementia or osteoporosis, and skills in rehabilitation and complex disease management.
- Geriatric care training participation for nurse students can be increased by sponsoring access to LTC education with the introduction of scholarships (Austria, Israel, and Japan), providing internship and mentorship opportunities (Canada and Korea) and development of "excellence

curricula" in LTC (Canada and Bulgaria), with new advanced professions for nurses (Ireland, Sweden, the Netherlands, the United Kingdom, and the United States).

- Increasing training participation, at least for some personal care workers, should help reaching the right mix of workers/competencies to LTC settings. On-the-job training participation among experienced workers could be increased with tailored learning programmes, financial support (Australia, Austria, Canada, Cyprus, Germany, Iceland, Korea, Latvia, Sweden, the United Kingdom and the United States), career progression perspectives and recognition of prior experience or learning (Australia, Denmark, France, Germany, Korea and the Netherlands).

3.2. While many tasks are low skilled, LTC jobs are more complex than often portrayed

Little is known about what LTC workers do across OECD countries when they provide care to elderly people. This section provides comprehensive mapping of their tasks and functions. It updates and expands previous analyses (Colombo et al., 2011[1]) using new information collected via an international survey specifically designed to map LTC workers' tasks and functions across 26 OECD countries (Box 3.1).

Box 3.1. LTC worker definition

LTC workers are individuals who provide care to recipients at home or in LTC institutions (other than hospitals). Following the OECD definition, formal LTC workers comprise two main professional categories: nurses and personal care workers. Personal care workers include formal workers providing LTC services at home or in institutions (other than hospitals) and who are not qualified or certified as nurses.

This chapter uses data from an LTC workforce questionnaire and a pilot study. Twenty-six OECD countries participated in the LTC workforce questionnaire: Australia, Austria, Belgium, Bulgaria, Cyprus, the Czech Republic, Denmark, Estonia, Germany, Hungary, Iceland, Israel, Japan, Korea, Latvia, Lithuania, Luxembourg, Malta, the Netherlands, Norway, Poland, Romania, Slovenia, Sweden, the United Kingdom and the United States. The survey focused on several themes: the different tasks provided by LTC workers, the professions that carry out LTC tasks, opportunities for task delegation between professionals, opportunities for career progression and raising status, the specificity of standards and regulations for LTC workers and the initial training and qualification levels in these professions.

This chapter also uses data from O*NET, which is a primary source of occupational information in the United States. The O*NET database contains standardised and occupation-specific descriptors on almost 1 000 occupations, covering the entire US economy. Although focusing on US workers, the O*NET data provide relevant information for other countries. Prior evidence suggests that these data are useful to map skills in other countries such as the United Kingdom or New Zealand (Qian et al., 2012[2]).

Moreover, US workers' main tasks are comparable to those performed in other countries. Note, however, that despite some similarities, these data cannot be interpreted as a direct measure of personal care workers' situation in each country for two main reasons. First, the US system is very focused on institutional care. Workers in countries with greater home-based supply may have to deal with different problems, which could add to the skill set that they require. Second, care workers in countries where the mean length of stay is higher than in the United States could be dealing with more frail individuals or those with more complex needs, which may influence the range of tasks they are expected to cover.

3.2.1. Personal care workers perform several functions and tasks beyond basic care

Personal care workers' activities can cover four main functions (Figure 3.1): i) providing assistance with activities of daily living (ADL) such as getting dressed and feeding; ii) helping with elderly people's instrumental activities of daily living (IADL) such as cooking; iii) communicating with care recipients and their families; and iv) performing health care monitoring. In most countries, they are central actors in preventing elderly people's loss of autonomy. The most common tasks within each function are also listed and include maintaining elderly people's hygiene standards, monitoring their health status evolution and response to care, transporting them from their home to outside places and providing psychological support (mainly through discussion).

Figure 3.1. Basic care, monitoring and communication are the most common functions of personal care workers

Personal care workers' functions and tasks

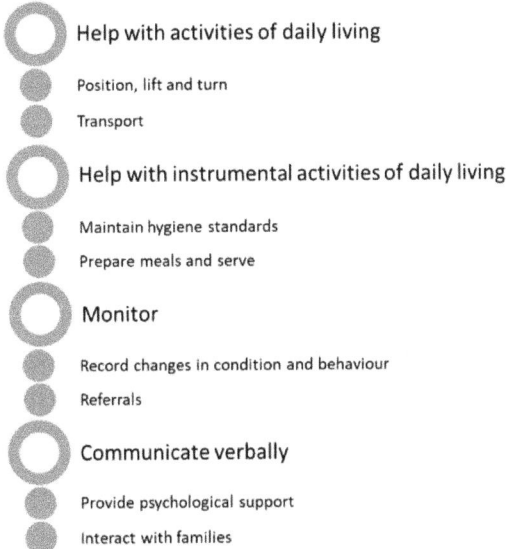

Note: The ranking of all tasks is provided in Figure 3.2. Each function (large circle) is followed by its two most common tasks (small circles).
Source: OECD LTC workforce survey (2018).

When investigating whether personal care workers' roles differ from one country to another, the ranking of tasks according to their frequency across the surveyed countries reveals three interesting results (Figure 3.2). First, personal care workers' main role across OECD countries is to provide basic care. The six most common tasks are centred on ADL and IADL provision. Helping elderly people perform their ADL represents the core of what personal care workers do. In most countries, this includes positioning, lifting and turning elderly people, transporting them (via wheelchairs, movable beds and/or motor vehicles) and assisting care recipients with personal hygiene, feeding and dressing. Another aspect of the job mostly involves maintaining environmental hygiene standards (e.g. changing bed linen, washing, cleaning), providing assistance with the planning, purchasing, preparing or serving of meals to meet nutritional requirements and prescribed diets, and accompanying elderly people on errands. Preparing care recipients for examination or treatment is a less common task that personal care workers provide; in some countries (Bulgaria, Estonia, Lithuania, Norway and the United States), they are not allowed to administer medications. Prior empirical work in Australian nursing homes shows that these activities represent more than half of personal care workers' total working time (Qian et al., 2012[2]).

Figure 3.2. Most common tasks of personal care workers involve hygiene, lifting and transporting elderly people

Ranking of personal care workers' tasks

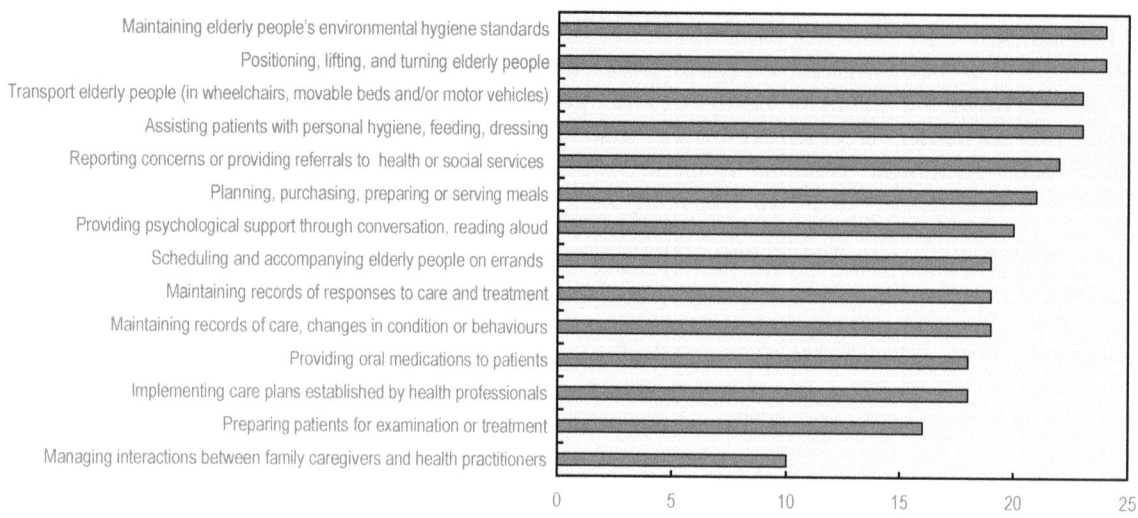

Source: OECD LTC workforce survey (2018).

Second, personal care workers actively collaborate with health care professionals, and this activity is a major component of their role in over 90% of surveyed countries. While they usually do not provide health care *per se*, personal care workers are involved in monitoring care recipients' health status. In almost all surveyed countries, they are in charge of reporting concerns about the care recipient's condition and (when possible) providing referrals to a health or social services professional. They compare the care recipient's evolution to a benchmark of healthy ageing – monitoring, for instance, weight loss or appetite loss, which are usually the first signs of frailty issues. In many countries, they can actively participate in the implementation of care plans designed by health care professionals. They may also have to maintain records of care, responses to care and treatment, and changes in condition or behaviours in many countries. This can involve locating care recipients' records, taking photos of elderly people, viewing results and identifying situations of distress. Being able to distinguish situations needing urgent health care assistance from non-urgent situations is therefore an important skill they need to master. In almost 40% of countries, personal care workers directly manage interactions between family caregivers and health practitioners. Empirical analyses show that in Australia documentation of activities and infection control together represent close to 10% of personal care workers' daily working time (Qian et al., 2012[2]).

Third, 80% of countries report that one of personal care workers' key tasks is communicating with elderly people and their families. In LTC provision, verbal communication is tremendously important to understand people's expectations, culture and habits, to stimulate them and to prevent their social isolation (which can be a risk factor for health deterioration). Communication between LTC workers and informal caregivers is also central for disabled elderly people, who often use a mixture of formal and informal care (Brunel, Latourelle and Zakri, 2018[3]; Bonsang, 2009[4]; Rapp et al., 2011[5]). Providing psychological support through conversation is a common task reported for personal care workers.

Two different models of personal care provision seem to emerge from an international comparison of the specific tasks provided (Table 3.1):

- A few countries seem to strictly limit the range of personal care workers' tasks. This is the case in Norway and Israel, where tasks mostly involve ADL support provision and verbal communication.

- Meanwhile, a larger group of countries (including, for instance, Canada, Korea, Japan, Belgium, Sweden and the Czech Republic) report that personal care workers perform all the listed tasks, and seem to have developed a model of LTC provision where they play a more comprehensive role. In Sweden, for instance, they commonly provide medications. In Korea and Japan, they may even act (and be considered) as case managers: professionals able to aggregate all the micro-services gravitating around elderly people (such as transportation, meals-on-wheels and so on).

Table 3.1. In most countries, personal care workers' tasks are diverse

	Positioning, lifting and turning elderly people	Transporting elderly people (via wheelchairs, movable beds and/or motor vehicles)	Assisting care recipients with personal hygiene, feeding and dressing	Maintaining elderly people's environmental hygiene standards	Planning, purchasing, preparing or serving meals	Scheduling and accompanying elderly people on errands	Preparing care recipients for examination or treatment	Providing oral medications to care recipients	Providing psychological support through conversation and reading aloud	Managing interactions between family caregivers and health practitioners	Maintaining records of care and changes in condition or behaviour	Maintaining records of responses to care and treatment	Reporting concerns or providing referrals to health or social services	Implementing care plans established by health professionals
Australia	●	●	●	●	●	●		●	●		●	●	●	●
Austria	●	●	●	●	●	●		●	●		●	●	●	●
Belgium	●	●	●	●	●	●		●	●	●	●	●	●	●
Bulgaria	●	●	●											
Canada	●	●	●	●	●	●	●	●	●		●	●	●	●
Cyprus	●		●				●		●					
Czech Republic	●	●	●	●	●	●	●	●	●	●	●	●	●	●
Estonia	●	●	●	●	●	●	●		●					
Germany	●	●	●	●	●	●	●	●			●		●	●
Hungary	●	●	●	●	●	●	●	●	●		●	●	●	●
Iceland	●	●	●	●	●	●		●	●				●	
Israel	●		●	●	●	●	●	●	●	●	●	●	●	●
Japan	●	●	●	●	●	●							●	
Korea	●	●	●	●	●	●	●	●	●		●	●	●	●
Latvia			●	●	●		●	●	●				●	
Lithuania	●	●	●	●	●		●	●	●	●	●	●	●	●
Luxembourg	●	●	●	●	●	●	●	●	●	●	●	●	●	●
Malta	●	●	●	●	●	●	●	●	●				●	
Netherlands	●		●	●	●		●	●					●	●
Norway		●	●	●	●	●	●	●	●	●	●	●	●	●
Romania	●	●	●	●	●		●	●	●	●	●		●	●
Slovenia	●	●	●	●	●		●	●	●	●	●	●	●	●
Sweden	●	●	●	●	●	●		●					●	
United Kingdom	●	●	●	●	●		●	●	●		●	●	●	●
United States		●	●	●	●		●	●	●				●	●

Note: Poland did not provide information for personal care workers. Dots indicate that personal care workers commonly provide the task.
Source: OECD LTC workforce survey (2018).

3.2.2. Nurses providing LTC are often involved in care co-ordination

Among nursing professionals, LTC can be perceived as less technical than hospital care and less attractive. However, evidence suggests that this perception of the role of nurses in LTC is under-rated, as it can involve complex functions and tasks. Figure 3.3 summarises what nurses do in most OECD countries when they work in the LTC sector. Nurses in LTC are in charge of four main functions: health care provision, health care monitoring, care co-ordination and communication with families. The bulk of nurses' tasks involve providing health care, including medication administration and health status monitoring. They also show the importance of teamwork, as nurses often have to implement care plans and supervise/evaluate the work provided by other staff. Reporting tasks usually require after-hours telephone communication with off-site physicians, during which nurses have to describe patient-related issues to physicians who often lack physical access to the patient and are not fully aware of their medical history (Whitson et al., 2008[6]).

These functions demand soft skills, such as being competent in social and interpersonal relations. They also require specific geriatric care expertise, such as understanding the LTC system as a whole and being able to identify the relevant service providers. In many countries, nurses providing LTC can act as case managers. Their role covers two of its most important aspects (as perceived by both elderly people and nurses): care co-ordination and provision of assistance in accompanying old people.

Figure 3.3. Beyond care provision, monitoring, care co-ordination and communication are also key functions for nurses

Nurses' functions and tasks when providing LTC

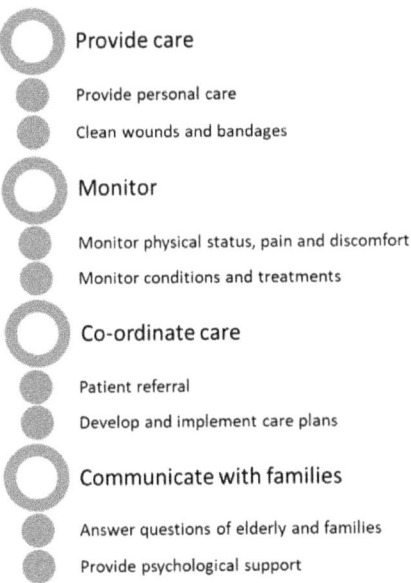

Note: the ranking of all tasks is provided in Figure 3.4. Each function (large circle) is followed by its two most common tasks (small circles)
Source: OECD LTC workforce survey (2018).

The ranking of nurses' tasks according to their frequency across OECD countries (Figure 3.4) shows two additional results. First, nurses may have less autonomy to provide medical treatments in some countries. While health care provision is also a key aspect of their job, it mostly involves cleaning wounds and applying surgical dressings and bandages. Again, countries have specificities. In Bulgaria and Lithuania, wound care is one of the main health care tasks provided by nurses, while Korean and Slovenian nurses are not supposed to perform this specific task. Administering medications is not a task performed by nurses in many eastern Europe countries (Bulgaria, Hungary, Lithuania and Slovenia) or Australia. Provision of treatment and personal health care is more frequent when included in a care plan that the nurse has to follow. Most of the role involves management of multiple comorbidities.

Second, the ranking confirms that nurses play a central role in care co-ordination in most OECD countries, often bridging health and social care provisions. Their common activities are associated with the updating, monitoring and record-keeping of care recipients' health status; co-ordination and supervision of care recipients' care plans; and interactions with care recipients, family caregivers, care providers and health care professionals. Care following hospital discharge needs specific monitoring and communication with hospital teams. Supervising and co-ordinating care recipients' care along with other health care and social care professionals is the most frequent co-ordination task provided by nurses (it is found in 19 countries). In Sweden, for instance, registered nurses provide continuous control of elderly people's adherence to pharmaceutical treatments, and act as "vigilant intermediaries" between physicians and pharmacists (Johansson-Pajala et al., 2016[7]).

Figure 3.4. Most common tasks for nurses include health monitoring and co-ordinating care

Ranking of nurses' tasks when providing LTC

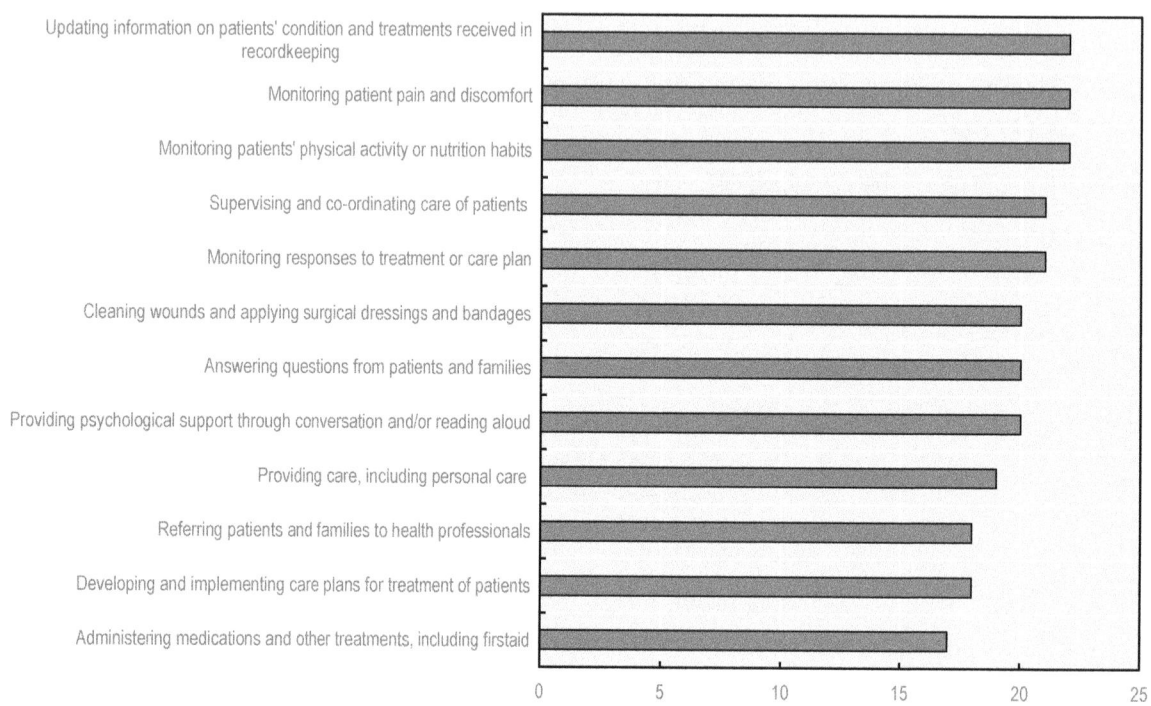

Source: OECD LTC workforce survey (2018).

It also appears that the role of nurses in LTC across OECD countries is more homogeneous than that of personal care workers (Table 3.2). Nevertheless, case management tasks seem to be undertaken less frequently in eastern Europe countries. Nurses do not provide care co-ordination support in Bulgaria, they do not participate in referrals of care recipients in Hungary, Lithuania or Romania and they are not in charge of developing or implementing care plans in the Czech Republic, Latvia or Slovenia. Note, however, that the definition and scope of the role can change if LTC reforms are implemented. In Germany, for instance, a change in needs assessment in 2017 led to a change in definition of what constitutes care, which has significant implications for the workforce. While before workers were focused on individual actions to be completed, a more comprehensive approach to care should now encourage workers to make full use of their competencies and think of what can be done to improve autonomy and self-reliance for the care recipient. Nurses can now act on a care plan rather than completing a number of set tasks, which makes better use of their qualifications.

Table 3.2. Nurses' tasks show little variation across OECD countries

	Providing psychological support through conversation and/or reading aloud	Answering questions from care recipients and families	Monitoring responses to treatment or a care plan	Monitoring care recipients' physical activity or nutrition habits	Monitoring care recipients' pain and discomfort	Updating information on care recipients' condition and treatments received in record-keeping	Developing and implementing care plans for treatment of care recipients	Referring care recipients and families to health professionals	Supervising and co-ordinating care of care recipients	Administering medications and other treatments, including first aid	Cleaning wounds and applying surgical dressings and bandages	Planning and providing care, including personal care
Australia	•	•				•	•	•	•			•
Austria	•	•	•	•	•	•	•	•	•	•	•	
Bulgaria	•	•	•	•	•	•				•	•	•
Canada		•	•	•	•	•	•	•	•	•	•	•
Cyprus		•	•	•	•	•	•	•	•	•	•	•
Czech Republic	•	•	•	•	•	•	•	•	•	•	•	•
Estonia	•	•	•	•	•	•	•	•	•	•	•	•
Germany	•	•	•	•	•	•	•	•	•	•	•	•
Hungary	•	•	•	•	•	•	•	•	•	•	•	•
Iceland		•	•	•	•	•	•	•	•	•	•	•
Israel	•	•	•	•	•	•	•	•	•	•	•	•
Korea	•	•	•	•	•	•	•	•	•	•	•	•
Latvia	•	•	•	•	•	•	•	•	•	•	•	•
Lithuania	•		•	•	•	•	•	•	•	•	•	•
Luxembourg	•	•	•	•	•	•	•	•	•	•	•	•
Malta		•	•	•	•	•	•	•	•	•	•	•
Netherlands	•	•	•	•	•	•	•	•	•	•	•	•
Norway	•	•	•	•	•	•	•	•	•	•	•	•
Poland	•	•	•	•	•	•	•	•	•	•	•	•
Romania		•	•	•	•	•	•	•	•	•	•	•
Slovenia	•	•	•	•	•	•	•	•	•	•	•	•
Sweden	•	•	•	•	•	•	•	•	•	•	•	•
United Kingdom	•	•	•	•	•	•	•	•	•	•	•	•
United States			•	•	•	•	•	•	•	•	•	•

Note: Japan did not provide information for nurses. Dots indicate that personal care workers commonly provide the task.
Source: OECD LTC workforce survey (2018).

3.3. Current training requirements may not always ensure care quality

3.3.1. Education and initial training requirements are low for personal care workers

A majority of LTC workers hold upper secondary educational qualifications or equivalent (medium education level) across OECD countries (63%). Across OECD countries, 63% of LTC workers have a high school diploma or attended vocational schools, while 16% have lower education and 21% higher education. In Canada and the United States, over 74% of LTC workers have a medium education level (see Figure 3.5). In Greece, Israel, Ireland and Japan, a higher share of LTC workers have high education levels, at around 40% or more.

Figure 3.5. Most LTC workers hold high school diplomas or vocational degrees

Composition of the LTC workforce, by education level, in 2016 (or nearest year)

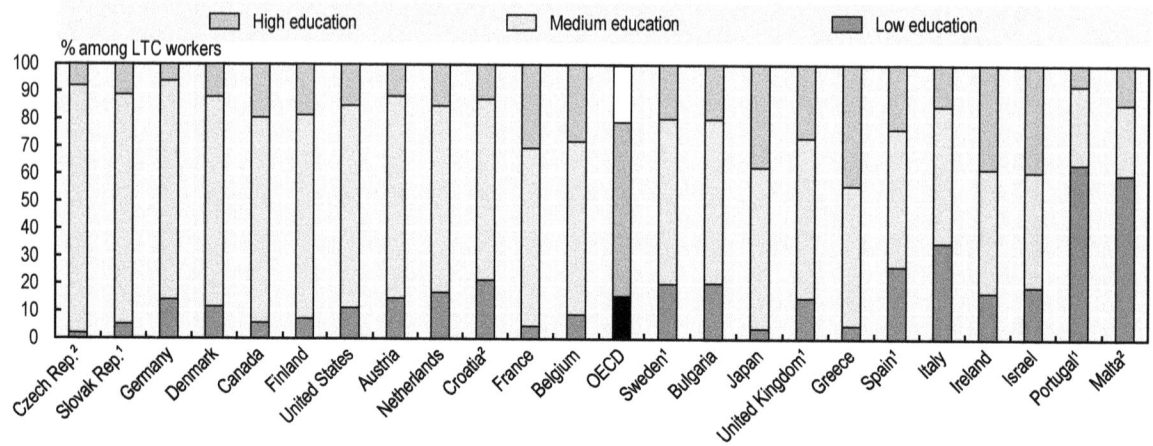

Note: The OECD data point is the unweighted average of the 21 countries shown in the chart. Education was categorised in three groups that follow international standard classification of education (ISCED) 99 code. Low education corresponds to a lower secondary education (ISCED 0-2), medium education to an upper secondary education or a post-secondary non-tertiary education – vocational schools (ISCED 3-4), and high education to tertiary level of education – university (ISCED 5-8). EU-Labour Force Survey data are based on the International Standard Classification of Occupations (ISCO) 4-digit codes and the Nomenclature Statistique des Activités Économiques dans la Communauté Européenne (NACE) 2-digit codes. For a detailed description of the data sources, see Annex 2.A in Chapter 2.
1. Data were calculated based on ISCO 3-digit and NACE 2-digit codes. 2. Data must be interpreted with caution, as sample sizes are small.
Source: EU-Labour Force Survey; the Annual Social and Economic Supplement of the Current Population Survey (ASEC-CPS) for the United States; Census 2016 for Canada; Labour Force Survey for Israel; Survey on Long-term Care Workers for Japan. Data refer to 2016 or nearest year.

The lower education levels among personal care workers drive down the overall LTC workforce's education level on average across OECD countries, since they represent the largest component of LTC workers in most countries. Figure 3.6 provides a comparison of the average education levels between nurses and personal care workers. Not surprisingly, nurses have higher education levels than personal care workers: almost half of nurses have high education levels. In contrast, almost 70% of personal care workers have medium levels of education and 17% have low education levels. The education differences between nurses and personal care workers are particularly large in some countries. In Sweden and Belgium, for instance, more than 80% of nurses participating in the LTC workforce have a high education, compared to less than 20% of personal care workers.

The educational levels of nurses in the LTC sector do not seem to be different from those of nurses working outside the sector (OECD, 2016[8]). Therefore, there does not seem to be selection into LTC among nurses, who receive standard nursing education before joining the LTC workforce.

Figure 3.6. Personal carers are more likely to have lower education levels than nurses

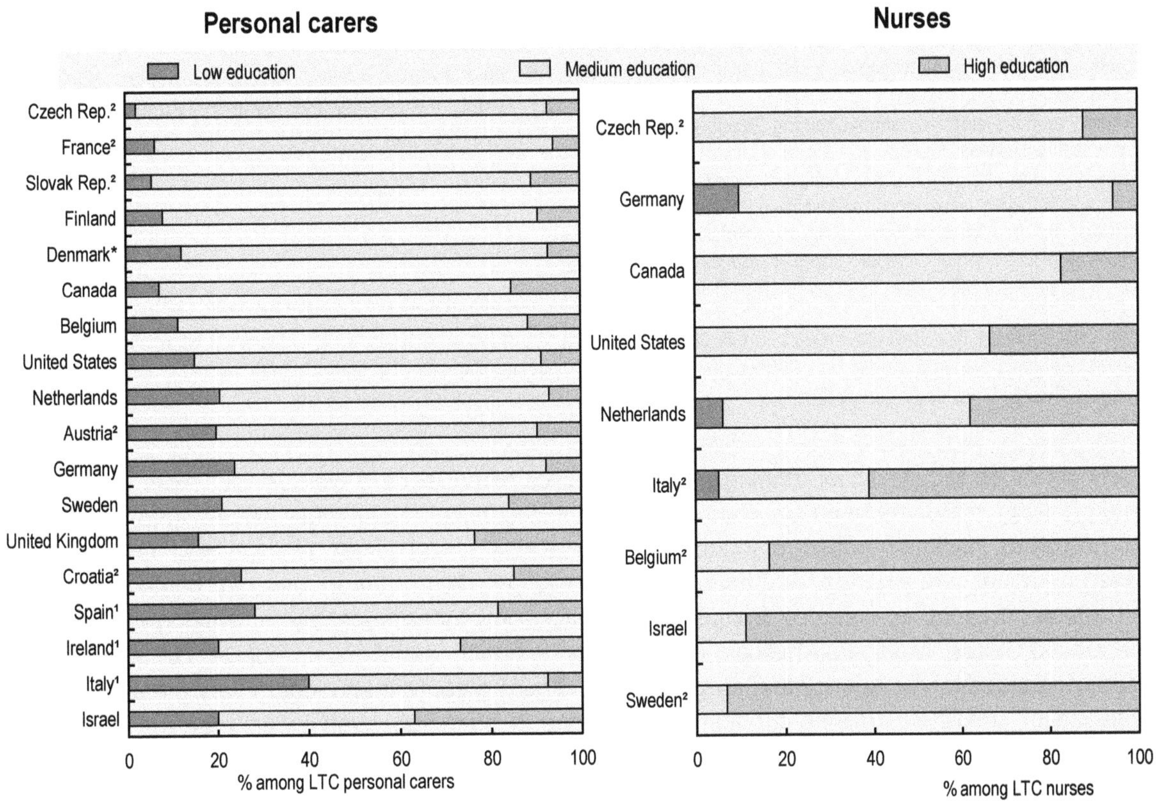

Note: Education was categorised in three groups that follow ISCED-99 code. Low education corresponds to a lower secondary education (ISCED 0-2), medium education to an upper secondary education or a post-secondary non-tertiary education – vocational schools (ISCED 3-4), and high education to tertiary level of education – university (ISCED 5-8). The number of countries is reduced for nurses because data for most countries were not reported as their sample sizes were too small. EU-Labour Force Survey data are based on the ISCO 4-digit codes and NACE 2-digit codes. For a detailed description of the data sources, see Annex 2.A in Chapter 2.
1. Data were calculated based on ISCO 3-digit and NACE 2-digit codes. 2. Data must be interpreted with caution, as sample sizes are small.
Source: EU-Labour Force Survey; ASEC-CPS for the United States; Census 2016 for personal carers and Health Workforce Database, Canadian Institute for Health Information for nurses for Canada; Labour Force Survey for Israel. Data refer to 2016 or nearest year.

Initial training policies for personal care workers are diverse

Minimum qualification requirements offer the guarantee that staff have sufficient knowledge, skills and competencies to provide care to frail elderly people. However, in most countries, almost anyone can become a personal care worker (Table 3.3). Indeed, less than half of the surveyed countries require personal care workers to hold a minimum education level. Among those that do, it varies from vocational training (Hungary, Luxembourg, the Netherlands and Latvia) to a high school diploma (Belgium and Sweden) or a technical degree after high school (Canada, Malta and Estonia after 2020). Conversely, nurses are required to hold high education levels (such as a bachelor's degree) in half of countries.

Table 3.3. Requirements for personal carers are low

LTC workers' minimum education requirements

Personal care workers	Nurses in the LTC sector
No minimum education level (Australia, Bulgaria, Czech Republic, Iceland, Israel, Japan, Korea, Norway, Romania, Slovenia, United Kingdom, United States) **High school diploma** (Belgium, Portugal, Sweden) **Technical degree after high school** (Austria, Canada, Estonia (after 2020), Malta) **Primary or intermediate vocational training** (Hungary, Latvia, Luxembourg, Netherlands) **Other** (40 hours of training in Lithuania, basic knowledge of Greek language in Cyprus, caregiver course/training in Croatia. In Germany, provided that the training for nursing assistants meets the mutually agreed minimum requirements of the federal states, a secondary school leaving certificate (nine-year general education) is a prerequisite for admission.)	**High school diploma** (Croatia) **Technical degree after high school** (Bulgaria, Canada, Hungary, Korea, Latvia, Luxembourg, Poland, Romania, United States) **Intermediate vocational training** (Netherlands) **Bachelor's degree** (Australia, Austria, Cyprus, Czech Republic, Estonia, France, Iceland, Israel, Malta, Norway, Slovenia, Sweden)

Note: Only countries that provided answers to this question are included in the table. Poland did not provide information for personal care workers. Lithuania, Portugal and the United Kingdom did not report training requirements for nurses in LTC.
Source: OECD LTC workforce survey (2018).

Many countries require initial training programmes for personal care workers but there is quite a lot of heterogeneity in the requirements. Training rules and organisation can differ according to the LTC setting (home-based, institution-based) or job title (e.g. nurse aide, social carer). Training often targets institution-based personal care workers, and training participation is often not mandatory for home-based workers. In Canada (Ontario), for instance, training is mandatory only for personal carers working in LTC homes. In the United States, Medicare/Medicaid-certified home health aides must receive 75 hours of training, usually provided by the agency that employs them. Training content and length vary greatly by state. The absence of consistent training for home care aides is observed even when they are paid by public programmes (Spetz and Dudley, 2019[9]). In Sweden, personal care workers can follow a three-year high school professional programme financed by public taxation. In Bulgaria, personal care workers are not obliged to pass or follow any training programme in elderly care, but training opportunities are provided by the National Agency for Vocational Education and Training. In Iceland, personal care workers can receive education or training specific to LTC. Courses take 2-3 months, part time alongside work. For social care workers, formal LTC education usually takes 2 years; for nurse aides, it usually takes 3-4 years. In Korea, a person without any job experience or licence can follow 240 hours of training, involving classroom learning (80 hours), practice sessions (80 hours) and on-the-job training (80 hours).

Less than half of the surveyed countries (Australia, Austria, Belgium, Canada (Ontario), Cyprus, Germany, Korea, Slovenia and the United States) require personal care workers to pass or hold a licence or a certification showing that they have the basic competencies and skills to work in health care and social services for elderly people. Table 3.4 provides examples of the situation in Canada, Romania, Korea, Belgium and the United Kingdom. Both government agencies and private institutions can be involved in the certification process. While the nature of the LTC job (which mainly remains low skilled) is such that many tasks do not require certification, certificates can offer some guarantees, not only for clients but also for workers, in terms of salary.

Table 3.4. Some countries provide certification for personal care workers

	Entities controlling and granting certification	Entities providing training for certification	Specific rules
Canada (Ontario)	Ministry of Training, Colleges and Universities, the National Association of Career Colleges, Ontario Community Support Association	LTC programmes for personal care workers offered in publicly funded colleges, private career colleges and as part of high school continuing education programmes	Ontario introduced a comprehensive mandatory personal support worker registry to ensure greater public protection and personal care worker accountability. Every licensee of an LTC home should ensure that on and after the first anniversary of the coming into force of this section, every person hired by the licensee as a personal support worker or to provide personal support services, regardless of title, has successfully completed a personal support worker programme that meets specific requirements. The registry only accepts workers who are deemed qualified to provide competent and safe care.
Romania	Ministry of Education, Ministry of Labour and Social Justice, and National Authority for Qualification, Order of Generalist Medical Assistants, Midwives and Medical Assistants	Private providers, employers	In Romania, while formal education is required to obtain certification of skills, caregivers in residential centres are not legally required to obtain specific certification before being hired. However, nursing aides have to obtain certification. Employers have to draw up an instructional and professional education plan for their employees, and must offer and facilitate training on a regular basis.
Belgium	Ministry of Employment of the region	Private providers, employers	Flanders has introduced minimum qualification requirements controlled by the region to be registered as a personal care worker. In Wallonia, the Ministry of Employment of the region provides registration and employers provide continuing training programmes.
Korea	Head of local government (metropolitan city mayor or do governor)	Licensed personal care worker education institutions	Different levels of training are often offered, ranging from basic to professional qualification training. The head of local government is in charge of checking that sufficient job training has been received before issuing the personal care worker certificate.
United Kingdom (England)	Care Certificate for National Vocational Qualification	Private providers, employers	The care certification is an entry-level certificate. Personal care workers have opportunities to develop and take further qualifications, varying according to the worker's profile and job role.

Source: OECD LTC workforce survey (2018).

3.3.2. Skills required are not necessarily guaranteed through initial LTC training

While the bulk of LTC work involves ADL (such as dressing, bathing, cooking) support and does not require a high level of training, some basic tasks (like, for instance, administering food) can become complex and require training when disabled elderly people have severe conditions (such as dementia). Analysis from O*NET based on US occupational data shows the top abilities, skills and knowledge required, and records the rating out of 100 for the importance given to each by employers, as well as level required to perform the occupation. For instance, it is important to employers that personal care workers are able to communicate verbally with others (importance of 69), but they are only required to have average levels (52) of communication abilities (Table 3.5).

Table 3.5. Personal care workers' top ability needs are comprehension and communication

Ability	Description	Importance (level)
Oral comprehension	The ability to listen to and understand information and ideas presented through spoken words and sentences	69 (52)
Oral expression	The ability to communicate information and ideas in speaking so others will understand	66 (48)
Problem sensitivity	The ability to tell when something is wrong or is likely to go wrong: this does not involve solving the problem, only recognising that there is a problem	63 (43)
Written comprehension	The ability to read and understand information and ideas presented in writing	53 (43)
Deductive reasoning	The ability to apply general rules to specific problems to produce answers that make sense	53 (43)
Near vision	The ability to see details at close range (within a few feet of the observer)	53 (43)
Written expression	The ability to communicate information and ideas in writing so others will understand	50 (41)
Inductive reasoning	The ability to combine pieces of information to form general rules or conclusions (includes finding a relationship among seemingly unrelated events)	50 (43)
Information ordering	The ability to arrange things or actions in a certain order or pattern according to a specific rule or set of rules (e.g. patterns of numbers, letters, words, pictures, mathematical operations)	50 (41)

Note: the data were collected in the United States, but strong similarities exist for other OECD countries. Since they are key LTC providers, this table focuses on personal and home care aides. This description targets workers whose job consists of assisting elderly people, convalescents or people with disabilities with ADL at the person's home or in a care facility. A score of 100 shows extreme importance or level requirement for the item, a score of 75 shows high importance/level, a score of 50 shows average importance/level, and a score of 25 shows below-average importance/level.
Source: O*NET data online accessed June 2019, https://www.onetonline.org/link/details/39-9021.00.

Similarly, social orientation and social perceptiveness skills are the two most important skills personal care workers need to have, but only average and below-average levels of these skills are required (Table 3.6). For several other skills of lower importance (e.g. decision-making and time management), below-average levels are required.

Table 3.6. Social and interpersonal skills are in demand for personal carers

Skill	Skill description	Importance (level)
Service orientation	Actively looking for ways to help people	72 (54)
Social perceptiveness	Being aware of others' reactions and understanding why they react as they do	66 (45)
Active listening	Giving full attention to what other people are saying, taking time to understand the points being made, asking questions as appropriate and not interrupting at inappropriate times	63 (41)
Speaking	Talking to others to convey information effectively	56 (41)
Monitoring	Monitoring/assessing performance of yourself, other individuals or organisations to make improvements or take corrective action	53 (45)
Critical thinking	Using logic and reasoning to identify the strengths and weaknesses of alternative solutions, conclusions or approaches to problems	50 (43)
Co-ordination	Adjusting actions in relation to others' actions	50 (41)
Instructing	Teaching others how to do something	50 (34)
Judgement- and decision-making	Considering the relative costs and benefits of potential actions to choose the most appropriate one	50 (36)
Time management	Managing one's own time and the time of others	50 (37)

Note: the data were collected in the United States, but strong similarities exist for other OECD countries. Since they are key LTC providers, this table focuses on personal and home care aides. This description targets workers whose job consists of assisting elderly people, convalescents or people with disabilities with ADL at the person's home or in a care facility. A score of 100 shows extreme importance or level requirement for the item, a score of 75 shows high importance/level, a score of 50 shows average importance/level and a score of 25 shows low importance/level.
Source: O*NET data online accessed June 2019 https://www.onetonline.org/link/details/39-9021.00.

Finally, while it is important that personal care workers have knowledge of customer and personal service provision, they are only required to have average levels of needs assessment, quality standards for services and evaluation of customer satisfaction (Table 3.7).

Table 3.7. Customer service, language and psychology are the top knowledge requirements for personal carers

Knowledge	Knowledge description	Importance (level)
Customer and personal service	Knowledge of principles and processes for providing customer and personal services, including customer needs assessment, meeting quality standards for services and evaluation of customer satisfaction	74 (59)
Language	Knowledge of the structure and content of the English language, including the meaning and spelling of words, rules of composition and grammar	58 (39)
Psychology	Knowledge of human behaviour and performance; individual differences in ability, personality and interests; learning and motivation; psychological research methods; and the assessment and treatment of behavioural and affective disorders	50 (48)
Administration and management	Knowledge of business and management principles involved in strategic planning, resource allocation, human resources modelling, leadership technique, production methods and co-ordination of people and resources	48 (29)
Transportation	Knowledge of principles and methods for moving people or goods by air, rail, sea or road, including the relative costs and benefits	43 (26)
Education and training	Knowledge of principles and methods for curriculum and training design; teaching and instruction for individuals and groups; and the measurement of training effects	42 (33)
Medicine	Knowledge of the information and techniques needed to diagnose and treat human injuries, diseases and deformities, including symptoms, treatment alternatives, drug properties and interactions, and preventive health care measures	40 (24)
Public safety and security	Knowledge of relevant equipment, policies, procedures and strategies to promote effective local, state or national security operations for the protection of people, data, property and institutions	40 (27)
Mathematics	Knowledge of arithmetic, algebra, geometry, calculus, statistics and their applications	37 (25)
Therapy and counselling	Knowledge of principles, methods and procedures for diagnosis, treatment and rehabilitation of physical and mental dysfunctions, and for career counselling and guidance	36 (30)

Note: the data were collected in the United States, but strong similarities exist for other OECD countries. Since they are key LTC providers, this table focuses on personal and home care aides. This description targets workers whose job consists of assisting elderly people, convalescents or people with disabilities with ADL at the person's home or in a care facility. A score of 100 shows extreme importance or level requirement for the item, a score of 75 shows high importance/level, a score of 50 shows average importance/level, and a score of 25 shows below-average importance/level.
Source: O*NET data online accessed June 2019 https://www.onetonline.org/link/details/39-9021.00.

It is not clear whether the levels of competency requirements are always sufficient to ensure the quality of LTC provision. The absence of minimum education requirements may not be a problem across all staff, as the bulk of personal care workers' roles involve low-skilled tasks. However, the absence of minimum qualifications could be of concern when workers are allowed to perform specific tasks that require a higher level of expertise and knowledge. Several factors may lead to the importance and level requirements of some of these competencies increasing in the future.

First, elderly people's disabilities may increase with population ageing. LTC provision can become complex for the most disabled elderly people, creating issues when workers lack competencies. This is, for instance, the case when personal care workers provide support to frail elderly people receiving palliative care or need to talk about death with care recipients, their informal care providers and other staff. It can represent an important part of the job, for which they often lack knowledge (Kaasalainen, Brazil and Kelley, 2014[10]). Even some of the most basic tasks (for instance, administering food to elderly people) can become complex and require more advanced competencies when disabled elderly people have severe conditions, such as dementia. LTC workers are likely to face situations requiring higher levels of competency. For instance, carers who deliver home-based care or work on night shifts must be prepared to manage stressful situations on their own, as events such as falls, fugues and strokes are common issues faced by disabled elderly people. Low levels of competency may be problematic when workers need to identify risks and reduce hazards in their daily jobs, especially when they have to provide care in dementia wards.

Substantial dementia training is rarely included in the minimum training requirements for care staff (OECD, 2018[11]). Although many OECD countries offer voluntary dementia-specific training programmes tailored for or including professional care staff, few countries have dementia-related requirements for training. Many people in care facilities have or will develop dementia, and may display behaviours that are challenging or risky to themselves and the people who care for them. Knowing how to manage these behaviours is crucial to providing high-quality and safe care, for both people with dementia and their carers.

Second, recent evidence suggests the need to raise workers' awareness about basic issues that can have dramatic consequences for frail elderly people. For instance, almost two-thirds of LTC workers surveyed in a large French study declared that they never get a flu shot (Truchot, 2018[12]), although flu can lead to serious health complications among frail and disabled elderly populations. A lack of knowledge of these consequences could be detrimental for the most disabled elderly people.

Third, personal care workers often have to handle many medical devices to manage specific issues that frail elderly people may encounter in their daily lives: back problems, muscular pain, hearing impairment issues, respiratory conditions, vascular issues and so on. Currently, many of these devices (bedpans, canes, back braces etc.) do not require advanced competencies, but the use of oxygen delivery equipment, automatic blood pressure machines or hearing aid devices can require more advanced abilities, skills and knowledge to guarantee their safety and/or effectiveness. The fact that personal care workers are only required to have lower levels of public safety and security knowledge may raise an issue that could grow in the future with the flow of more complex technological innovations in ageing care (discussed in Chapter 6).

Finally, the absence of minimum qualifications and the low levels of competency among personal care workers could be of concern when they are allowed to perform specific tasks that require higher levels of expertise and knowledge. For instance, some countries (Australia, the Czech Republic, Japan, Korea and the United Kingdom) have no educational requirements for personal care workers, even though they commonly allow them to provide oral medication, maintain records of care and treatment, and implement care plans. This may indicate a potential need for training to increase the level of competency among personal care workers involved in these tasks.

Table 3.8. Personal care workers are asked to use many technical tools

Category
Back or lumbar or sacral orthopaedic soft goods
Bedpans for general use
Blood pressure cuff kits
Braille devices for physically challenged people
Canes or cane accessories
Crutches or crutch accessories
Electric vibrators for rehabilitation or therapy
Electronic blood pressure units
Electronic medical thermometers
Glucose monitors or meters
Hearing aids for physically challenged people
Lower extremity prosthetic devices
Medical acoustic stethoscopes or accessories
Oxygen therapy delivery system products, accessories or supplies
Paging controllers
Patient bed or table scales for general use
Patient lifts or accessories
Patient shifting boards or accessories
Shower or bath chairs or seats for physically challenged people
Specimen collection containers
Mobile operating system and touchscreen display
Upper extremity prosthetic devices
Vascular or compression apparel or supports
Voice synthesisers for physically challenged people
Walkers or rollators

Note: the data were collected in the United States, but strong similarities exist for other OECD countries. Since they are key LTC providers, this table focuses on personal and home care aides. This description targets workers whose job consists of assisting elderly people, convalescents or people with disabilities with ADL at the person's home or in a care facility.
Source: O*NET data online accessed June 2019, https://www.onetonline.org/link/details/39-9021.00.

Nurses sometimes lack sufficient geriatric training

In most countries, nurses usually have high education, with several years of training in general nursing, but they do not necessarily have to participate in specialised geriatric care training. Therefore, they may lack some of the specific skills needed in LTC. Given the tasks provided by nurses, training programmes increasingly need to focus on several new aspects of LTC provision: using telemedicine and eHealth, performing preventive actions (especially concerning nutrition) and developing networking skills (in particular to accommodate informal caregivers' needs). In the LTC sector, good knowledge of complex geriatric conditions, caring needs following hospital discharge, case management, bereavement coping and prevention is crucial.

Prior work underlines the need to develop age-appropriate care for chronic diseases in the elderly population (dementia, stroke, chronic obstructive pulmonary disease and vision impairment), with more effective primary, secondary and tertiary prevention targeting older people (Prince et al., 2015[13]). In addition, the increasing prevalence of frailty requires development of screening measures to detect and monitor frailty risks in the elderly population and disability risks in the frail elderly population (Clegg et al., 2013[14]). Nurses can play a major role in improving care recipients' health literacy on important issues, such as flu vaccination for the elderly population (Ellen, 2018[15]). These issues are likely to increase geriatric training needs.

Palliative care issues are not usually taught in general nurse training, while LTC workers increasingly need to master these skills. Palliative care involves discussions with care recipients, their family members and formal caregivers to promote a positive perspective on death (Kaasalainen et al., 2013[16]). Prior work suggests that LTC workers do not always have sufficient knowledge to provide end-of-life care, which usually requires advanced training (Carlson and Bengtsson, 2014[17]).

Finally, it is expected that future LTC reforms will change nurses' roles, requiring further skills. As healthy ageing becomes a policy priority in many countries (see Chapter 6), nurses will increasingly have to learn how to evaluate the overall efficacy of the care provided to elderly people, using evidence-based outcomes, such as changes in grip strength loss, body mass index or walking speed, and signs of exhaustion. They will also have to learn how to monitor and assess the level of burden among family caregivers, to evaluate the risks of emergencies within informal care networks.

Only a few countries include geriatric care training in general nursing curricula, or require nurses to follow such training when working in the LTC sector. In Iceland, training programmes in geriatric care are part of the basic education for all nurses. In Israel, registered nurses receive post-basic one-year training in geriatrics, after which they have to pass a simulation-based registration exam. In Sweden, there is a general university degree for nurses, but students have to choose a specialisation (postgraduate diploma in specialist nursing) in special care for elderly people when they work in LTC. In Estonia, nurses have to spend at least 60 hours per year on training specialising in geriatric care when working in the LTC sector. In Poland, depending on the form of postgraduate education, the time allocated to geriatric care training varies between 1 and 20 months. In Malta, at present, a general degree in nursing is sufficient, but a new degree in LTC nursing has been launched, and it is expected that this will be required in the future to become an LTC nurse.

Most countries offer the option of a geriatric care specialisation for nurses during initial training. In more than half of the surveyed countries (Australia, Bulgaria, Canada, Croatia, Hungary, the Czech Republic, Luxembourg, Cyprus, Latvia, Korea, Portugal, Slovenia, Estonia, Iceland, the United States, the Netherlands and Norway), there is no national curriculum for LTC nurses, and geriatric care training remains optional. In these countries, it is therefore not guaranteed that nurse graduates working in the LTC sector have had any geriatric care training. Recent evidence suggests that participation rates can be low. For instance, a recent survey of a sample of Norwegian nurses showed that less than a quarter of those providing elderly care had received geriatric care training during their nurse curriculum (Sunde, Øyen and Ytrehus, 2017[18]). Nurses in Australia do not have to pass formal education/training in geriatric care, but they have to receive registration from the Nursing and Midwifery Board of Australia and to complete a minimum of 20 hours of continuing professional development per registration period of 12 months. However, it is not guaranteed that they follow geriatric training courses.

3.4. Better training policies can address the shortfall in skills

While in the future the largest share of LTC needs should be addressed with personal care workers providing many low-skilled tasks (such as washing and helping to dress), the LTC workforce will also have to rely on some workers equipped with more advanced geriatric care competencies. Increasing geriatric care training participation for nurse students and experienced workers should help achieve the right mix of workers/competencies in LTC settings.

3.4.1. Nurse students could benefit from improving geriatric care training

Geriatric care curricula are not always attractive to nurse students. They suffer from comparisons with other health care sectors (such as paediatrics or hospital-based practice), which have a better image and different practice environment (including greater team working and technology use). Low training participation can also be explained by the fact that career progression prospects after graduation can be low, even among nurses with substantial experience.

Various measures have been implemented to increase students' participation in LTC training (Table 3.9). Several initiatives have been developed to increase exposure to geriatric care during nursing training, with the objective of helping students shift their impressions of future career prospects from the start and giving them a better understanding of the realities of the job and the opportunity to acquire specific skills. These initiatives are very important, as geriatric care exposure was found to increase interest in geriatric care professions (Meiboom et al., 2015[19]). Nurse students who go on to specialise in LTC often declare that they were sensitive to the pedagogical atmosphere (personal interactions with the staff), the leadership of the ward manager, and supervisors' attitudes to mentoring (Carlson and Idvall, 2015[20]).

Several countries have provided additional funds for education and/or are redesigning degrees. Germany, Japan, Austria and Israel have sponsored access to LTC education with the introduction of scholarships. Sweden, Canada and Korea have developed internship opportunities and mentorship programmes for nurse students. Germany has completely abolished school fees in their nursing education. In Germany, new legislation will merge three specialised nursing education streams (general, geriatric, paediatric) into a general one from 2020. As the country is expecting a large shortage of nurses, the change in the nursing degree was a move to make the profession more attractive. It is hoped that the new degree will open up career opportunities by being more general, so that nurses can switch between types of practice (working in hospitals, with children and with elderly people) and define which specialisation fits them better. In the United States, the Veterans Health Administration, a large LTC service provider, offers geriatric scholars programmes (Spetz and Dudley, 2019[9]).

Increasing exposure to research and developing excellence programmes is another way of increasing students' interest in LTC professions. Canada and Bulgaria are supporting the development of "excellence curricula" in LTC. In the United States, the implementation of a research internship programme for nursing students successfully raised interest in geriatric care among participants (Mewshaw et al., 2017[21]). Exposure to a research project provided students with an opportunity to learn directly from specialists and gain more field experience. Close interactions with nursing staff also provided a great opportunity to develop interpersonal skills, which are very important in LTC professions. Note that these programmes require some flexibility (both students and mentors have to adapt to each other's schedule) and some commitment from staff to provide mentorship. This requires careful selection of applicants with sufficient motivation and organisational skills to succeed.

Several countries (the United States, the Netherlands, Ireland, the United Kingdom and Sweden) have introduced advanced nurse practitioners, whose role is to be responsible for case management (Ljungbeck and Sjögren Forss, 2017[22]). They are trained to deliver specific LTC tasks of key importance, such as monitoring care plans provided to frail elderly people; managing interactions between frail elderly people, informal care providers, social care workers and health care workers; and detecting loss of autonomy among frail elderly people.

Table 3.9. Several measures could improve initial training for nurses

Measure	Examples
Scholarships for nurses specialising in geriatric care, and funding for training	- In Israel, "perseverance grants" are scholarships for nurses who will work in the LTC sector for four years - In Japan, financial support is given to students applying for certified nursing and LTC training for beginners. - In Korea, the second LTC master plan (2018-22) compensates for training time. - In Austria, training for LTC workers is fully covered by governments and employers.
Adapting nursing degrees to allow students more exposure to geriatric care	- The Netherlands is developing dual-track programmes (including a general nurse and a geriatric nurse track), which are helpful solutions to give students better understanding of the realities of the job and allow them to acquire specific skills. - In Germany, new legislation will merge three specialised nursing education streams (general, geriatric, paediatric) into a general one from 2020. - In Canada (Ontario), in 2016-17, over 100 student received internship initiatives in nursing home placements via the Centres for Learning, Research and Innovation (CLRIs). Over 600 hours of coaching were given to LTC homes, and over 180 LTC homes received formal coaching.
Developing research, innovation and excellence programmes	- In Canada (Ontario), the CLRIs promote a "teaching nursing home" programme model that is unique among OECD countries. In 2016-17, over 360 students participated in programmes made available in LTC teaching nursing home environments, and over 3 800 staff received training/education from the CLRIs. This quality-based programme focuses on resident-centred care issues, such as responsive behaviours, falls prevention, peritoneal dialysis and obstructive sleep apnoea. While successful, however, this programme gives rise to important costs. In 2017/18, the Ontario authorities announced base funding for the CLRIs, representing between USD 2.35M and USD 3.1M each year until 2021. Additional investment in training and education in LTC will relate to: i) new dedicated staff training funding to support medically complex residents, which will also focus on falls prevention, behavioural support, palliative and end-of-life care and medication management; ii) the design of an LTC educational framework aimed at promoting legislative and regulatory compliance, practice excellence and an informed and engaged sector and public; and iii) support of education and training for the provision of culturally appropriate services. - In Bulgaria, the University of Veliko Tarnovo introduced a Master's degree programme on social work in LTC that provides profiled knowledge needed for the profession of social worker in the field of social services for people with special needs. The graduates can become leading specialists and managers in the structures of social services. Their training allows professional recognition in European and international social organisations and specialised social services. Graduates of the programme can apply for doctoral training. - The Norwegian government introduced an ambitious programme to redefine professional roles by 2020. This inter-ministerial established new guidelines for health and social care education with 12 learning outcomes, aiming in particular to increase competences in managing and developing technology and soft skills. One important aspect is teamwork skills to favour inter-disciplinary work (e.g. soft skills, identifying people's needs and case management). This reform applies to nurses, not assistant nurses.

Source: OECD (2018) LTC workforce pilot survey and review of the literature.

3.4.2. Several countries are improving initial and on-the-job training for personal care workers

Given the heterogeneity of skills levels, training requirements and mobility for personal care workers across countries, there is also scope for ensuring better international recognition of qualifications. This could be facilitated by more referencing of the qualifications in the LTC sector (as opposed to the nursing sector) to national qualifications frameworks, and/or at a global level (for instance, in European countries, to the European Qualifications Framework) (Cedefop, 2018[23]). This could include a common understanding of the skills required, preparing curricula for the sector and even for assessment purposes. Some initiatives already exist and could be pursued or adapted to the LTC sector. For instance, the European Care Certificate initiative was developed as a basic entry certificate for the care sector. This created a set of learning outcomes covering essential knowledge that any worker new to care needs to know to work safely and in line with person-centred values. The eight basic European social care learning outcomes covered in the certificate have been shown reliably to cover this essential knowledge. Yet more could be done in this area because it only covers 16 countries and initial entry knowledge. Some other countries are developing initiatives in that direction. For instance, in collaboration with stakeholders, Canada (Ontario) is developing an LTC educational framework, with priorities and demonstration projects to improve skills training and fulfil future staffing needs. In the United States, a recent task force on the LTC workforce recommends creation of a work group, through which several LTC sector representatives (home care aides, home care agencies, home health nurses etc.) should define standards for future curricula to train home care aides (Spetz and Dudley, 2019[9]).

On-the-job training options may not be always affordable, especially because of high opportunity costs. LTC workers can lack time to pursue education, for work or personal reasons, especially when they face important commuting times or difficult working schedules. In Austria, training in the LTC workforce is provided during working time, and the ten weeks of education required to participate in the LTC workforce can be provided on-site, in schools or in universities. In Germany, the education and training initiative for elderly care implemented between 2012 and 2015 extended existing options for shortening training when applicants have relevant knowledge and contributed to an increase in the number of trainees in geriatric care.

Governments can provide financial incentives to both employers and employees. More specifically, they can provide financial support to individuals, encourage the development of training facilities and work with employers' associations and trade unions to make it easier for LTC workers to undertake training. In Austria, Canada, Sweden, Cyprus, Australia and Latvia, continuing training programmes for LTC workers are sponsored by government funding. Agreements between employers and unions can ease access to training (as in the United States, Iceland and the United Kingdom). In 2014, Korea implemented a continuing education programme for personal care workers, which is covered by government funds and employment insurance schemes. Personal care workers must receive continuous training offered by licensed institutions; the programme length depends on the worker's experience. In Iceland, short training is mostly covered by unions or employers, and workers are often allowed to take part of it within working time.

In Norway, the government has strengthened efforts to promote competency-building for personal care workers with formal education in health and social care by increasing funding for basic and continuing education. Specific grants are available for municipalities willing to develop education programmes for personal care workers. The purpose of the funding is to increase recruitment to the sector; stabilise the personnel situation; raise the level of expertise in the services, including in the areas of dementia, geriatrics, mental health and substance abuse; implement life-long learning; and anticipate future needs. In Australia, following the Aged Care Workforce Strategy, the Aged Services Industry Reference Committee is examining how to reform the national training package qualifications and skill sets needed for LTC, as well as new approaches to career structuring and progression in the sector and scoping opportunities for collaboration across vocational education training, higher education and industry.

In addition, measures have been introduced across OECD countries to make on-the-job training easier for low-skilled workers, which may benefit personal care workers (OECD, 2019[24]). Measures include, for instance; personal training accounts, which open an internet-based account presenting workers' rights for training; personal objectives; training searches results (France); degree study allowances (Estonia); and training vouchers available for specific vocational training programmes (United States). These existing measures may help personal care workers access training and acquire some of the basic competencies they may lack. Also, legal rights for education and training leave represent an important policy tool to guarantee low-skilled workers' rights to training when they need it (OECD, 2019[25]).

Another legal, pivotal policy tool can be comprehensive safety standards, including those mandated through accreditation process, as they can help ensure that minimum standards are met with regard to LTC workers qualifications, whether through initial or on-the-job trainings. In addition, improving qualifications would also contribute to foster higher safety standards for workers and patients – adequate qualifications are intimately linked to safer care. Numerous studies show that adverse events, such as infections or injuries, are not only widespread but also preventable (de Bienassis, Llena Nozal and Klazinga, forthcoming[26]). For instance, a study in Medicare patients in LTC in the United States found that over half of events were preventable, and the majority of these would have been prevented if not for substandard care and medical errors (OIG, 2018[27]).

To make training programmes more attractive, the return to training in terms of salaries and career progression also needs to improve. Indeed, the return on investment is likely to decline for older workers who are facing retirement. This is particularly important in the LTC workforce, which is mainly composed of middle-aged workers, and which has aged over the past decade (see Chapter 2). It is also very important in countries like the United States, where the rate of return on acquiring any college education in terms of additional wages for personal care workers is low: it represents 9% higher earnings for each additional year of schooling compared with 45% for other employees in the United States (Osterman, 2017[28]).

Examples of career perspectives provided by training programmes include access to managerial roles for personal care workers, or access to nurse diplomas for nurse aides willing to progress (Denmark, Germany). In France, a recent report recommends the introduction of a new profession for personal care workers for elderly people and notes that frailty detection should be included in initial training programmes (Libault, 2019[29]). An intermediate professional level to advance the roles of personal carers with specific qualifications would add value to the profession and increase remuneration, and potentially improve retention rates. Korea plans to have more training for personal care workers in the future and to offer a managerial role.

Easing training entry requirements to broaden recognition of prior experience or learning, which can be very valuable for personal care workers, is also a critical issue. However, while some programmes exist in most OECD countries, accessing such initiatives can prove difficult for personal care workers owing to complex procedures or to the courses' duration, which can be perceived as too long. Facilitating personal care workers' take-up of these programmes should therefore be promoted through initiatives like the *validation des acquis* in France, or the *Qualifica Centres* in Portugal, which target low-qualified adults and accompany them throughout the skills recognition procedures (OECD, 2019[24]). For low-skilled workers, strong career guidance is often needed. Indeed, recent OECD work shows that while individual learning accounts are a way of empowering low-skilled workers in their own training decisions, these schemes should be complemented by face-to-face support with specialists. Specifically, specialised career guidance officers could be trained to provide this comprehensive approach and inform workers about the needs of the LTC sector, alongside suggesting the best training options for them. Some countries promote policies increasing training participation among older adults through career transition advice (Australia, the

Netherlands) or programmes encouraging employers to train older workers or low-skilled workers (like the *WeGebAU* programme in Germany).

Even when training is sponsored by governments or employers, there can be a lack of meaningful training options among experienced workers. The heterogeneity of cases makes it difficult to match training to their expectations because their needs are often case-specific. A systematic review of the literature (Surr et al., 2017[30]) underlines that successful programmes for the health and social workforce in dementia care are tailored to participants' experience; involve active and experience-driven participation; and rely on mixed material (such as written material reviews and face-to-face interactive activities). Active participation means listening to workers' specific needs in order to adjust the training length according to their experience, seniority and profile. Several options can be used to expand training options: specialised university training, specific courses from accredited programmes, participation in professional traineeships, practical training in a special social institution and training events and conferences.

Modern learning programmes promote three dimensions of flexibility: time, location and content. They combine a choice of timelines for training receipt, are closely linked to the working environment (residences, homes, care centres) and target workers' specific needs. They are centred on caregivers' specific needs (e.g. language, communication), and the learning activities support the application of training into practice. They provide diversified forms of training (theoretical, practical), with several ways of obtaining credits (course exams, conference participation, training), and provide practical tools to solve daily issues. For instance, use of case studies can provide decision support tools to groups of workers at risk of facing specific issues (such as crisis or death). They promote training with active participation, which is encouraged through small or large group face-to-face learning.

Tailoring learning programmes for experienced workers may not necessarily be expensive or burdensome. For instance, in the United States, a programme implemented through telephone conversations (the Communicating Health Assessments by Telephone Project) to aid LTC nurses with symptom assessment and communication of health information was successful while inexpensive (Whitson et al., 2008[6]). The individualised training sessions providing decision support tools to nurses improved the quality of their communications with off-site physicians.

Table 3.10. Enhanced training for personal care workers is available in some countries

Measure	Examples
Provide career perspectives to strengthen the motivation of professionals willing to progress.	• In Denmark, experienced personal care workers willing to provide more advanced care and become health assistants have the opportunity to follow a two-year programme and pass a different national examination. • In Norway, assistant nurses are offered numerous ways to specialise after high school. Training courses run for between six months and three years, and can be organised part time. Participants can become registered nurses if, after vocational training, they attend a one-year general study course to access nursing education. • In Korea, the "Centres for LTC workers" provide various services, including counselling, training and job information. • In Germany, one of the aims of new legislation to reform education and training for nurses is to increase the opportunities for further career progression via further training at the university level through bachelor's degrees. The Nursing Profession Act provides comprehensive crediting options of equivalent qualifications for the duration of nursing training. For example, a one-year training programme for nursing assistants can be fully credited towards training of specialists, which is thereby shortened from three to two years. In addition, the Nursing Care Reform Act ensures that retraining for nurses, health and child nurses and geriatric nurses is made possible by employment agencies and job centres.
Flag experience and prior learning recognition	• In Korea, the Ministry of Health and Welfare plans to build a career ladder for personal care workers by creating a new profession of personal care worker manager. This will allow personal care workers to take a position of director of home care facilities once they have more than five years' job experience in the LTC field. • In France, elderly care training programmes to become an LTC nurse are open to people with a baccalaureate, with at least three years of professional experience in health care or with five years of professional experience in another sector (in which case they need to pass an exam). Applicants who hold an *aide soignante* diploma and have three years of professional experience (working full time) are eligible to take an exam (a written exam looking at three case studies) to determine whether they can access the LTC nurse training programme. Physicians, midwifes, physiotherapists and massage therapists, or medical degree students, are eligible to access elderly care training without having to pass an exam. • In Portugal, the *Qualifica Centres* target low-qualified adults and accompany them throughout the skills recognition procedures.

Source: OECD (2018) LTC workforce pilot survey, and review of the literature.

Moreover, enhancing the use of digital training methods could represent an interesting solution to improve training flexibility without increasing its costs. Online courses could have the advantage of bringing training into nursing homes or wherever the professional is located, and require low equipment needs (a TV or computer screen and an internet connection). Moreover, these courses can be taken whenever workers are ready. Note however, that while Massive Open Online Courses open many opportunities, they are still widely underused because of a perception of low quality. In addition, this type of training can hardly be done for more practical, hands-on subjects such as communication skills. Thus, certification and quality assurance for such courses is important (OECD, 2018[31]). In the United States, internet-based dementia training programmes with video-situation testing improved personal care workers' knowledge, attitudes, self-efficacy and behavioural intentions (Irvine et al., 2012[32]), and allowed them to deal more effectively with aggressive behaviour among nursing home residents with dementia (Irvine et al., 2012[33]).

3.5. Conclusion

While for many tasks LTC jobs require a low level of skill, LTC workers perform a variety of tasks that are more complex. This chapter underlines two important conclusions. First, there is a need to provide basic support to personal care workers; for example, in the form of training. Second, it is also crucial to ensure that in the future part of the LTC workforce will be able to focus increasingly on outcomes (such as disability prevention, re-enablement and healthy ageing) rather than mainly focusing on outputs (such as the day-to-day tasks that cover elderly people's immediate needs). For instance, disability prevention among frail elderly people will represent a growing issue in the future, in which some LTC workers will have a central role to play (see Chapter 6). Thus, there is a need for better training to enable some LTC workers to take on a more advanced role.

Better understanding of the skills and qualifications of LTC workers helps to formalise their role in the sector and should lead to proper career prospects and structures. Many countries need to have a broad strategy to identify the skills needed among LTC workers and to define a common approach to guarantee that the need for low-skilled task provision is fulfilled while some workers focus more on outcomes. This will help to ensure that most LTC workers receive basic training and promote an advanced role for the most experienced or trained workers. While all these actions contribute to increasing the attractiveness of on-the-job training, they may also contribute to increased service costs in LTC. At the same time, implementation of on-the-job training could be staggered.

References

Bonsang, E. (2009), "Does informal care from children to their elderly parents substitute for formal care in Europe?", *Journal of Health Economics*, Vol. 28/1, pp. 143-154, http://dx.doi.org/10.1016/j.jhealeco.2008.09.002. [4]

Brunel, M., J. Latourelle and M. Zakri (2018), "Un senior à domicile sur cinq aidé régulièrement pour les tâches du quotidien", *Études et Résultats*, Vol. 1103, https://drees.solidarites-sante.gouv.fr/etudes-et-statistiques/publications/etudes-et-resultats/article/un-senior-a-domicile-sur-cinq-aide-regulierement-pour-les-taches-du-quotidien. [3]

Carlson, E. and M. Bengtsson (2014), "The uniqueness of elderly care: Registered nurses' experience as preceptors during clinical practice in nursing homes and home-based care", *Nurse Education Today*, Vol. 34/4, pp. 569-573, http://dx.doi.org/10.1016/j.nedt.2013.07.017. [17]

Carlson, E. and E. Idvall (2015), "Who wants to work with older people? Swedish student nurses' willingness to work in elderly care – a questionnaire study", *Nurse Education Today*, Vol. 35/7, pp. 849-853, http://dx.doi.org/10.1016/j.nedt.2015.03.002. [20]

Cedefop (2018), "Analysis and Overview of NQF Level Descriptors in European Countries", No. 66, Publications Office of the European Union, Luxembourg, http://data.europa.eu/doi/10.2801/566217. [23]

Clegg, A. et al. (2013), "Frailty in elderly people", *The Lancet*, Vol. 381/9868, pp. 752-762, http://dx.doi.org/10.1016/S0140-6736(12)62167-9. [14]

Colombo, F. et al. (2011), *Help Wanted? Providing and Paying for Long-Term Care*, OECD Health Policy Studies, OECD Publishing, Paris, http://dx.doi.org/10.1787/9789264097759-en. [1]

de Bienassis, K., A. Llena Nozal and N. Klazinga (forthcoming), "The Economics of Patient Safety Part III: Long-Term Care", *OECD Health Working Papers*, OECD Publishing, Paris. [26]

Ellen, M. (2018), "Factors that influence influenza vaccination rates among the elderly: nurses' perspectives", *Journal of Nursing Management*, Vol. 26/2, pp. 158-166, http://dx.doi.org/10.1111/jonm.12528. [15]

Irvine, A. et al. (2012), "Use of a dementia training designed for nurse aides to train other staff", *Journal of Applied Gerontology*, Vol. 32/8, pp. 936-951, http://dx.doi.org/10.1177/0733464812446021. [32]

Irvine, B. et al. (2012), "An internet training to reduce assaults in long-term care", *Geriatric Nursing*, Vol. 33/1, pp. 28-40, http://dx.doi.org/10.1016/j.gerinurse.2011.10.004. [33]

Johansson-Pajala, R. et al. (2016), "Nurses in municipal care of the elderly act as pharmacovigilant intermediaries: a qualitative study of medication management", *Scandinavian Journal of Primary Health Care*, http://dx.doi.org/10.3109/02813432.2015.1132891. [7]

Kaasalainen, S., K. Brazil and M. Kelley (2014), "Building capacity in palliative care for personal support workers in long-term care through experiential learning", *International Journal of Older People Nursing*, Vol. 9/2, pp. 151-158, http://dx.doi.org/10.1111/opn.12008. [10]

Kaasalainen, S. et al. (2013), "Role of the nurse practitioner in providing palliative care in long-term care homes", *International Journal of Palliative Nursing*, Vol. 19/10, pp. 477-485, http://dx.doi.org/10.12968/ijpn.2013.19.10.477. [16]

Libault, D. (2019), *Concertation: Grand âge et autonomie*, Ministère des Solidarités et de la Santé, Paris, https://solidarites-sante.gouv.fr/IMG/pdf/rapport_grand_age_autonomie.pdf. [29]

Ljungbeck, B. and K. Sjögren Forss (2017), "Advanced nurse practitioners in municipal healthcare as a way to meet the growing healthcare needs of the frail elderly: a qualitative interview study with managers, doctors and specialist nurses", *BMC Nursing*, Vol. 16, p. 63, http://dx.doi.org/10.1186/s12912-017-0258-7. [22]

Meiboom, A. et al. (2015), "Why medical students do not choose a career in geriatrics: a systematic review", *BMC Medical Education*, Vol. 15, p. 101, http://dx.doi.org/10.1186/s12909-015-0384-4. [19]

Mewshaw, J. et al. (2017), "A novel program for ABSN students to generate interest in geriatrics and geriatric nursing research", *Journal of Nursing Education and Practice*, Vol. 7/6, pp. 96-99, http://dx.doi.org/10.5430/jnep.v7n6p95. [21]

OECD (2019), *Getting Skills Right: Future-Ready Adult Learning Systems*, Getting Skills Right, OECD Publishing, Paris, https://dx.doi.org/10.1787/9789264311756-en. [25]

OECD (2019), *OECD Employment Outlook 2019: The Future of Work*, OECD Publishing, Paris, https://dx.doi.org/10.1787/9ee00155-en. [24]

OECD (2018), *Care Needed: Improving the Lives of People with Dementia*, OECD Health Policy Studies, OECD Publishing, Paris, https://dx.doi.org/10.1787/9789264085107-en. [11]

OECD (2018), *OECD Employment Outlook 2018*, OECD Publishing, Paris, http://dx.doi.org/10.1787/empl_outlook-2018-en. [31]

OECD (2016), *Health Workforce Policies in OECD Countries: Right Jobs, Right Skills, Right Places*, OECD Health Policy Studies, OECD Publishing, Paris, https://dx.doi.org/10.1787/9789264239517-en. [8]

OIG (2018), *Adverse Events in Long-Term-Care Hospitals: National Incidence Among Medicare Beneficiaries*, https://oig.hhs.gov/oei/reports/oei-06-14-00530.pdf (accessed on 5 October 2019). [27]

Osterman, P. (2017), *Who Will Care for Us? Long-term Care and the Long-term Workforce*, Russell Sage Foundation, New York, http://www.jstor.org/stable/10.7758/9781610448673. [28]

Prince, M. et al. (2015), "The burden of disease in older people and implications for health policy and practice", Vol. 385/9967, pp. 549-562, http://dx.doi.org/10.1016/S0140-6736(14)61347-7. [13]

Qian, S. et al. (2012), "The work pattern of personal care workers in two Australian nursing homes: a time-motion study", *BMC Health Services Research*, Vol. 12/1, http://dx.doi.org/10.1186/1472-6963-12-305. [2]

Rapp, T. et al. (2011), "Public financial support receipt and non-medical resource utilization in Alzheimer's disease results from the PLASA study", *Social Science and Medicine*, Vol. 72/8, pp. 1310-1316, http://dx.doi.org/10.1016/j.socscimed.2011.02.039. [5]

Spetz, J. and N. Dudley (2019), "Consensus-Based Recommendations for an Adequate Workforce to Care for People with Serious Illness", *Journal of the American Geriatrics Society*, Vol. 67/S2, pp. S392-S399, http://dx.doi.org/10.1111/jgs.15938. [9]

Sunde, O., K. Øyen and S. Ytrehus (2017), "Do nurses and other health professionals' in elderly care have education in family nursing?", *Scandinavian Journal of Caring Sciences*, Vol. 32/1, pp. 280-289, http://dx.doi.org/10.1111/scs.12459. [18]

Surr, C. et al. (2017), "Effective dementia education and training for the health and social care workforce: a systematic review of the literature", *Review of Educational Research*, Vol. 87/5, pp. 966-1002, http://dx.doi.org/10.3102/0034654317723305. [30]

Truchot, D. (2018), *Rapport de recherche sur la santé des soignants*, Laboratoire de psychologie, Université Bourgogne-Franche Comté, https://www.asso-sps.fr/assets/rapport-de-recherche-sur-la-sante-des-soignants---pr-didier-truchot.pdf. [12]

Whitson, H. et al. (2008), "A quality improvement program to enhance after-hours telephone communication between nurses and physicians in a long-term care facility", *Journal of the American Geriatrics Society*, Vol. 56/6, pp. 1080-1086, http://dx.doi.org/10.1111/j.1532-5415.2008.01714.x. [6]

4 Addressing retention by creating better-quality jobs in long-term care

This chapter reports new analysis on tenure and working conditions for long-term care (LTC) workers. It highlights in particular the fact that LTC workers tend to have lower than average tenure, and quantifies the extent of non-standard work, low pay and health problems among LTC workers in OECD countries. The chapter also identifies policy options to address challenges in working conditions that may thereby contribute to retaining workers in the LTC sector. These include measures on wages, social dialogue, occupation health and improving workers' autonomy.

4.1. Many more quality jobs are needed

Over recent decades, low retention in the LTC workforce has been an important topic and is one of the main policy challenges encountered in OECD countries. Difficult working conditions, such as low competitiveness of wages, precarious job status, demanding jobs with high exposure to physical and mental risk factors and low job satisfaction – driven by low support and autonomy – explain why it is difficult to retain workers in LTC (OECD, 2019[1]; Osterman, 2017[2]). The Norwegian Nurses Organisation reports that one nurse in five quits the LTC workforce within the first five years of their employment, mainly because of the working conditions affecting their work-life balance and health.

Addressing future LTC needs of the ageing population will not be possible unless more is done to make the sector more attractive and to improve working conditions. Turnover in health facilities reduces the effectiveness and productivity of delivering care (Squillace, 2008[3]). For instance, a 10% increase in turnover was associated with an increase in mortality among nursing home care residents and a decrease in the quality of care measured by the physical environment and infection control, among others (Akosa Antwi and Bowblis, 2016[4])

High rates of staff turnover generate not only a poorer quality of care but also higher costs. Turnover requires hiring replacement staff, which entails recruitment costs and generates periods of understaffing. In addition, newly hired personnel require training in the facility's policies and work procedures. A US study found that the marginal cost savings associated with a ten percentage point increase in turnover for an average facility was 3% of annual total costs (Mukamel, 2009[5]).

The objective of this chapter is to document the working conditions driving poor retention in the LTC workforce across OECD countries and explore policies that could be implemented. The remaining sections are organised as follows. Section 4.2 shows that LTC workers do not stay long with their employers. Section 4.3 shows that LTC workers face low job quality. Section 4.4 investigates how countries are seeking to improve working conditions in the LTC sector. Section 4.5 provides a short conclusion.

Key findings

- Tenure in the LTC workforce is low: LTC workers do not stay long with their employers. The average tenure is two years lower in the LTC than in the overall workforce, and fewer workers consider a long career in LTC work than in hospital work.
- LTC is predominantly a low-paid sector: wages are low, especially for personal care workers. Across 11 OECD countries, LTC workers receive EUR 9 per hour (median wage), compared to EUR 14 for hospital workers.
- LTC job quality is low. Non-standard employment is high in the LTC sector: temporary employment is almost twice as high as in the hospital sector. Half of LTC workers do shift work and 45% work part time. In several countries, part-time workers wish to increase their hours but are not offered longer schedules.
- LTC workers face important work-related health issues. Exposure to risk factors for mental well-being and for physical health issues is high among LTC workers, explaining why sickness leave is high in the profession in many countries. Poor work organisation leads to a lack of job satisfaction and increased stress among workers, and reduces opportunities to maintain a good work-life balance.
- It is unlikely to be possible to attract and retain sufficient workers in LTC to meet the growing demand unless pay and working conditions change. Improving LTC jobs would also improve quality of care and reduce turnover costs.

- More than half of OECD countries implemented measures to improve working conditions and address retention in the past decade. Many measures led to positive results, including improving working arrangements, such as introducing flexible workforce arrangements or increasing autonomy; reducing undeclared work through service vouchers or tax credits; workplace interventions; and improving safety at work.
- Some measures to improve working conditions are promising but have not yet been evaluated: providing longer working hours for involuntary part-time workers (Germany, Portugal), developing coaching programmes (Netherlands) to promote prevention of accidents and burnout in the workforce.
- More than half of OECD countries implemented measures to upgrade wages and benefits in the past decade. Evaluations suggest that while increasing wages influences turnover, the effect is small and, in some cases, may lead to more precarious employment, reduced hours or increased workload, unless accompanied by sufficient funding. Collective bargaining and social dialogue can help to implement comprehensive policy measures, including on pay, training and working conditions.

4.2. LTC workers do not stay long in the sector

This section documents the extent of challenges to address retention among LTC workers. Identifying LTC workers in data sources to have comprehensive picture of their working conditions is not straightforward. Using specific surveys on the sector precludes comparison with other sectors, and such surveys are not always performed on a regular basis across a number of countries. In order to identify LTC workers in routinely collected data, it is necessary to cross-reference information on the specific occupation and industry with a high level of detail (Box 4.1).

Box 4.1. Identifying LTC workers: Data sources

LTC workers are individuals who provide care to LTC recipients at home or in LTC institutions (other than hospitals). Following the OECD definition, formal LTC workers comprise two main professional categories: nurses and personal care workers. Personal care workers include formal workers providing LTC services at home or in institutions (other than hospitals) who are not qualified or certified as nurses.

Few reports provide international comparisons of the working conditions of LTC workers. Routinely collected surveys of workers can be used to explore the characteristics of the LTC workforce, but in order to identify LTC workers, such data sources need to have a high level of detail in terms of occupation (at the 3- or 4-digit level) and need to cross-reference that information with the industry code (at the 2-digit level) to make sure that such nurses and personal care workers are in institutions or homes and not in other health sectors.

For European countries, this chapter relies on the European Union Labour Force Survey (EU-LFS). Identification is based on the Nomenclature des Activités économiques dans la Communauté Européenne [Classification of economic activities of the European community] (NACE) 2-digit (88 social work activities without accommodation and 87 residential care activities) and the International Standard Classification of Occupations (ISCO) 4-digit codes (2221 for professional nurses, 3221 for associate professional nurses, 5322 for home-based personal care workers, and 5321 for health care assistants). In addition, information on wages for Europe comes from the 2014 European Union Structure of Earnings Survey (EU-SES). For health-related information, the 2013 ad hoc module of the LFS includes data on accidents at work and other work-related health problems.

In the United States, the March supplement of the Annual Social and Economic Supplement of the Current Population Survey (ASEC-CPS) is used. The cross-referencing of industry and occupation is based on the North American Industry Classification System (NAICS) codes (8170 for home health care services, 9290 for private households health services, 8270 for nursing care facilities, and 8290 for residential care facility without nursing) and the Standard Occupational Classification (SOC) codes (3130 and 3255 for registered nurses, 3258 for nurse practitioners, 3500 for licensed practical and licensed vocational nurses, 3 600 for nursing, psychiatric and home health aides, and 4610 for personal and home care aides).

In addition, Australia's data were based on the Australia Aged Care Workforce 2016 report, published by the Department of Health of the Australian Government. For Canada, the source was the Census survey of 2016. Israel's data were based on their national LFS. For Japan, the source was the survey on Long-term Care Workers FY2016. For Korea, the source was the National Health Insurance Survey's database for the registry of LTC providers, using the Long Term Care Provider Report for Registration. New Zealand's data were based on the New Zealand Aged Care Workforce 2016 report, published by the New Zealand Work Research Institute.

4.2.1. Addressing retention issues is a top policy priority

Almost two-thirds of OECD countries identified LTC worker retention as one of the highest political challenges within the LTC agenda (Figure 4.1) Failing to address this has implications for both quantity and quality of LTC. High turnover can reduce quality of work, as new workers need to learn the care recipients' preferences; this disrupts elderly people and results in a waste of resources from employers who need to spend time on recruitment and training efforts.

Figure 4.1. Many countries rank retention as a challenge of high importance within the LTC agenda

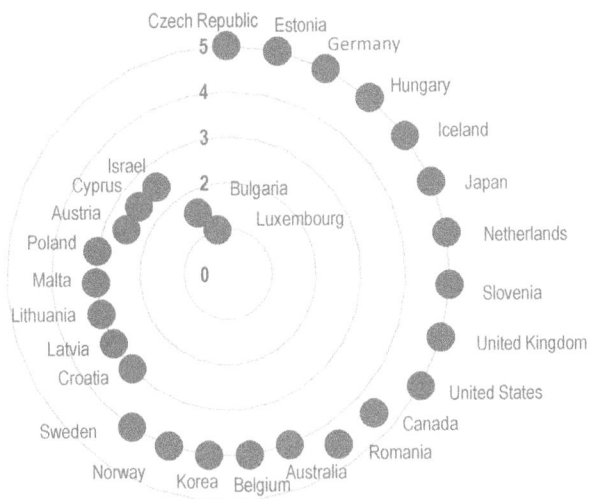

Note: Countries answered the following question: "On a scale between 1 (low-level) and 5 (high-level), what is the challenge faced to retain LTC workers into the LTC workforce in your country?"
Source: 2018 OECD LTC workforce survey.

Most OECD countries face high turnover, with workers leaving the sector after a few years. In countries for which data are available, it is estimated that turnover issues affect between one-quarter and one-third of LTC workers. For instance, in the United States, turnover in the overall LTC workforce is a challenging issue: in 2013, 13% of LTC workers were entrants while 21% were LTC sector leavers (OECD, 2019[1]). In

Germany, estimates based on the German Socio-economic Panel show that on average only 68% of LTC workers in a given year keep participating in the LTC workforce the following year. This holds true for people who have recently completed their training, according to the German Institute for Employment Research. However, after that high turnover in the first professional year, the loyalty to the profession remains relatively constant in the following years. Reasons for the high turnover in the first professional year. In Australia, recent evidence shows that, in 2017, 94% of LTC employers had to recruit personal care workers just to cope with turnover issues (compared to 88% in 2014) (Mavromaras et al., 2017[6]). In France, about 20% of home-based positions were estimated to be vacant in 2018 and over 80% of institutions reported at least one vacant position in 2015, the position of personal care workers being the most difficult position to fill in institutions. Overall, it was estimated that 60 000 positions were unfilled in 2019 (El Khomri, 2019[7]). In addition, results from the last wave of the survey on LTC institutions (Enquête auprès des établissements d'hébergement pour personnes âgée/EHPA) survey show that, in 2015, 34.6% of institution-based workers were interim workers (Muller, 2017[8]). In the United Kingdom, the mean turnover rate among care workers between 2008 and 2010 was 23% (Hussein, Ismail and Manthorpe, 2016[9]).

European data show that more workers are looking for another job in the LTC workforce than in the hospital workforce, reflecting either dissatisfaction with the work or a lack of job security (Figure 4.2). In the United Kingdom, almost 10% of LTC workers are actively looking for another job, compared to 6% in the hospital workforce. In Spain, the equivalent proportions are 9% (LTC) and 2% (hospital); in France, they are 6% (LTC) and 2% (hospital). In Scandinavian countries (Finland, Denmark and Sweden), the proportions of LTC workers looking for new job opportunities are also high but are close to the hospital workforce proportions. A large share of care workers (one-third to almost one-half) in Scandinavian countries reported that they had seriously considered quitting; this increased between 2005 and 2015 (Rostgaard et al., 2019[10]).

Figure 4.2. More workers are looking for another job in the LTC than in the hospital workforce

Share of workers reporting looking for another job, by sector, 2016

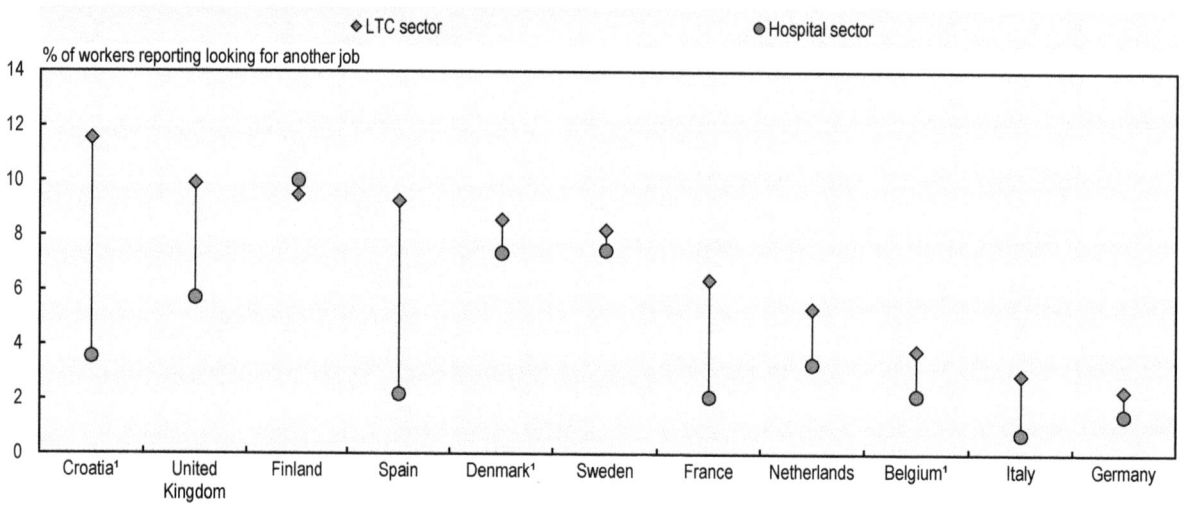

Note: Data were calculated based on ISCO 3-digit and NACE 2-digit codes. For a description of the methodology to identify workers, see Annex 2.A in Chapter 2.
1. Data must be interpreted with caution, as sample sizes are small.
Source: EU-LFS (data refer to 2016).

4.2.2. Tenure is low in the LTC workforce

In most OECD countries, the average tenure[1] rate in the LTC sector is lower than in the overall working population (Figure 4.3), with an overall difference of two years. The exceptions are the Netherlands and Norway, where the average tenure rates in the LTC workforce (11 and 10 years respectively) are 1 year higher than in the overall working population. Since 2011, both countries have implemented a comprehensive strategy to develop their LTC workforces, involving policies to improve co-ordination, retention, prevention and use of technology, as well as recruitment programmes targeting new groups of workers, which may explain in part why tenure is higher.

Figure 4.3. Tenure is lower in the LTC workforce than in the overall workforce

Average tenure of LTC workforce, by sector, 2016

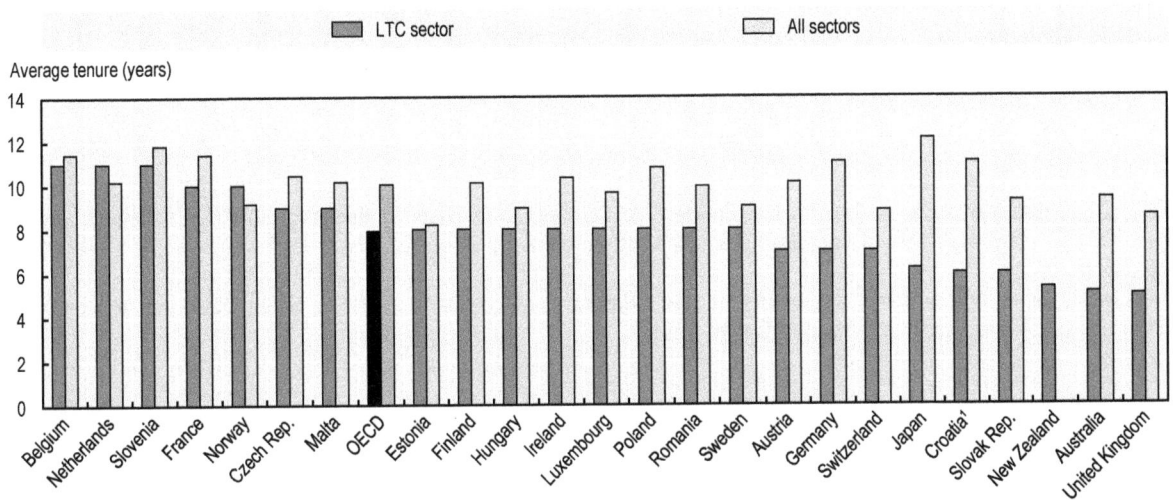

Note: The OECD data point is the unweighted average of the 21 OECD countries shown in the chart. EU-LFS data were based on ISCO 3-digit and NACE 2-digit codes. For a description of the methodology to identify workers, see Annex 2.A in Chapter 2.
1. Data must be interpreted with caution, as the sample size is small.
Source: EU-LFS; Survey on Long-term Care Workers for Japan; OECD estimates based on national sources for Australia and New Zealand; OECD Database. Data refer to 2016.

In addition to mean tenure, looking at median data provides a better understanding of tenure, in particular if there are many low values because of people leaving the sector early. In OECD countries, the median tenure rate is five years, which is lower than average and confirms that many LTC workers have low tenure (Figure 4.4). Again, there are large differences across countries: median tenure ranges between two years in Korea and eight years in the Netherlands.

Note, however, that because of data limitations, the tenure rates presented in Figure 4.3 and Figure 4.4 aggregate nurses and personal care workers, who often have different tenure rates. In Norway and the Netherlands, nurses have lower median tenure rates than personal care workers, and both countries report that the challenge associated with nurses' retention is higher than the challenge associated with personal care workers' retention. In other countries, such as Austria and Belgium, nurses have a lower median tenure than personal care workers.

Figure 4.4. The median tenure in the LTC workforce varies across OECD countries

Median tenure of LTC workforce, by country, 2016

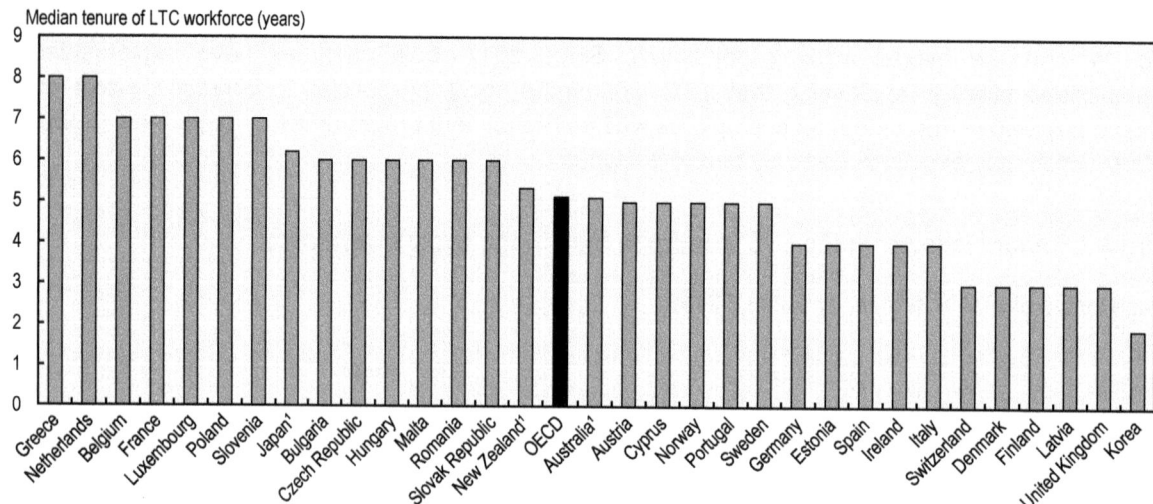

Note: The OECD data point is the unweighted average of the 29 OECD shown in the chart. For European countries, data refer to personal carers and nurses not working in hospital. For a description of the methodology to identify workers, see Annex 2.A in Chapter 2. 1. Data refer to average tenure.
Source: EU-LFS; Survey on Long-term Care Workers for Japan, National Health Insurance System for Korea, OECD estimates based on national sources for Australia and New Zealand. Data refer to 2016.

Figure 4.5 shows the correlation between median tenure rates and the LTC supply per 100 people aged 65 and over. Four groups of countries can be identified:

- In some countries (Luxembourg, the Netherlands, Sweden and Norway), the supply of LTC workers is high, and workers' tenure is greater than or equal to five years. In these countries, both recruitment and retention rates are among OECD's highest. They have been able to develop their LTC workforce successfully since 2011 (both number of workers and experience).

- In some countries (including Estonia, Germany, Finland and Denmark), the supply of LTC workers is larger than or close to the OECD average, but the number of years LTC workers spend with their employer is lower. Therefore, these countries seem mainly to face retention issues.

- In some countries (including France, Slovenia, the Czech Republic and Poland), LTC workers' tenure is greater than the OECD average, but the number of LTC workers per 100 people aged 65 and over is much lower. These countries seem to face greater recruitment than retention issues.

- Finally, certain countries (including the United Kingdom and Italy) face both lower supply and lower tenure of LTC workers than most OECD countries.

Figure 4.5. Tenure and size of the workforce differ across countries

Number of LTC workers per 100 individuals aged 65 and over and median tenure, 2016 (or nearest year)

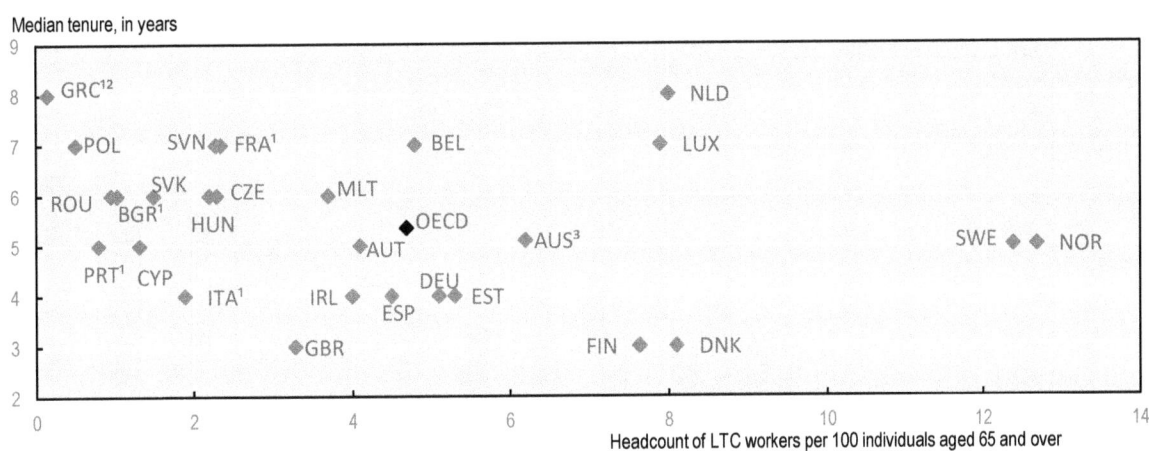

Note: The OECD data point is the unweighted average of the 23 OECD countries shown in the chart. EU-LFS data are based on ISCO 4-digit and NACE 2-digit codes. A list of country abbreviations is provided in Annex 4.A.
1. Data are based on ISCO 3-digit and NACE 2-digit codes. 2. Data must be interpreted with caution, as sample sizes are small. 3. Data refer to average tenure.
Source: EU-LFS, Quarterly Labour Force Survey for the United Kingdom, ASEC-CPS for the United States, OECD Health Statistics 2018, https://doi.org/10.1787/health-data-en, Eurostat for population demographics; OECD tenure estimate based on national source for Australia. Data refer to 2016 or nearest year.

4.3. Low pay and poor job quality prevail in LTC

4.3.1. LTC is predominantly a low-paid sector

Current wages in the LTC workforce are low, especially for personal care workers, who often have lower salaries than nurses (Figure 4.6). In several countries, personal care workers are paid the minimum wage. In Portugal, for instance, the average annual salary of a personal care worker is around EUR 600 monthly, roughly the minimum wage (based on 12 monthly payments), while nurses are paid EUR 900. In Ireland, personal care workers (health care assistants) receive an average of EUR 10.40 per hour in the private LTC sector, which represents a wage 6% above the minimum wage but 23% lower than in the public LTC sector.

Earnings in the LTC workforce are significantly lower than in the hospital sector when comparing workers in the same broad occupations (Figure 4.7). Across 11 EU countries, LTC workers received EUR 9 per hour (median wage), compared to EUR 14 for hospital workers. This wage difference contributes to explaining why hospital jobs are more attractive than LTC jobs. The wage difference can be large in some OECD countries (such as Israel, Canada and the United Kingdom).

Figure 4.6. Salaries in the LTC workforce tend to be low

Average gross monthly earnings in EUR, 2017 (or nearest year)

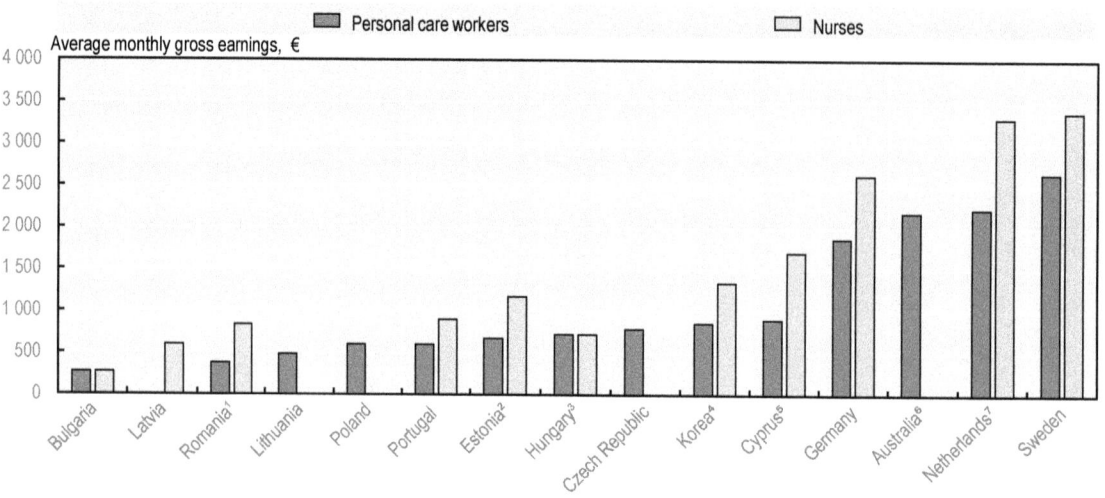

Note: For a description of the methodology to identify workers, see Annex 2.A in Chapter 2.
1. Data for personal carers and nurses refer to an average based on different qualifications. 2. Data for personal carers refer to an average based on different qualifications. 3. Breakdown is not available. 4. Data for nurses refer to an average based on different qualifications. 5. Data refer to the public sector. 6. Data refer to the median gross monthly earnings in residential aged care for personal carers. 7. Data for personal carers refer to an average based on different qualifications and data for nurses, excluding irregular earnings.
Source: OECD LTC workforce survey 2018 (data refer to 2017 or nearest year).

Figure 4.7. Workers are paid less in the LTC than the hospital sector

Median hourly gross earnings, population aged 20-59, 2014 (or nearest year)

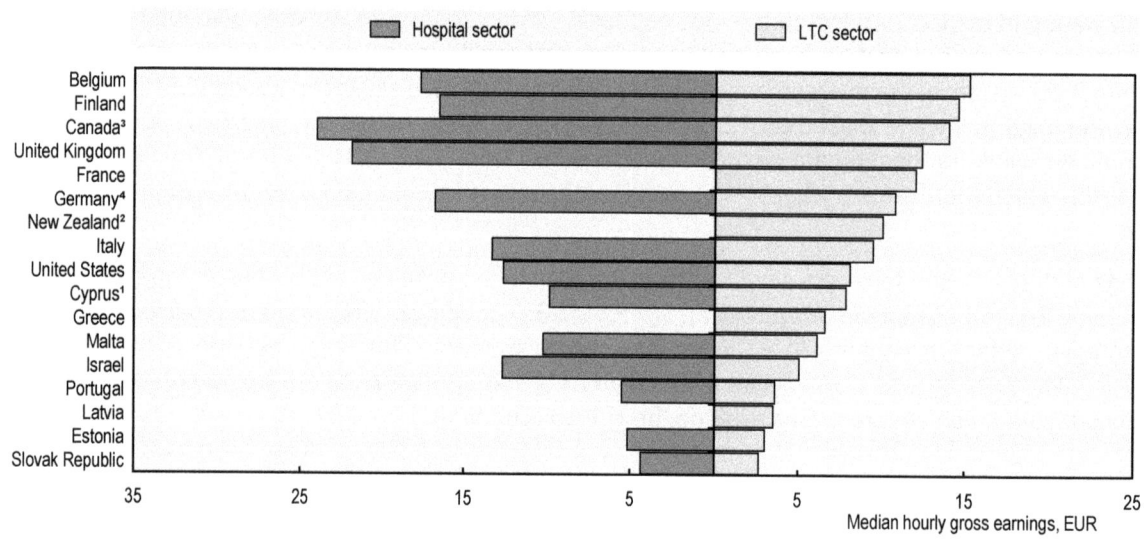

Note: Data cover those aged between 20 and 59 years old. For a description of the methodology to identify workers, see Annex 2.A in Chapter 2.
1. Data refer to 2010 and must be interpreted with caution, as the sample size is small. 2. Data refer only to personal carers. 3. Data cover those working full time, full year. 4. Data on the hospital sector cover those working full-time and assume an equal distribution of nurses and personal carers.
Source: European Union Structure of Earnings Survey (2014), OECD questionnaire (2018) for Latvia, ASEC-CPS (2015) for the United States, Census 2016 for Canada, OECD estimate based on national source for New Zealand (2016). Data refer to 2014 or nearest year.

Low wages in some countries are explained by the fact that certain parts of the sector are not fully covered by regulations on wage agreements or fall under special regulations. In the United Kingdom, the Low Pay Commission has flagged social care as a sector of concern due to non-compliance with the national minimum wage. The difficulty of solving underpayment issues (low wages, non-payment of the national minimum wage) has been a factor explaining why the home care sector experiences the highest turnover and vacancy rates in adult social care in England, United Kingdom (Hussein, Ismail and Manthorpe, 2016[9]). In England, between 9% and 13% of care jobs are estimated to pay below the national minimum wage, mostly because of unpaid time, which includes travelling time, training time and "on-call" hours (Gardiner, 2015[11]). Similarly, a study of home care of elderly people in England found widespread use of zero-hours contracts[2] and paid hours restricted to time with patients, with staff uncompensated for travel time (Rubery et al., 2015[12]). In France, the wage agreements for home-based LTC workers, established in 2010, set a gross minimum wage that is now below the national minimum wage (EUR 1 452.6 per month and EUR 1 521.22 per month respectively in 2019) (El Khomri, 2019[7]).

Cost-cutting measures in countries facing LTC system financing constraints can also lead to downward pressure on wages in the formal LTC sector, or lower employment. This is, for example, the case in the Netherlands, where a 2015 reform transferred the LTC insurance budget management to municipalities, which are now in charge of paying LTC workers mostly for household tasks such as cleaning and cooking. The reform was associated with a EUR 0.5 billion budget cut (Maarse and Jeurissen, 2016[13]), which decreased substantially the funds allocated to municipalities, to the detriment of the workforce and employers. It led municipalities negotiating lower tariffs with LTC providers. Providers of domestic help complain that this has led to lower prices per hour for services, resulting in providers going bankrupt, lay-offs, low wages and temporary contracts and/or contracts for short hours.

4.3.2. Non-standard work can affect work-life balance and job security

Non-standard employment is high in LTC

Part-time employment is sizeable in the LTC workforce. It is on average twice as high as the average rate in the economy. Figure 4.8 shows that 45% of LTC workers work part time in OECD countries. In northern and central European countries, more than half of the workers have part-time jobs. In most countries, personal care workers and home-based workers are more likely to work part time than nurses and residential-based workers.

While working part time can be a choice, especially among workers wanting a better work-life balance, high rates of part-time work are also due to use of LTC services for reduced hours at specific times of the day. Consequently, part-time contracts usually result in short-hour contracts of 12-18 hours per week; these are often for morning and evening hours to provide help with getting out of bed, going to bed and feeding and washing. In France, for instance, half of the elderly population with LTC needs receive one hour and 10 minutes per day of professional help (Brunel, Latourelle and Zakri, 2018[14]) and almost 80% of home-based LTC employees work part-time (El Khomri, 2019[7]) In this respect, involuntary part-time work can be an issue in the sector. For instance, almost one-third of workers in Australia report that they want to work more hours (Meagher, Szebehely and Mears, 2016[15]). Involuntary part-time work has also been recorded as an issue in Scandinavian countries, especially in Norway, using Nordcare surveys. Part-time work can also affect take-home pay, especially if travel time is not fully compensated for. In the United States, personal care workers wish to work more hours and have to work with multiple clients or agencies to earn sufficient income (Osterman, 2017[2]). LTC work can also be part time because of the heavy workload, which is often cited as a reason to limit working hours.

Figure 4.8. About 45% of LTC workers hold part-time positions across OECD countries

Share of the workforce reporting working part time, 2016

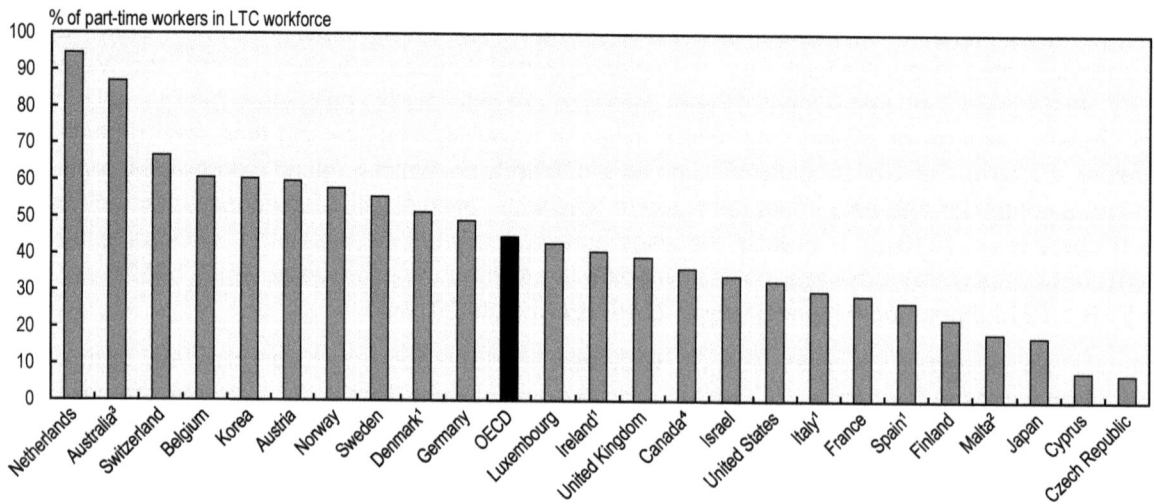

Note: The OECD data point is the unweighted average of the 22 OECD countries shown in the chart. EU-LFS data are based on ISCO 4-digit and NACE 2-digit codes. For a description of the methodology to identify workers, see Annex 2.A in Chapter 2.
1. Data are based on ISCO 3-digit and NACE 2-digit codes. 2. Data must be interpreted with caution, as sample sizes are small. 3. Data cover only those with a permanent position. 4. Data cover only those working mostly full time or mostly part time.
Source: EU-LFS; ASEC-CPS for the United States; Census 2016 for Canada; Labour Force Survey for Israel; Survey on Long-term Care Workers for Japan; National Health Insurance System for Korea; OECD estimate based on national source for Australia. Data refer to 2016 or nearest year.

Figure 4.9. Half of carers work shifts on average in OECD countries

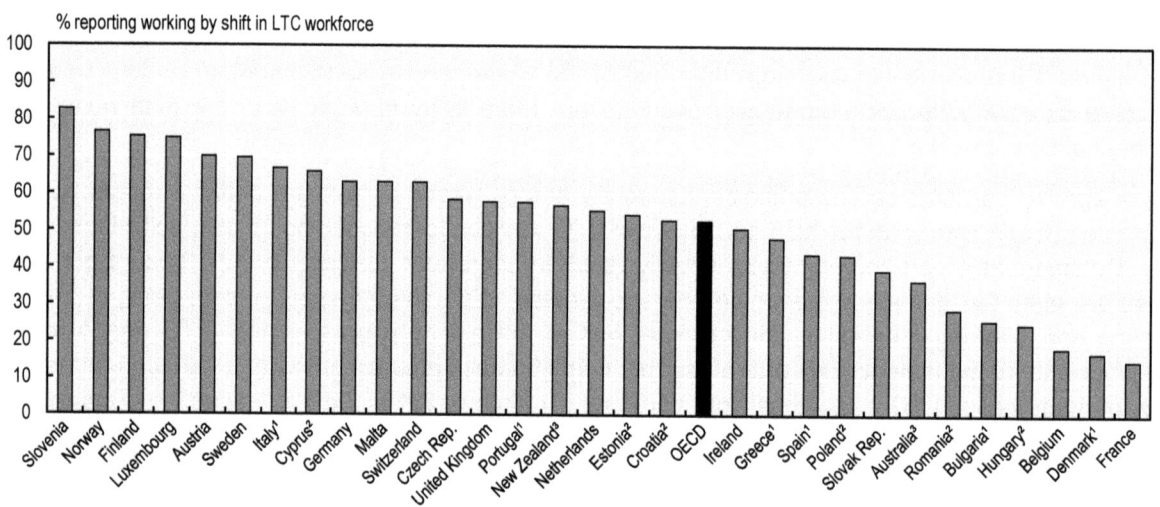

Note: The OECD data point is the unweighted average of the 25 OECD countries shown in the chart. EU-LFS data are based on ISCO 4-digit and NACE 2 digit codes. For a description of the methodology to identify workers, see Annex 2.A in Chapter 2.
1. Data are based on ISCO 3-digit and NACE 2-digit codes. 2. Data must be interpreted with caution, as sample sizes are small. 3. Data refer to those who do not work regular daytime shifts.
Source: EU-LFS; OECD estimates based on national sources for Australia and New Zealand.

Shift work[3] is widespread in the LTC sector (Figure 4.9): half of LTC workers work shifts across OECD countries, although there are large differences across countries. In Scandinavian and central European countries, more than 70% of LTC workers work shifts, while the figure is less than one-quarter in Belgium, Denmark and France. A large body of evidence suggests that shift work is associated with a wide range of health risks such as anxiety, burnout and depressive syndromes (Saint-Martin, Inanc and Prinz, 2018[16]).

Large differences also exist within the LTC workforce. Compared to home-based carers, those working in institutions are 80% more likely to work shifts on average (in the 14 countries for which data are available). Again, there are large differences across countries. In Finland, Norway, Sweden and Germany, more than half of home-based carers work shifts, while the figure is less than 40% in the United Kingdom and the Slovak Republic.

In addition, LTC workers are also more likely to work on weekends compared to other medical or social professions. For instance, a survey of 6 066 French LTC workers showed that 92.9% of personal care workers and 85.1% of nurses regularly work during weekends, compared to 42% of general practitioners and 35.6% of speech therapists (Truchot, 2018[17]).

Three models of working arrangements in the LTC sector can be identified. In the first, the LTC workforce market relies on high levels of part-time and shift work (Netherlands, Switzerland, Austria, Norway, the United Kingdom and Sweden). In the second, working arrangements mix low levels of part-time work with high levels of shift work (Italy, Denmark and Finland). In the third, working arrangements involve low levels of part-time and shift work (France, Spain and Ireland).

Temporary contracts and new forms of employment raise concerns for job security

The share of temporary employment is high in the LTC sector compared with the hospital sector (and with the average in the economy). This situation reduces job security and career prospects among workers. In the 20 OECD countries for which data were available, 19% of LTC workers on average have temporary contracts (Figure 4.10). This share reaches 30% or more in Poland and Spain, while it is 10% or less in Belgium, the Slovak Republic, Ireland and the United Kingdom. In comparison, the share of temporary hospital workers is 11% on average in the 20 countries. In many countries, temporary workers face a wage penalty and their contracts are not stepping stones to permanent jobs (OECD, 2015[18]).

New forms of employment (such as zero-hours contracts and temporary agency work), while not yet widely used, appear to be prominent in some countries, generating more job insecurity in the sector. In France, institutions employ a great proportion of temporary agency (interim) workers: results from the last wave of the survey on LTC institutions (EHPA) show that, in 2015, 41.1% of institutions and 33.3% of long-stay facilities faced recruitment issues, and 34.6% of institution-based workers were interim workers (Muller, 2017[8]). In England, United Kingdom, the share of workers on zero-hours contracts represents a quarter of the entire workforce in the sector (Eurofound, 2015[19]). In the Netherlands, workers providing domestic help are sometimes hired as "false" self-employed workers, as they typically work for a single employer. This is a means of avoiding social security obligations, since employers do not have to contribute to disability insurance and pensions. In the United States, 10% of personal care workers are self-employed and thus do not have the same access to collective bargaining rights and social protection as those with employment contracts (Osterman, 2017[2]).

Figure 4.10. Temporary contracts are more common in the LTC than the hospital sector

Share of temporary workers in LTC sector and hospital sector, 2017 (or nearest year)

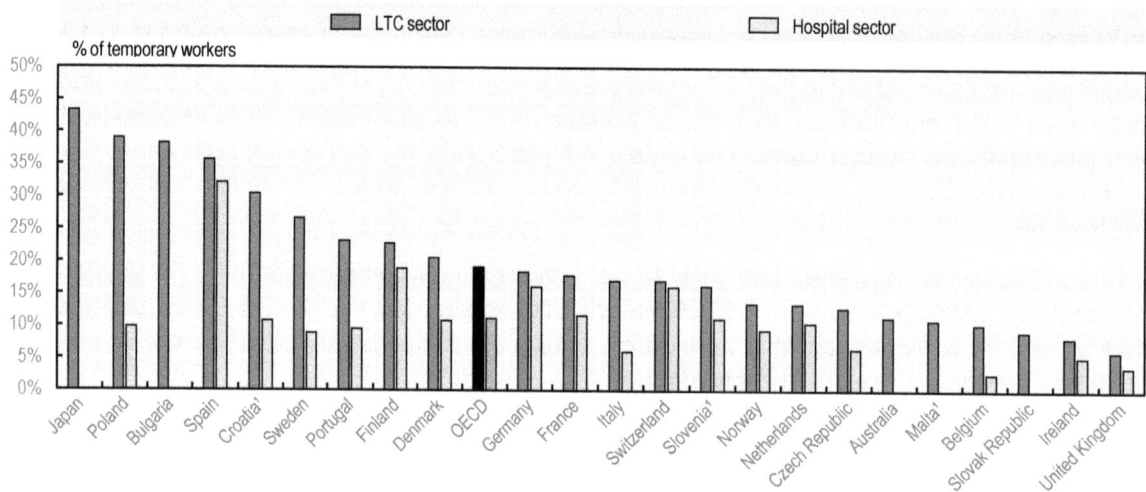

Note: The OECD data point is the unweighted average of the 20 OECD countries shown in the chart. Data are based on ISCO 3-digit and NACE 2-digit codes. For a description of the methodology to identify workers, see Annex 2.A in Chapter 2.
1. Data must be interpreted with caution, as sample sizes are small.
Source: EU-LFS; Survey on Long-term Care Workers for Japan; OECD estimate based on national source for Australia. Data refer to 2016 or nearest year.

Undeclared work employment is also a concern in the LTC workforce. Undeclared workers are often irregular migrant workers hired privately by households. In the United States, there is also a so-called grey market, where consumers hire and pay LTC workers under the table; this is estimated to include about 300 000 personal care workers, or an additional 20% (Osterman, 2017[2]). In Spain and Italy, the widespread undeclared status of workers can lead to abusive situations, including long working hours and low wages, and a lack of training opportunities (Casanova, Lamura and Principi, 2017[20]). Undeclared workers in LTC are often migrants, and guaranteeing fair working conditions for migrant workers is a major challenge. A particular issue is that undocumented people may often enter the country with a tourist or student visa and perform illicit work as domestic workers but fail to access social security benefits (Luppi et al., 2014[21]). In Latin American countries, such as Colombia, in some cases workers perform their duties following a verbal agreement and work without a contract, without minimum standards.

4.3.3. Work-related health issues are important

Care workers say that their work is often rewarding but emotionally and physically demanding. Between one-third and just under one-half of LTC workers in Scandinavian countries report being usually physically exhausted after a work day (Rostgaard et al., 2019[10]). This figure is comparable to the share of home care workers in Austria (41%) but among residential care workers in Austria the proportion who report being physically exhausted after a work day is 68% (Bauer, Rodrigues and Leichsenring, 2018[22]). This may help to explain why the prevalence of health issues related to work is slightly higher in the LTC than in the hospital sector (Figure 4.11).

Over 25% of LTC workers in Finland and Sweden report at least one work-related health problem. Among southern European countries, Italy, Spain and Portugal have lower rates, ranging from 7% to 11%. Across OECD countries, 15% of LTC workers reported work-related health issues on average, compared to 12% of hospital-based workers. In comparison, 7.9% of people across all 28 EU countries reported experiencing work-related health problems in the past 12 months, showing that in most countries LTC workers face larger risks than the overall population.

In some countries (Sweden, the Czech Republic, Switzerland, the United Kingdom and Denmark), work-related issues are less prevalent in the LTC than in the hospital workforce. In these countries, differences are small, except in Sweden, where the difference is six percentage points (26% for LTC workers and 32% for hospital-based workers).

Figure 4.11. Over 15% of LTC workers report work-related health problems

Share of workers reporting physical or mental health problems suffered in the previous 12 months caused or made worse by work, excluding accidents at work, by sector, 2013

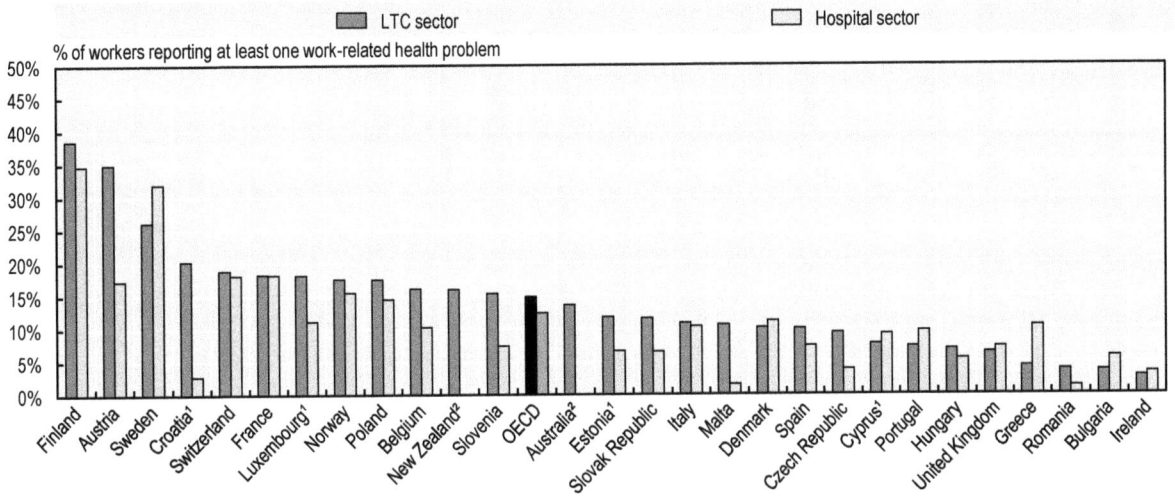

Note: The OECD data point is the unweighted average of the 23 OECD countries shown in the chart. EU-LFS data were calculated based on ISCO 3-digit and NACE 2-digit codes. For a description of the methodology to identify workers see Annex 2.A in Chapter 2.
1. Data must be interpreted with caution, as sample sizes are small. 2. Data refer to those reporting back pain in New Zealand and those reporting at least one illness or injury in Australia.
Source: Ad hoc module EU-LFS (data refer to 2013); OECD estimates based on national sources for Australia and New Zealand (data refer to 2016).

LTC workers have a higher risk than hospital workers of experiencing accidents at work leading to injuries (Figure 4.12). Available data show that the rate varied from 20% in Japan to 1% in the Czech Republic and Slovak Republic. In Scandinavian countries, more than 6% of carers suffer from accidents at work on average. In the United Kingdom and in Spain, the rate was 5%.

Figure 4.12. Accidents at work leading to injuries are higher in LTC than in hospitals

Share of workers reporting at least one accident at work resulting in injury in the previous 12 months, by sector, 2013 (or nearest year)

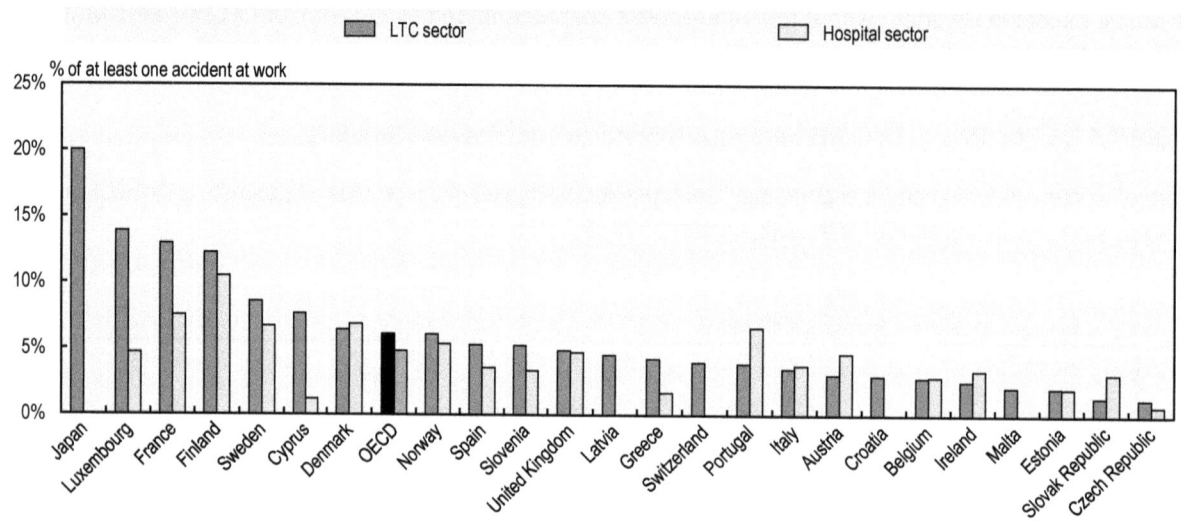

Note: The OECD data point is the unweighted average of the 21 OECD countries shown in the chart. EU-LFS data were calculated based on ISCO 3-digit and NACE 2-digit codes. For a description of the methodology to identify workers, see Annex-2.A in Chapter-2.
Source: Ad hoc module EU-LFS (data refer to 2013); Survey on Long-term Care Workers for Japan (data refer to 2014).

Countries with a high share of accidents also show high rates of health complications. Figure 4.13 shows that the association between accidents at work resulting in injuries and work-related health problems is important (correlation of +0.18). Countries such as France and Finland have the highest shares of LTC workers reporting accidents at work and work-related health problems. In France, the social health insurance (*Caisse nationale d'assurance maladie*) counted in 2017 that 24 000 accidents, 2 000 transport accidents linked to work and 1 200 work-related illnesses occurred in institutions and that another 19 000 accidents happened at homes when working (El Khomri, 2019[7]).

Sickness absence tends to be high in the LTC sector. In Norway, close to 10% of the municipal workforce experienced sick leave, representing 8 million work days annually. Although this figure includes all workers, data show that health care workers are one of the largest groups of sick leave users, so the Norwegian Association of Local and Regional Authorities suggests that extra efforts are needed to reduce sick leave rates in order to meet the 6.7% target defined by the Inclusive Workplace Agreement signed by the Norwegian government and social partners (2014-18). In the Netherlands, sickness absence in the sector is twice the national average. In France, on average, personal care workers take 24 days of sick leave (Truchot, 2018[17]), which is greater than the French average (14.2 days in 2016). LTC, together with health care, has been identified as a sector of priority in Australia to reduce the high rate of work-related injuries and diseases. It ranks high in terms of the numbers of serious worker compensation claims, especially because of muscular stress while handling objects, lifting or moving elderly people.

Figure 4.13. Work-related health problems and accidents at work tend to be correlated

Share of LTC workers reporting at least one accident at work resulting in injury in the previous 12 months and share of workers reporting physical or mental health problems suffered in the previous 12 months caused or made worse by work, excluding accidents at work, 2013

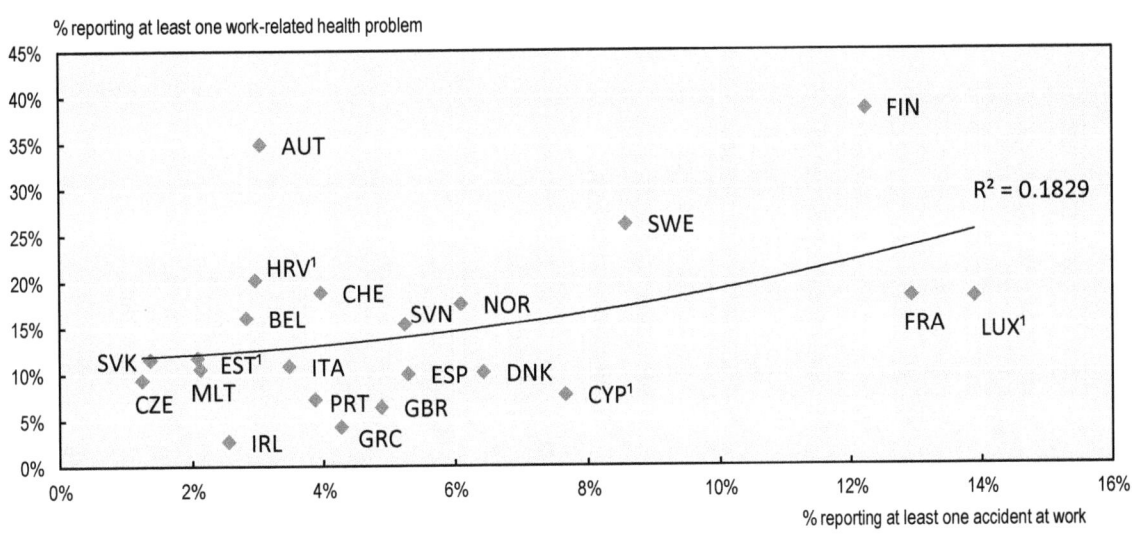

Note: Data were calculated based on ISCO 3-digit and NACE 2-digit codes. For a description of the methodology to identify workers, see Annex 2.A in Chapter 2. A list of country abbreviations is provided in Annex 4.A.
1. Data must be interpreted with caution, as sample sizes are small.
Source: Ad hoc module EU-LFS (data refer to 2013).

LTC workers often face both physical and mental health risk factors

Almost two-thirds (64%) of LTC workers experience physical risk factors across European countries (Figure 4.14), including difficult work postures and handling of heavy loads. The share of LTC workers reporting exposure to physical risk factors varies markedly between countries, from 94% in France to 17% in Romania. Workers in the LTC sector report being as exposed to physical risk factors as hospital-based workers on average across European countries. In half of the countries considered, LTC workers report being slightly more exposed.

Figure 4.14. About 64% of LTC workers report exposure to physical risk factors across OECD countries

Share of workers reporting exposure at work to risk factors that can affect physical health, by sector, 2013

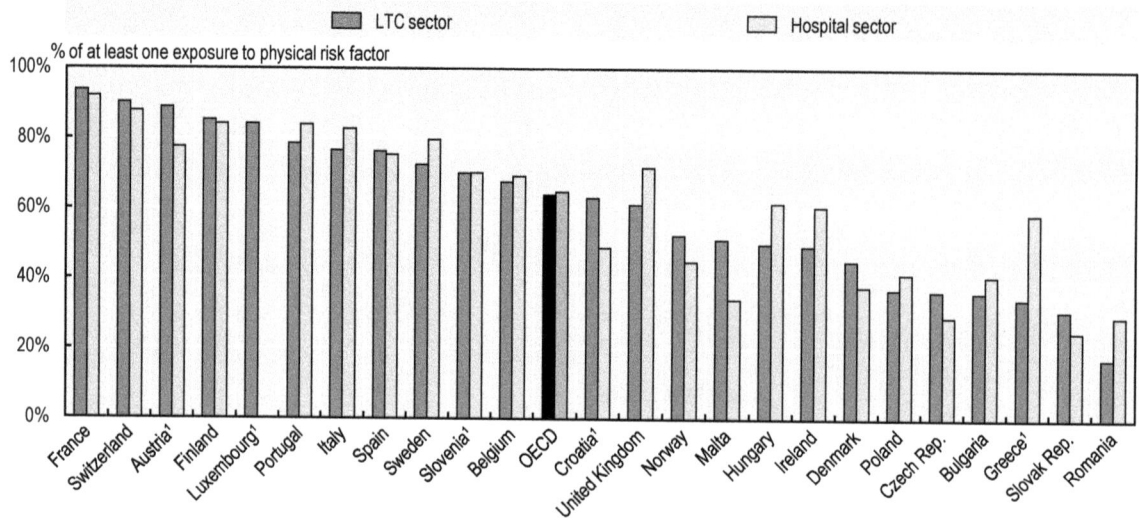

Note: The OECD data point is the unweighted average of the 20 OECD countries shown in the chart. Data were calculated based on ISCO 3-digit and NACE 2-digit codes. For a description of the methodology to identify workers, see Annex 2.A in Chapter 2. Physical risk factors cover difficult work postures or work movements, handling of heavy loads, noise or strong vibration, chemicals, dust, fumes, smoke or gases, strong visual concentration and risk of accidents.
1. Data must be interpreted with caution, as sample sizes are small.
Source: Ad hoc module EU-LFS (data refer to 2013).

Such high rates of physical risk exposure are explained by the nature of the daily tasks LTC workers have to provide, which often require physical efforts (see Chapter 3). For instance, tasks such as lifting patients and bending over a bed when providing care contribute to develop health problems (Kromark et al., 2009[23]; Dulon et al., 2007[24]). This issue is growing in countries like the United States, where obesity rates in the elderly population are growing. Among physical health problems, those related to musculoskeletal conditions such as back pain are widespread (Simon et al., 2008[25]; Evanoff et al., 2003[26]; Needham et al., 2005[27]; Miranda et al., 2011[28]).

On average just under half (46%) of LTC workers in OECD countries are exposed to mental well-being risk factors on average (Figure 4.15), including severe time pressure or overload of work, violence or threat of violence, harassment or bullying. Exposure to mental well-being risk factor also concerns over half of hospital-based workers across European countries. In most countries, risks to mental well-being are reported more frequently, or at least as often, among hospital-based workers than LTC workers.

These data are in line with previous evidence showing the importance of burnout risks in the LTC workforce (Rai, 2010[29]). In France, for instance, a recent survey (Truchot, 2018[17]) shows that nurses and personal care workers are more likely to face sleep deprivation than other professions (such as doctors and speech therapists). Indeed, 28.8% of nurses and 36.4% of personal care workers face difficulties sleeping almost every night of the week. More than 11% declare that they take sleeping pills at least once a week.

Figure 4.15. About 46% of LTC workers report exposure to mental well-being risk factors across OECD countries

Share of workers reporting exposure at work to risk factors that can affect mental well-being, by sector, 2013

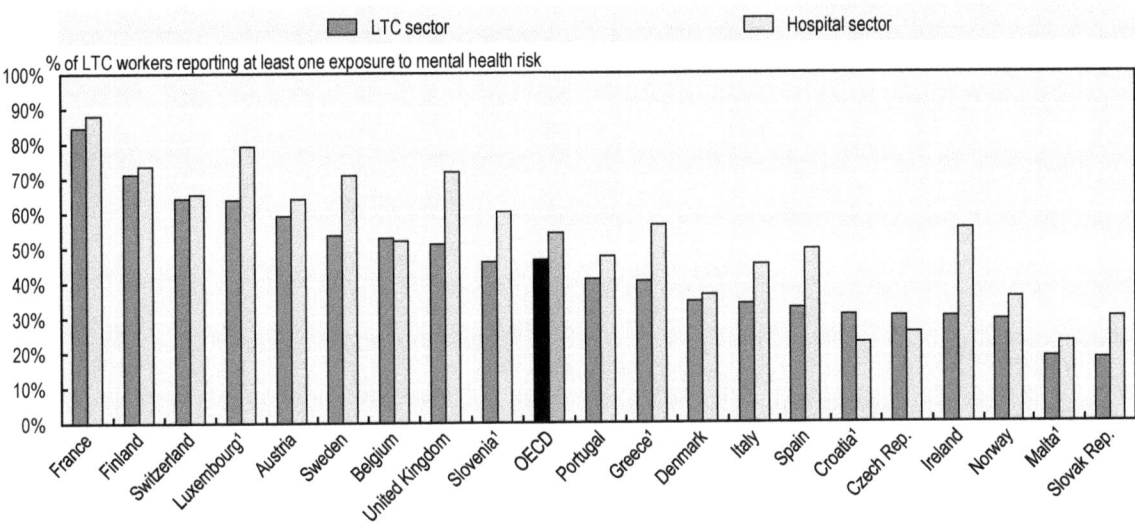

Note: The OECD data point is the unweighted average of the 18 OECD countries shown in the chart. Data were calculated based on ISCO 3-digit and NACE 2-digit codes. Mental well-being risk factors cover: severe time pressure or overload of work, violence or threat of violence, harassment or bullying. For a description of the methodology to identify workers, see Annex 2.A in Chapter 2.
1. Data must be interpreted with caution, as sample sizes are small.
Source: Ad hoc module EU-LFS (data refer to 2013).

Violence perpetrated by a resident or a resident's visitor is common in the LTC sector, which may further contribute to mental and physical health risks at work. In the United States, a study showed that 48% of institution-based workers had been assaulted at least once in the last three months, 26% had been assaulted 1-2 times and 22% had been assaulted at least three times (Miranda et al., 2011[28]). Both institution-based and home-based workers are exposed to violence from patients, co-workers, patients' families and management, which can include intimidation, degradation, humiliation, verbal abuse, physical abuse and/or constant criticism (Fasanya and Dada, 2016[30]). Moreover, workers are exposed to sexual harassment and sexual aggression, resulting in greater stress, depression, sleep problems and burnout (Perrin et al., 2015[31]). Often, workers do not report this violence because they are afraid of losing their jobs and/or fear retaliation (Fasanya and Dada, 2016[30]). For home-based workers, these issues are more likely to be observed in consumer-driven programmes than in agency-based home care models, because the level of monitoring and supervision is often lower in consumer-driven models (Perrin et al., 2015[31]).

Assaulted LTC workers can experience physical reactions, such as fatigue, sleep problems, headaches and musculoskeletal pain (low back, shoulder, wrist, hand and knee pain) resulting from scratches, cuts and bruises. They can also have emotional reactions, such as anger, sadness, frustration, irritability, fear, self-blame and depression (Needham et al., 2005[32]; Miranda et al., 2011[28]).

Figure 4.16 shows that in most countries the association between mental and physical health risks is strong (correlation of +0.59). LTC workers report the highest exposure to physical and mental health risk factors in France, Finland and Switzerland. In Spain, Italy and Portugal, about 80% of LTC workers report exposure to physical risks, while about 40% report exposure to mental well-being risk factor. In Denmark and Norway, about 50% of LTC workers report exposure to physical risk factors, and about 32% LTC workers report exposure to mental well-being risk factor.

Figure 4.16. Association between mental and physical risk factors is strong for LTC workers

Share of LTC workers reporting exposure at work to risk factors that can affect mental well-being and physical health, 2013

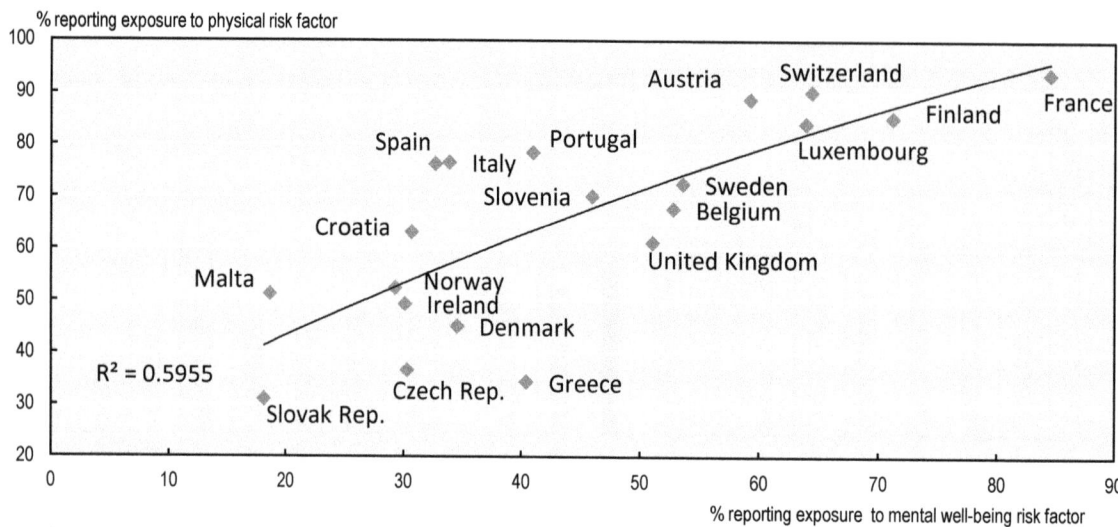

Note: Data were calculated based on ISCO 3-digit and NACE 2-digit codes, leading to the inclusion of midwives working at home. Mental well-being risk factors cover severe time pressure or overload of work, violence or threat of violence, harassment or bullying. Physical risk factors cover difficult work postures or work movements, handling of heavy loads, noise or strong vibration, chemicals, dust, fumes, smoke or gases, strong visual concentration and risk of accidents. Data on mental risk factors for Croatia, Greece, Luxembourg, Malta and Slovenia must be interpreted with caution, as sample sizes are small. Data on physical risk factors for Austria, Croatia, Greece, Luxembourg and Slovenia must also be interpreted with caution, as sample sizes are small. For a description of the methodology to identify workers, see Annex 2.A in Chapter 2.
Source: Ad hoc module EU-LFS (data refer to 2013).

4.3.4. The LTC workforce does not have a high-quality work environment

A poor work environment – characterised by intensive job demands with insufficient job resources (e.g. feedback and support) – reduces worker well-being, weakens worker engagement and productivity, and increases the risk of physical and mental health problems (Saint-Martin, Inanc and Prinz, 2018[16]).

LTC workers face high demands on their time but lack support

LTC workers often complain of high caseloads and limited time with care recipients, which generates a feeling of frustration and overload. Administrative regulations and organisational processes might also restrict autonomy in decision-making.

Table 4.1 outlines the main concerns about the work environment in LTC. Recurrent issues include regulations that constrain workers' capacity to deliver care according to their best judgement; shortage of workers, which reduces their capacity to deliver patient-centred care; an absence of support from the management hierarchy for the challenges they face on a daily basis (such as changes in regulations, conflicts with other care providers); and the difficulty they face in maintaining an adequate work-life balance (especially when they have to travel long distances from their home to work). These issues are likely to drive job satisfaction down and increase workers' intention to leave their current employment (Kim and Kim, 2017[33]).

Table 4.1. Managerial issues explain in part low workforce retention in LTC

Reason LTC workers leave the workforce	Description of common issues
Regulations are too constraining and they are unable to use their professional judgement.	Constraining rules and regulations often dictate care. LTC staff have low autonomy in decision-making about the best care solution for the elderly person, and are unable to rely on their professional judgement to deliver patient-centred care. For instance, Canadian regulations require that elderly people dine in formal dining places, while this does not necessarily match residents' expectations.
Residences do not always have enough funding to meet patients' caring needs.	Both limited budgets and a lack of flexibility in budget allocation reduce LTC workers' capacity to deliver patient-centred care.
Supportive leadership is absent.	There is a general lack of recognition of LTC workers' performance. Most LTC workers deal with a crisis environment and have to deal with several conflicts (such as with families, staff, regulations, budgets).
It is difficult to maintain an adequate work-life balance.	Personal factors such as children and workplace proximity to home reduce participation. Commuting time is particularly difficult, as most LTC workers have to juggle multiple part-time jobs.

Source: Adapted from McGilton et al. (2014[34]), "Making tradeoffs between the reasons to leave and reasons to stay employed in long-term care homes: perspectives of licensed nursing staff", http://dx.doi.org/10.1016/j.ijnurstu.2013.10.015; Chamberlain et al. (2016[35]), "Individual and organizational predictors of health care aide job satisfaction in long term care", http://dx.doi.org/10.1186/s12913-016-1815-6.

LTC workers face three main stressors. First, they often face conflicting demands: they receive contradictory orders, their work lacks co-ordination with other workers and they risk conflicts with co-workers with whom they may have issues of communication. For example, half of LTC workers in Austria assess that the number of people they have to care for is too high (Bauer, Rodrigues and Leichsenring, 2018[22]). Second, they often have to cope with patients' difficult behaviours, including a lack of respect, physical aggression, excessive demands (from patients and their families) and a lack of adherence to medical advice. Third, their workload can be high because of emergencies (exacerbated by insufficient staffing); for instance, a recent French survey shows that almost half of nurses and personal care workers rarely or never have time to sit down for lunch (Truchot, 2018[17]).

These stressors contribute to reduce LTC workers' perceptions of job control, which increases their intention to leave. Prior work shows that among German nurses working in for-profit care, those in nursing homes have a higher intention to leave than those in home care because they have lower job control (Wendsche et al., 2016[36]). In particular, time pressures and social conflicts were found to mediate workers' intention to leave (Rahnfeld et al., 2016[37]). Similarly, LTC workers in Scandinavian countries are more willing to stay in the job and less likely to quit if they have more autonomy, more support from their managers and an appropriate workload (Trydegard, 2012[38]).

In addition, increased LTC budget constraints are likely to increase pressure on workers, and thus change the way they deliver care. In the Netherlands and Scandinavian countries, reforms have increased monitoring of LTC workers' activities. LTC workers complain about the increasing importance of administrative tasks in their jobs. Because they spend long hours on reporting, they often lack time for more qualitative activities with care recipients (such as cooking, discussions and so on).

In Scandinavian countries and Austria, pressure is on the rise for LTC workers: since 2005, working conditions have worsened, with an increase in work intensity, less time to carry the work out and less time allocated to each elderly care recipient (Bauer, Rodrigues and Leichsenring, 2018[22]). For instance, the share of workers reporting that they have too much to do and too little discretion to perform their tasks, lack support from their supervisor and lack time to discuss work with colleagues increased between 2005 and 2015 (Rostgaard et al., 2019[10]). In the United States, personal care workers suffer from isolation, especially when working at home: they help elderly people on a regular basis but do not meet nurses or other support people, sometimes for six months at a time, and care coordinators who could provide advice are overloaded (Osterman, 2017[2]).

LTC workers struggle to maintain a good work-life balance

Difficult working conditions (shift work, night work etc.) and important commuting times often reduce LTC workers' capacity to maintain a good work-life balance. In particular, the availability of childcare for those on shift work can be problematic, and the lack of capacity to work regular hours in order to spend mornings and evenings with the family may discourage workers. Figure 4.17 shows that half of LTC workers have children in their household, and micro-econometric analyses confirm that having children is associated with lower workforce participation. In the United States and the United Kingdom, the number of LTC workers' children is associated with a significant decrease in their working hours and tenure (Box 4.2).

Figure 4.17. The majority of LTC workers have children

Share of LTC workers with children, 2016 (or nearest year)

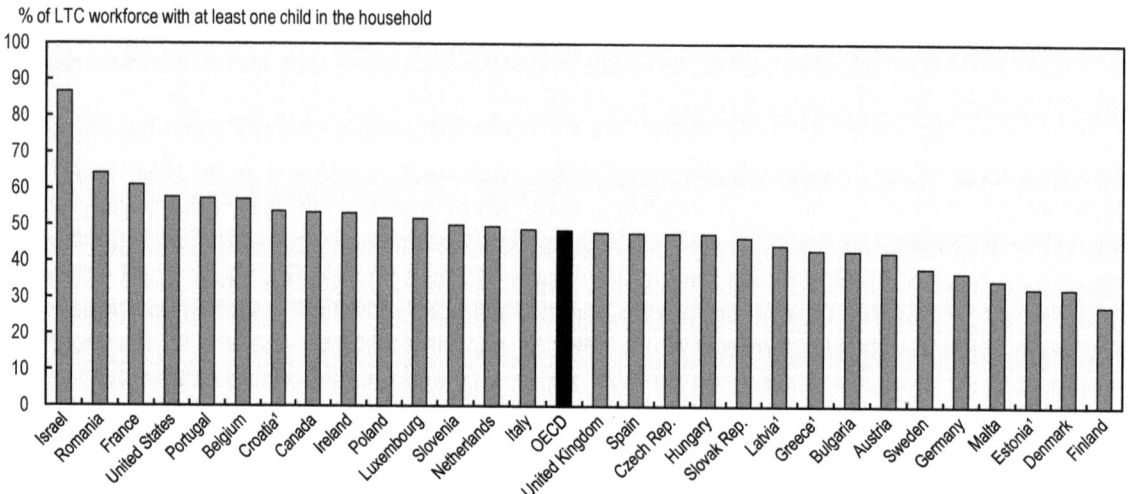

Note: The OECD data point is the unweighted average of the 26 OECD countries shown in the chart. EU-LFS data are based on ISCO 3-digit and NACE 2-digit codes. For a description of the methodology to identify workers, see Annex 2.A in Chapter 2.
1. Data must be interpreted with caution because of small samples.
Source: EU-LFS; ASEC-CPS for the United States; Census 2016 for Canada; LFS for Israel. Data refer to 2016 or nearest year.

Box 4.2. Having children is associated with lower participation in the LTC workforce: examples from the United States and the United Kingdom

In the United States and the United Kingdom, 58% and 48% of LTC workforce participants have children respectively. Regression results suggest that a greater number of children is associated with lower work supply: in the United States, LTC workers with four or more children work on average 11.8% fewer hours than LTC workers with no children (Table 4.2). An increased number of children is associated with a reduced probability of working full time: -3.2 percentage points when the worker has one child, -8.7 percentage points when the worker has four or more children. Finally, having four or more children is associated with a 4.9 percentage points decrease in the probability of staying two consecutive years in the LTC workforce.

In the United Kingdom, a greater number of children is also associated with a reduced number of hours worked per week. For instance, LTC workers with four or more children work 34% fewer hours than LTC workers with no children. Having four or more children also reduces the probability of working full time by 37.8 percentage points. There is no significant association between the number of children and the probability of staying two consecutive years with the same employer.

Results were estimated using regressions that included variables on age, age-squared, education categories (low vs. medium, low vs. high), foreign-born status (yes vs. no), number of children (0 vs. 1, 0 vs. 2, 0 vs. 3 and 0 vs. 4+), gender, ethnicity (white vs. other) and year dummies. In the model exploring the correlation between age and hours worked per week, the dependent variable was log-transformed. The two other models were linear probability models.

Table 4.2. Correlation between the number of children and LTC workforce participation

Results from multivariate analyses, estimations among samples of LTC workers

	No child vs. 1	No child vs. 2	No child vs. 3	No child vs. 4+
Average effect on the number of hours worked per week				
United Kingdom	-0.167*** (0.024)	-0.243*** (0.027)	-0.316*** (0.045)	-0.340*** (0.068)
United States	-0.010 (0.026)	-0.011 (0.028)	-0.024 (0.036)	-0.118** (0.051)
Effect on probability of working full time				
United Kingdom	-0.191*** (0.027)	-0.293*** (0.030)	-0.336*** (0.045)	-0.378*** (0.070)
United States	-0.032*** (0.010)	-0.043*** (0.011)	-0.072*** (0.014)	-0.087*** (0.019)
Effect on probability of staying at least two consecutive years				
United Kingdom	0.019 (0.024)	0.016 (0.027)	0.014 (0.040)	0.045 (0.060)
United States	-0.003 (0.009)	-0.011 (0.010)	-0.019 (0.013)	-0.049*** (0.018)

Note: * p<0.10, ** p<0.05, *** p<0.01. Robust standard errors are in parentheses. In the United States, regressions estimate the probability of staying two consecutive years in the LTC workforce, while in the United Kingdom, regressions estimate the probability of staying two consecutive years with the same employer. All regressions for the United Kingdom control for a dichotomous variable, describing whether the worker lives in Great Britain or in Northern Ireland. All regressions for the United States control for state-level fixed effects.
Source: Pooled cross-sections of UK-LFS (2012 to 2016) and ASEC-CPS (2012 to 2016).

4.4. Improving working conditions will contribute to reducing turnover

4.4.1. Compensation upgrades and improved social dialogue are often first on the list of policies

Wage improvements are likely to retain workers

Table 4.3 shows that since 2011 OECD countries have been implementing three main policies to improve earnings in the LTC workforce: wage improvements or guarantees, overtime and travel time pay, and tax benefits/financial incentives.

Table 4.3. Policies improving quality of earnings in the LTC workforce have been implemented since 2011 in some countries

Policy	Countries	Impact
Wage improvements	Austria, Czech Republic, Hungary, Korea, Malta, Poland, Germany, Romania, Slovenia, United Kingdom, United States, Netherland	Empirical evidence suggests a positive impact on retention in the United States and Czech Republic.
Overtime and travel time pay	Netherlands, United States	The scheme has not yet been evaluated.
Tax benefits and financial incentives	Korea	Allowances have reduced the turnover rate in Korea.

Source: OECD LTC workforce survey 2018 and literature review.

Various measures have been implemented to set minimum thresholds in order to improve wages. Changes in minimum wages (access or thresholds) have been an effective way of increasing pay in the LTC sector (Vadean and Allan, 2017[39]; Osterman, 2017[2]). Note, however, that in the United Kingdom, the introduction of the National Living Wage in 2016 may have contributed to an increase in the use of zero-hours contracts (Vadean and Allan, 2017[39]). In the United States, the Department of Labor issued a new regulation in 2013 extending the Fair Labor Standards Act protections (e.g. the right to a minimum wage) to unlicensed home care workers, who had previously been classified as "companion caregivers". The rule became effective in 2015. In Malta, all salaries in the LTC sector are aligned with public services salaries to ensure that private providers receive the same benefits. In Korea, care facilities are legally required to meet the minimum ratio of labour costs, according to the Policy Rule for Long Term Care Insurance Reimbursement Schedule. The purpose of this regulation is to encourage care facilities to pay fair wages to LTC workers. Germany introduced incentives for adequate salaries for LTC staff in 2010, with the introduction of a minimum wage in the sector, and has reinforced them since 2017 with a guarantee to reimburse collectively agreed wages in fee negotiations. In France, a recommendations for a new legislation proposal include the re-evaluation of minimum wages in the sector to the level of the national minimum wage (SMIC) and that minimum wages become automatically adjusted to the SMIC when the latter increases (El Khomri, 2019[7]).

Several countries have increased overall salaries in the LTC sector. In Hungary, LTC salaries increased by 62% between 2013 and 2018. In Romania, wage increases for LTC workers were included in a more general law (153/2017) on the salaries of employees in public institutions. Wage increases for nurses were implemented in 2018, and for personal care workers in institutions they will be implemented in 2022. In the Czech Republic, substantial increases in the salaries of personal care workers were achieved (with a 4% increase in November 2016, a 23% increase in July 2017 and a 10% increase in January 2017). These have contributed to stabilising the LTC workforce at 100 000 people. In Austria, the professional Association of Austrian Social and Health Companies negotiated wages increases of 3.2% in 2019 in the collective agreements. Norway introduced a new minimum wage for nurses with 10 years' seniority in the sector, representing a wage increase of 12% for them.

Compensating workers for overtime and travel time is another way a few OECD countries have improved earnings quality (especially for home-based workers). In the United States, the Fair Labor Standards Acts protections give unlicensed home-based workers access to overtime pay: LTC workers who do more than 40 hours per week have the right to be paid for extra hours. The Act also allows travel time compensation. In 2017, Korea introduced an allowance to support transportation costs. Note, however, that this policy aims to improve service quality for service users, rather than support LTC workers.

Finally, some countries (Slovenia and Korea) enhanced benefits and financial incentives for LTC workers to improve income or savings. In Slovenia, adoption of regulations governing compulsory pension, health and unemployment insurances for family (home care) assistants, who represent 7% of the total LTC workforce, is pending. In Korea, LTC workers (including temporary workers who work more than 60 hours per month) contribute to national pension plans, health insurance plans, employment insurance plans and accident compensation insurance plans.

Prior research shows that wages and benefits in the LTC sector influence recruitment and retention. Higher wages are a predictor of longer job tenure among home care aides (Butler et al., 2014[40]), while increased incidence of real pay below minimum wage levels contributes to explaining significant increases in turnover rates (Hussein, Ismail and Manthorpe, 2016[9]). In the United States, the Medicaid Wage-Pass-Through programmes increased wages, which had a positive (although small) influence on retention: a USD 1 increase in hourly wage reduced LTC workers' propensity to leave the workforce by 2% for a given month (Baughman and Smith, 2012[41]). Similarly, Korea reported that the introduction of specific allowances increasing personal care workers' wages and improving their benefits reduced turnover rates in the LTC workforce. In France, a study focusing on institution-based workers found that an increase in personal care workers' wages was associated with a 1.2-1.3% decrease in the probability of leaving the institution. However, wage increases were not associated with turnover among nurses (Martin and Ramos-Gorand, 2017[42]).

At the same time, initial wage increases are not the sole or only solution. Recognising experience in wage levels is also important. Previous work shows that in countries where agreements differentiate pay scales to years of experience, such as Belgium, the Netherlands and Sweden, retention is higher (Colombo et al., 2011[43]).

Collective bargaining and social dialogue help with pay, training and working conditions

The extent of unionisation levels and social dialogue is uneven across countries in the LTC sector. Home care workers are less likely to be organised and unionised. In Germany, private for-profit providers do not always have collective agreements. Many central and eastern European countries lack appropriate representative employers' organisations in the sector, which renders the social dialogue process more difficult. In the United States, home care workers in Illinois and California won the right to bargain directly with these states, which are considered to be the "employer for the purpose of bargaining", and have achieved wage increases.

Differences in the degree of collective bargaining are leading to different solutions to improve wages and working conditions across countries. In some countries, such as the Netherlands, the major employer and workers' organisations decide on sector-wide national agreements. The most recent one (for 2018-19) agreed a 4% increase in wages in late 2019 for the entire sector to address the issue of low pay. In Finland, public LTC services comply with municipal service agreements. In Portugal, wages in the LTC sector follow salary tables negotiated between the three main unions of providers and the Instituto de Seguranca Social, according to education and experience, but they only cover the non-profit sector. In Austria, collective agreements are carried out at the company level – regularly between management and the work council, and at national levels of industry during annual negotiations or joint professional events (e.g. on working hours, internships). In 2019, the negotiation led to a 3.2% increase in wages for the overall workforce, and also led to paid leave agreements. In the future, unions are planning to negotiate that LTC workers should reduce their working time to 35 hours a week while maintaining their full salary (currently, they work 38 hours a week).

In contrast, in Bulgaria, the Czech Republic and Poland, collective agreements are conducted at the enterprise level and very few agreements exist compared with the extent of the sector. Such firm-level bargaining, without co-ordination within and across sectors, tends to be associated with somewhat poorer labour market outcomes (OECD, 2018[44]). There is thus a need to have well organised social partners in the sector or well tailored administrative extensions of collective agreements.

Beyond social dialogue, New Zealand provides an interesting example of a new wage structure in the sector achieved through a pay equity settlement. Trade unions lodged a claim with the Employment

Relations Authority, maintaining that there was systemic undervaluation of care and support work because it was mainly carried it out by women. The Ministry of Health started to implement new wage rates, which increased the pay scale in the sector in 2017, leading to a rise of between 15% and 50% in hourly wages. At the same time, the way the funding was implemented has led to negative consequences in terms of reduced hours, increased workload and duties, and sometimes reduced quality of care (Douglas and Ravenswood, 2019[45]). In this sense, higher reimbursement rates for LTC services are necessary to guarantee wage rises and increases in quality of care through having more skilled LTC workers (Hackmann, 2019[46]).

Collective bargaining is also needed to ensure that LTC workers receive proper training and have improved working conditions. A large proportion of the LTC workforce is in temporary employment and may not always benefit from the same training opportunities as permanent workers and employees (OECD, 2019[1]). Non-discrimination rules are central to guarantee that temporary LTC workers have equal treatment. Several countries (Poland, Greece, Germany, Belgium and France) have introduced such rules. However, even despite this, significant challenges remain in most OECD countries to ensuring equality of rights and entitlement to training, as LTC workers often lack representation and therefore have little collective bargaining power to negotiate better conditions. For instance, there is a need to adapt the legislative and collective bargaining framework to the increasing importance of own-account self-employed workers who deliver LTC at home. In Austria, collective bargaining in LTC led to the approval of improved working conditions: more vacation and free weekends were negotiated in the collective agreement, along with compulsory supervision in the care sector.

4.4.2. Improved retention will also come from better working conditions and lower health risks

Better organisation of working time is one of the prime demands

Introducing flexible working time arrangements with choice of hours can help to address work-life balance concerns and improve job satisfaction. Switching to self-scheduling, which enables shift workers to have control over which shifts they work, when they start work or when their rest days occur, is associated with improvements in health, work-life balance and organisational effectiveness (Costa, Cesana and Kogi, 1990[47]; Gauderer and Knauth, 2004[48]; Wortley and Grierson-Hill, 2003[49]). Moreover, prior work shows that more flexibility in work schedules is likely to enable better retention, while fuller workloads lead to early retirement (Uthaman, Chua and Ang, 2015[50]). Legislative approaches to guarantee employer provision of some flexible working arrangements, promoting social dialogue on employee-friendly working time and helping companies to adapt work organisation and managerial practice, have proved to be useful in ensuring better work-life balance. In Australia, a new management model (Table 4.3) in nursing homes has contributed to reducing turnover rates among LTC workers. These flexible management models provide LTC workers with more opportunities to control their work-life balance. Better organisation of daily work and planning shifts and teams are cited as important elements for job satisfaction by workers in Austria, the Netherlands and Portugal.

Adapting working hours to caregivers' profiles could also contribute to addressing concerns about older workers who are not able to continue to perform the same physical tasks. While its effect remains untested, Dutch unions are suggesting implementation of a generation pact that would allow workers aged 45 and over to work 15% less while keeping pension contributions at 100%, and would increase by 15% the work provided by the young generations. A more promising solution would be to adapt caregivers' tasks according to their age profile, in which older workers would coach new recruits rather than providing tasks that are physically difficult directly (such as lifting or carrying elderly people).

Given the high rate of part-time work, especially for low hours of care per week, additional solutions to give workers the option to increase working hours would be suitable. In Germany and Portugal, some companies motivate part-time workers to increase their working hours, or combining different jobs in various nursing homes, or home care and day care in order to reduce involuntary part-time jobs. In the Netherlands, a combination of hospital and LTC work is put forward as a way to increase working hours for those with very low part-time hours. The main trade unions in the LTC sector in Norway have a goal of developing a culture of full-time employment and work at the local level to organise longer shifts, increase the number of weekend hours and fill additional part-time positions through existing part-time employees, among other solutions. Furthermore, to make work more attractive on the weekend there are new minimum rates in Norway for Saturday and Sunday supplements.

Finally, LTC workers' tasks increasingly involve administrative duties (reporting budget use and activities provided on a daily basis, for instance), which are time-demanding. Organisational innovations should allow their timetables to be reorganised so that they have dedicated time for administration, such as during the afternoon when care needs are low. The use of new technologies (tablets, smartphones) is likely to improve work organisation (see Chapter 6). Moreover, the implementation of a unique electronic record should allow better articulation of the health and social care provision, and better record-keeping of the care recipient's health details and circumstances.

Box 4.3. The Adards management model in Australia

In 1991, Adards, a nursing home in Tasmania, Australia, implemented an original management model for dementia care, based on flexibility (Cohen-Mansfield and Bester, 2006[51]). The average annual worker turnover and absenteeism rates in this facility are very low (10% and 0.6% respectively), compared with those observed in other settings, showing the success of this approach. The model underlines four main advantages to flexibility regarding the number of hours worked per shift and per week: it tailors staffing levels to resident care needs, reduces potential burnouts and the caregiving burden, improves LTC workers' work-life balance and attracts employees who would not otherwise have participated in the LTC workforce.

While the shift lengths vary from four to eight hours, the staffing schedule remains constant to ensure that patients' needs are met. Morning and evening shifts are the most demanding. Flexible staff rotation allows LTC workers to change their schedule according to their personal needs. It also ensures that all LTC workers know all the residents. The median number of working hours for Adards employees is 21 per week. Five main principles aim to prevent burnouts and maximise worker satisfaction: shifts must be shorter than eight hours; weekly schedules must be shorter than 40 hours; shifts can be exchanged at LTC workers' convenience; LTC workers alternate three days on duty with three days off; and two shifts concentrate most of the teams' efforts (morning and evening).

Reducing incentives for undeclared work will benefit both workers and care recipients

Many countries face the existence of undeclared private work, which is often the case for foreign workers, especially if undocumented. Individuals under these work arrangements are not eligible for social protection or fail to build up substantial entitlements because of intermittent working patterns and frequent transitions.

A variety of approaches is available to prevent undeclared work and transform it into declared work. The main objective of the approaches consists of making declared work more beneficial and easier, through simplification procedures and help with record-keeping, direct tax and social security incentives. This is often done using service vouchers or tax credits. In France, service vouchers for elderly care are subsidised via the Personalised Autonomy Allowance. Families can use the universal voucher to buy personal care and home help. In Finland, 20% of the wage paid, including social security contributions, or 50% of the work compensation paid to an entrepreneur or enterprise, is tax deductible. Similarly, the tax deduction for household services in Sweden applies to 50% of labour costs and has led to a decline of 10% in undeclared work in all activities (Williams, 2018[52]). Such schemes need to be designed carefully to avoid partial displacement of workers from the regular market.

Training programmes and improved inspection create a healthier work environment

Good workplace safety not only improves the health of LTC workers but also decreases their intention to leave. Prior work shows that in Sweden work-related exhaustion is one of the strongest predictors of low workplace satisfaction, among both home-based and institution-based workers (Hasson and Arnetz, 2008[53]). In the United States, people reporting that they worked in a less safe environment, in institutions, were almost twice as likely to consider leaving their job in the next two years, compared to those working in a good safety climate (Miranda et al., 2011[28]).

Countries can follow several strategies to promote a healthier work environment, through training but also through a safety culture. Some countries have implemented coaching programmes, especially for stress management. The Dutch government introduced a programme providing 20 000 coaches in the workplace to create a healthy working environment. In the United States, LTC workers (personal care workers or nurses) who work for an agency are likely to have a supervisor or care manager who is in charge of providing mentoring or support. Japan arranges counselling services through professional agencies to provide advice on how to improve employment management in LTC. The Province of Saskatchewan in Canada offers transferring, lifting and repositioning training to reduce the risk of injuries.

Fostering a healthier work environment is also intimately linked to a safety culture, and especially a patient safety culture. Numerous studies show the empirical relationship between patient safety culture, workers injuries and psychological well-being. Creating a safer work environment requires from countries to know how they are performing on worker and patient safety in order to appropriately identify where improvements can be made. As an example, countries can develop and implement appropriate safety standards for institutions to measure patient and worker safety (de Bienassis, Llena Nozal and Klazinga, forthcoming[54]).

Second, prevention tools to improve safety at work and prevent musculoskeletal disorders exist and have proved to be effective. Knowledge of workplace guidelines and management support (for instance, protocols that incorporate requirements on safe patient handling) were associated with sustained use of technical devices (Evanoff et al., 2003[26]). For instance, environmental interventions such as appropriate seat heights to aid sit-to-stand transfers can reduce staff injury and are more effective than training (Coman, Caponecchia and McIntosh, 2018[55]). Workplace interventions including ergonomics, physical training and cognitive behavioural therapy in Norway have proved to be very successful against low back pain for personal care workers who perform physically demanding jobs (Rasmussen et al., 2013[56]). In the Netherlands, the introduction of mechanical lifts reduced musculoskeletal injuries and lost days in several institutions.

Third, countries have implemented measures reinforcing control over working conditions. Effective prevention requires labour inspectorates, occupational health services and general practitioners to work closely with employers and workers' representatives, to create a culture of health in the workplace. With the renewed spread of non-standard forms of work, including (dependent) self-employment, temporary and casual work arrangements in many OECD countries, the need for credible and far-reaching initiatives to promote health at work has never been so strong. Korea is considering extending the Occupational Safety and Health (OSH) Act so that all working people, including non-regular workers are protected. Other countries (including the United Kingdom, Ireland, Canada and Australia) have OSH regulations for employers that are broad enough to cover more than just the traditional employment relationship.

Finally, workplace violence should be prevented by implementation of preventive safety training programmes, along with procedures protecting LTC workers who face these issues (Perrin et al., 2015[31]). In particular, protocols and training should focus on effective prevention and harassment response. These issues should be identified early on (during the recruitment process) and receive constant follow-up with the development of the care relationship between workers and patients. Such policies should include setting a zero-tolerance rule, clear sanctions against the use of threats, violence and harassment, and implementation of reporting procedures. Finally, workers should be able to leave the patient's home when facing workplace violence without facing the threat of being pursued for abandonment when the patient requires constant care.

4.4.3. The challenge of high demand and reduced support can be addressed by developing teamwork and autonomy

Improved teamwork and leadership in LTC can create a better-quality work environment

High rates of shift work may prevent the development of work relationships between care providers. Indeed, a Swedish study revealed that nurses value the long-term relationships built with patients and staff, and that loneliness may in some cases overcome the positive feeling associated with independence of home-based work (Carlson et al., 2014[57]).

Developing teamwork and engaging all care providers in decision-making are two key strategies to increase job satisfaction. A Canadian study also found that relationships with other staff and professional development opportunities influenced a decision to stay for nurses working in nursing homes (McGilton et al., 2014[34]). This effect could be mediated through reduced levels of emotional exhaustion and higher levels of personal accomplishment. Finally, an Italian study of 28 nursing homes provided evidence that support from colleagues has a positive impact on LTC work engagement (Sarti, 2014[58]). In France, an improvement to LTC worker mentoring was associated with lower turnover among LTC workers in institutions (Martin and Ramos-Gorand, 2017[42]).

Private providers in some countries try to increase job motivation by creating opportunities for different work. In Portugal, for instance, some nursing homes organise teamwork in an innovative manner. Teams are composed of three members at the same level of competence with different titles and roles – a manager, first assistant and second assistant – who rotate roles within this hierarchy. Each team is composed of at least one male worker, as they tend to stay longer in the job. Nursing homes often provide home care services and allow people to switch from one service to the other to allow for diversity in careers.

Prior work also shows that nursing home leadership, in particular from the director of nursing, influences staff tenure (Hunt et al., 2012[59]). Leaders that display individualised consideration towards employees provide intellectual stimulation, act as role models and inspire workers (Atwell, 2011[60]). Encouraging discussion, involving employees in problem-solving to improve resident care committees for informal learning and developing skills are some ways to stimulate employees in LTC. The use of such leadership styles is also associated with improved resident outcomes, such as reduction in pressure ulcers and falls; further, it makes workers feel valued and empowered in their work. In 2018, Hungary introduced a new training system, including specific management training for leaders in LTC work. Its goal is to prepare leaders to practise effective leadership according to new and emerging needs and challenges in the field, in a changing legal environment. In Norway, the government is sponsoring a Master's degree in leadership skills for nurses working in LTC.

LTC workers can benefit from more autonomy to decide on tasks

Scandinavian countries are strengthening highly educated nurses' roles by giving them more capacity to manage budgets and organise LTC. In Norway, nurses are becoming increasingly specialised and taking more leadership roles, especially in conducting assessment needs for services, based on a standardised assessment form that all municipalities are required to use. Nurses are being given more autonomy to decide on the type but also amount of care needed by each client. They are also taking decision-making roles when it comes to managing municipalities' budgets for LTC.

Self-managing or self-organising teams are ways of working without traditional management hierarchies. The Buurtzorg model is a well known example of self-managed teams of nurses, which has attracted interest and been replicated in several countries. The teams, often composed of up to 12 nurses, support 50-60 patients at a time. The nurses provide a wide range of care; they also try to mobilise the client's social network and work closely with general practitioners and other community health care workers. Providing more autonomy to LTC workers can contribute to increasing their satisfaction. In the United States, a survey of health care aides working in LTC found that a greater sense of autonomy leads to longer job retention (Butler et al., 2014[40]). Autonomy may be a particular issue for less senior staff, such as certified nursing aides, who report frequent exclusion from team communication and decision-making. Since 2011, the Israeli government has promoted a policy targeting empowering of nurses, to increase their independent practice in community care and home-based care.

Teams can be self-managed in the sense that they are operationally autonomous and self-governing. Self-managing teams have leadership tasks and operational tasks, resulting in a higher degree of decision-making autonomy and more task variety; supervision is focused on coaching colleagues in tasks. The teams can decide on a range of actions such as hiring and firing, the number of patients served, rostering, planning, individual and team performance monitoring, professional development and care delivery. Everyone in the self-managing team holds a main role and roles are rotated regularly. Coaches are available to solve problems for each team. There is flexibility in work arrangements to meet both nurses' and patients' needs (Box 4.4).

Evidence suggests that self-managed teams led by nurses may be a cost-effective way of delivering LTC services at the community level. A comparison of the Buurtzorg model with another 600 homecare providers showed that this model ranked among the top ten for client satisfaction, annual costs per client were lower (EUR 6 428 compared to the average of all others at EUR 7 995) and around four in five nurses and nurse assistants considered this model attractive (Box 4.4). In addition, costs are 40% lower than other home care organisations, thanks to reduced administration, because at 8% of total costs it has lower overhead costs than other organisations (Ernst & Young, 2009[61]). Compared with other district nurse types of model, self-managed teams have proved better for patient care continuity, multiple long-term conditions and proactive care. From the staff perspective, the opportunity to make decisions and operate as a team helped in supporting service access, response and efficiency, and made the job more attractive (Drennan et al., 2018[62]). Satisfaction among nurses facilitates the recruitment of talented staff as well as reducing absenteeism and turnover (Gray, Sarnak and Burgers, 2015[63]).

> **Box 4.4. The Buurtzorg model: self-managed home care teams**
>
> The Buurtzorg (neighbourhood care) model was initiated in 2006 in the Netherlands. It is an innovative approach for home care service delivery. The main rationale for its creation was to eliminate bureaucracy and hierarchy, and instead focus on building meaningful relationships between caregiver and client.
>
> Decisions are made together: for a solution to be adopted, it is enough that nobody has a principled objection. Team members are responsible for organising work, recruiting staff and determining the best approach to care without a manager. An initial schedule for shifts is made by a co-ordinator and circulated to team members, who are asked to fill it in. The process is repeated until it is acceptable to team members. They are supported by a tailored technology structure, composed of a web server and intranet health care platform that connects teams and ensures knowledge sharing. Time spent on administrative work is monitored, as teams should minimise it as possible. Teams must be available 24 hours a day, seven days a week. Individual team members are expected to meet a productivity

target, which is monitored centrally, the goal being that 60% of time is spend directly with clients. A regional coach – senior nurse – is available for questions.

To ensure effective collaboration and decision-making, new teams receive training on self-management (i.e. group decision-making, conducting meetings, conflict resolution and problem-solving) as well as peer coaching.

The seven roles of Buurtzorg's self-managed teams are: 1) the main role, 2) the housekeeper, 3) the informer, 4) the developer, 5) the planner, 6) the team player and 7) the mentor. Employees decide on their roles. There were 15 coaches for 700 teams in 2015 to provide advice about patient care.

While evaluations of clinical results are not yet available, since its inception in the Netherlands, the Buurtzorg model has been replicated in the United States, Japan, Finland and Sweden.

Source: Rosengren et al. (2017[64]) "Buurtzorg – an innovative model for caring elderly at home", http://www.karelia.fi/ikanyt/2017 13 November/buurtzorg-an-innovative-model-for-caring-elderly at-home/; Sheldon (2017[65]), "Buurtzorg: The district nurses who want to be superfluous", https://doi.org/10.1136/bmj.j3140; Drennan et al. (2018[62]), "Tackling the workforce crisis in district nursing: Can the Dutch Buurtzorg model offer a solution and a better patient experience? A mixed methods case study", https://doi.org/10.1136/bmjopen-2018-021931.

4.5. Conclusion

The increase in home-based LTC delivery drives the need for tailored solutions to meet the specific needs of each person. However, the current working conditions prevent the delivery of a more elderly person-centred LTC. Working arrangements – which are predominantly shifts, part-time arrangements and temporary contracts – and frequently low compensation schemes lead workers to try to deliver as much care as possible in a small amount of time. The current shortages in the LTC market dramatically increase the pressure on workers, who have to multiply basic and repetitive tasks, and cannot promote people-centred LTC. New LTC market trends could increase that tendency. In the future, policies will be needed to guarantee workers' rights and working conditions, but also to make sure that they provide services centred on elderly people's needs. However, these policies are likely to raise costs, although this should also be compensated in part by reducing the turnover costs.

References

Akosa Antwi, Y. and J. Bowblis (2016), *The Impact of Nurse Turnover on Quality of Care and Mortality in Nursing Homes:Evidence from the Great Recession*, MI: W.E. Upjohn Institute for Employment Research. [4]

Atwell, R. (2011), "Implementing transformational leadership in long-term care", *Geriatric Nursing*, Vol. 32/3, pp. 212-219, http://dx.doi.org/10.1016/j.gerinurse.2011.02.001. [60]

Bauer, G., R. Rodrigues and K. Leichsenring (2018), *Working Conditions in Long-term Care in Austria: The Perspective of Care Professionals*, Vienna: European Centre, https://www.euro.centre.org/publications/detail/3283. [22]

Baughman, R. and K. Smith (2012), "Labor mobility of the direct care workforce: Implications for the provision of long-term care", *Health Economics (United Kingdom)*, Vol. 21/12, pp. 1402-1415, http://dx.doi.org/10.1002/hec.1798. [41]

Brunel, M., J. Latourelle and M. Zakri (2018), "Un senior à domicile sur cinq aidé régulièrement pour les tâches du quotidien", *Études et Résultats*, Vol. 1103, https://drees.solidarites-sante.gouv.fr/etudes-et-statistiques/publications/etudes-et-resultats/article/un-senior-a-domicile-sur-cinq-aide-regulierement-pour-les-taches-du-quotidien. [14]

Butler, S. et al. (2014), "Determinants of longer job tenure among home care aides: What makes some stay on the job while others leave?", *Journal of Applied Gerontology*, Vol. 33/2, pp. 164-188, http://dx.doi.org/10.1177/0733464813495958. [40]

Carlson, E. et al. (2014), "Registered nurses' perceptions of their professional work in nursing homes and home-based care: a focus group study", *International Journal of Nursing Studies*, Vol. 51/5, pp. 761-767, http://dx.doi.org/10.1016/j.ijnurstu.2013.10.002. [57]

Casanova, G., G. Lamura and A. Principi (2017), "Valuing and integrating informal care as a core component of long-term care for older people: a comparison of recent developments in Italy and Spain", *Journal of Aging and Social Policy*, Vol. 29/3, pp. 201-217, http://dx.doi.org/10.1080/08959420.2016.1236640. [20]

Chamberlain, S. et al. (2016), "Individual and organizational predictors of health care aide job satisfaction in long term care", *BMC Health Services Research*, Vol. 16/1, p. 577, http://dx.doi.org/10.1186/s12913-016-1815-6. [35]

Cohen-Mansfield, J. and A. Bester (2006), "Flexibility as a management principle in dementia care: The Adards example", *Gerontologist*, Vol. 46/1, pp. 540-544, http://dx.doi.org/10.1093/geront/46.4.540. [51]

Colombo, F. et al. (2011), *Help Wanted? Providing and Paying for Long-Term Care*, OECD Health Policy Studies, OECD Publishing, Paris, http://dx.doi.org/10.1787/9789264097759-en. [43]

Coman, R., C. Caponecchia and A. McIntosh (2018), "Manual handling in aged care: impact of rnvironment-related interventions on mobility", *Safety and Health at Work*, Vol. 9/4, pp. 372-380. [55]

Costa, G., G. Cesana and K. Kogi (1990), *Shiftwork : Health, Sleep, and Performance*, Proceedings of the IX International Symposium on Night and Shift Work, Verona, Italy, 1989, Peter Lang Publishing, Bern, https://www.peterlang.com/view/product/42902. [47]

de Bienassis, K., A. Llena Nozal and N. Klazinga (forthcoming), "The Economics of Patient Safety Part III: Long-Term Care", *OECD Health Working Papers*, OECD Publishing, Paris. [54]

Douglas, J. and K. Ravenswood (2019), *The Value of Care: Understanding the Impact of the 2017 Pay Equity Settlement on the Residential Aged Care, Home and Community Care and Disability Support Sectors*, New Zealand Work Research Institute, Auckland, https://workresearch.aut.ac.nz/__data/assets/pdf_file/0019/258130/Pay-Equity-Report_Digital_final.pdf. [45]

Drennan, V. et al. (2018), "Tackling the workforce crisis in district nursing: Can the Dutch Buurtzorg model offer a solution and a better patient experience? A mixed methods case study", *BMJ Open*, Vol. 8/6, p. e021931, http://dx.doi.org/10.1136/bmjopen-2018-021931. [62]

Dulon, M. et al. (2007), "Prevalence of skin and back diseases in geriatric care nurses", *International Archives of Occupational and Environmental Health*, Vol. 81/8, pp. 983-992, http://dx.doi.org/10.1007/s00420-007-0292-y. [24]

El Khomri, M. (2019), *Plan national en faveur de l'attractivité des métiers du grand-âge 2020-2024*, Ministère des Solidarités et de la Santé, Paris, https://solidarites-sante.gouv.fr/IMG/pdf/rapport_el_khomri_-_plan_metiers_du_grand_age.pdf. [7]

Ernst & Young (2009), *Maatschaappelijke business case Buurtzorg (Social business case: Buurtzorg)*, https://transitiepraktijk.nl/files/maatschappelijke%20business%20case%20buurtzorg.pdf. [61]

Eurofound (2015), *New forms of employment*, European Foundation for the improvement of living and working conditions, Dublin, https://www.eurofound.europa.eu/publications/report/2015/working-conditions-labour-market/new-forms-of-employment. [19]

Evanoff, B. et al. (2003), "Reduction in injury rates in nursing personnel through introduction of mechanical lifts in the workplace", *American Journal of Industrial Medicine*, Vol. 44/5, pp. 451-457, http://dx.doi.org/10.1002/ajim.10294. [26]

Fasanya, B. and E. Dada (2016), "Workplace violence and safety issues in long-term medical care facilities: nurses' perspectives", *Safety and Health at Work*, Vol. 7/2, pp. 97-101, http://dx.doi.org/10.1016/j.shaw.2015.11.002. [30]

Gardiner, L. (2015), "The Scale of Minimum Wage Underpayment in Social Care", *Resolution Foundation, London*, https://www.resolutionfoundation.org/publications/the-scale-of-minimum-wage-underpayment-in-social-care. [11]

Gauderer, P. and P. Knauth (2004), "Pilot study with individualized duty rotas in public local transport", *Le Travail Humain*, Vol. 67/1, p. 87, http://dx.doi.org/10.3917/th.671.0087. [48]

Gray, B., D. Sarnak and J. Burgers (2015), "Home care by self-governing nursing teams: the Netherlands' Buurtzorg model", *The Commonwealth Fund Case studies, New York*, Vol. 14, https://www.commonwealthfund.org/publications/case-study/2015/may/home-care-self-governing-nursing-teams-netherlands-buurtzorg-model. [63]

Hackmann, M. (2019), "Incentivizing better quality of care: the role of Medicaid and competition in the nursing home industry", *American Economic Review*, Vol. 109/5, pp. 1684-1716. [46]

Hasson, H. and J. Arnetz (2008), "Nursing staff competence, work strain, stress and satisfaction in elderly care: a comparison of home-based care and nursing homes.", *Journal of Clinical Nursing*, Vol. 17/4, pp. 468-481, http://dx.doi.org/10.1111/j.1365-2702.2006.01803.x. [53]

Hunt, S. et al. (2012), "Registered nurse retention strategies in nursing homes", *Health Care Management Review*, Vol. 37/3, pp. 246-256, http://dx.doi.org/10.1097/HMR.0b013e3182352425. [59]

Hussein, S., M. Ismail and J. Manthorpe (2016), "Changes in turnover and vacancy rates of care workers in England from 2008 to 2010: panel analysis of national workforce data", *Health and Social Care in the Community*, Vol. 24/5, pp. 547-556, http://dx.doi.org/10.1111/hsc.12214. [9]

Kim, Y. and C. Kim (2017), "Impact of job characteristics on turnover intention and the mediating effects of job satisfaction: experiences of home visiting geriatric care workers in Korea", *Asia Pacific Journal of Social Work and Development*, Vol. 27/2, pp. 53-68, http://dx.doi.org/10.1080/02185385.2017.1331459. [33]

Kromark, K. et al. (2009), "Back disorders and lumbar load in nursing staff in geriatric care: a comparison of home-based care and nursing homes", *Journal of Occupational Medicine and Toxicology*, Vol. 4/1, p. 33, http://dx.doi.org/10.1186/1745-6673-4-33. [23]

Luppi, M. et al. (2014), *Report on the Legal-sociological Analysis of Discrepancies and Dilemmas in Care Workers' Rights*, Centre for Social Policy and Intervention Studies, Utrecht, https://www.uu.nl/en/research/beucitizen-european-citizenship-research/publications. [21]

Maarse, J. and P. Jeurissen (2016), "The policy and politics of the 2015 long-term care reform in the Netherlands", *Health Policy*, Vol. 120/3, pp. 241-245, http://dx.doi.org/10.1016/j.healthpol.2016.01.014. [13]

Martin, C. and M. Ramos-Gorand (2017), "High turnover among nursing staff in private nursing homes for dependent elderly people (EHPADS) in France: Impact of the local environment and the wage", *Economie et Statistique*, Vol. 2017/493, pp. 53-70, http://dx.doi.org/10.24187/ecostat.2017.493s.1912. [42]

Mavromaras, K. et al. (2017), *The Aged Care Workforce, 2016*, Department of Health, Canberra, https://agedcare.health.gov.au/sites/g/files/net1426/f/documents/03_2017/nacwcs_final_report_290317.pdf. [6]

McGilton, K. et al. (2014), "Making tradeoffs between the reasons to leave and reasons to stay employed in long-term care homes: perspectives of licensed nursing staff", *International Journal of Nursing Studies*, Vol. 51/6, pp. 917-926, http://dx.doi.org/10.1016/j.ijnurstu.2013.10.015. [34]

Meagher, G., M. Szebehely and J. Mears (2016), "How institutions matter for job characteristics, quality and experiences: a comparison of home care work for older people in Australia and Sweden", *Work, Employment and Society*, Vol. 30/5, pp. 731-749, http://dx.doi.org/10.1177/0950017015625601. [15]

Miranda, H. et al. (2011), "Violence at the workplace increases the risk of musculoskeletal pain among nursing home workers", *Occupational & Environmental Medicine*, Vol. 68/1, pp. 52-57, http://dx.doi.org/10.1136/oem.2009.051474. [28]

Mukamel, D. (2009), "The costs of turnover in nursing homes.", *Medical care*, Vol. 47/10, pp. 1039–1045, http://dx.doi.org/doi:10.1097/MLR.0b013e3181a3cc62. [5]

Muller, M. (2017), *L'accueil des personnes âgées en établissement : entre progression et diversification de l'offre*, DREES, Paris. [8]

Needham, I. et al. (2005), "Non-somatic effects of patient aggression on nurses: a systematic review", *Journal of Advanced Nursing*, Vol. 49/3, pp. 283-296, http://dx.doi.org/10.1111/j.1365-2648.2004.03286.x. [27]

Needham, I. et al. (2005), "Non-somatic effects of patient aggression on nurses: a systematic review", *Journal of Advanced Nursing*, Vol. 49/3, pp. 283-296, http://dx.doi.org/10.1111/j.1365-2648.2004.03286.x. [32]

OECD (2019), *OECD Employment Outlook 2019: The Future of Work*, OECD Publishing, Paris, https://dx.doi.org/10.1787/9ee00155-en. [1]

OECD (2018), *OECD Employment Outlook 2018*, OECD Publishing, Paris, https://dx.doi.org/10.1787/empl_outlook-2018-en. [44]

OECD (2015), *In It Together: Why Less Inequality Benefits All*, OECD Publishing, Paris, https://dx.doi.org/10.1787/9789264235120-en. [18]

Osterman, P. (2017), *Who Will Care for Us? Long-term Care and the Long-term Workforce*, Russell Sage Foundation, New York, http://www.jstor.org/stable/10.7758/9781610448673. [2]

Perrin, N. et al. (2015), "Workplace violence against homecare workers and its relationship with workers health outcomes: a cross-sectional study", *BMC Public Health*, Vol. 15, p. 11, http://dx.doi.org/10.1186/s12889-014-1340-7. [31]

Rahnfeld, M. et al. (2016), "Uncovering the care setting–turnover intention relationship of geriatric nurses", *European Journal of Ageing*, http://dx.doi.org/10.1007/s10433-016-0362-7. [37]

Rai, G. (2010), "Burnout among long-term care staff", *Administration in Social Work*, Vol. 34/3, pp. 225-240, http://dx.doi.org/10.1080/03643107.2010.480887. [29]

Rasmussen, C. et al. (2013), "Prevention of low back pain and its consequences among nurses' aides in elderly care: a stepped-wedge multi-faceted cluster-randomized controlled trial", *BMC Public Health*, Vol. 13/1, http://dx.doi.org/10.1186/1471-2458-13-1088. [56]

Rosengren, Å. et al. (2017), "Buurtzorg – an innovative model for caring elderly at home", *IkäNYT!*, Vol. 2, http://www.karelia.fi/ikanyt/2017/11/13/buurtzorg-an-innovative-model-for-caring-elderly-at-home/. [64]

Rostgaard, T. et al. (2019), *Changes in Nordic care work and their effects on work related problems for workers in long-term care*, The Danish Center for Social Science Research. Copenhagen. [10]

Rubery, J. et al. (2015), "'It's all about time' : time as contested terrain in the management and experience of domiciliary care work in England", *Human Resource Management*, Vol. 54/5, pp. 753-772, http://dx.doi.org/10.1002/hrm.21685. [12]

Saint-Martin, A., H. Inanc and C. Prinz (2018), "Job Quality, Health and Productivity: An evidence-based framework for analysis", *OECD Social, Employment and Migration Working Papers*, No. 221, OECD Publishing, Paris, https://dx.doi.org/10.1787/a8c84d91-en. [16]

Sarti, D. (2014), "Job resources as antecedents of engagement at work: Evidence from a long-term care setting", *Human Resource Development Quarterly*, Vol. 25/2, pp. 213-237, http://dx.doi.org/10.1002/hrdq.21189. [58]

Sheldon, T. (2017), "Buurtzorg: The district nurses who want to be superfluous", *BMJ*, Vol. 358, p. j3140, http://dx.doi.org/10.1136/bmj.j3140. [65]

Simon, M. et al. (2008), "Back or neck-pain-related disability of nursing staff in hospitals, nursing homes and home care in seven countries – results from the European NEXT-Study", *International Journal of Nursing Studies*, Vol. 45/1, pp. 24-34, http://dx.doi.org/10.1016/J.IJNURSTU.2006.11.003. [25]

Squillace, M. (2008), *An Exploratory Study of Certified Nursing Assistants' Intent to Leave*, U.S. Department of Health and Human Services, Office of Disability, Aging and Long-Term Care Policy. Washington DC. [3]

Truchot, D. (2018), *Rapport de recherche sur la santé des soignants*, Laboratoire de psychologie, Université Bourgogne-Franche Comté, https://www.asso-sps.fr/assets/rapport-de-recherche-sur-la-sante-des-soignants---pr-didier-truchot.pdf. [17]

Trydegard, G. (2012), "Care work in changing welfare states: Nordic car workers' experiences", *Eurjopean Journal of Ageing*, Vol. 9, pp. 119-129. [38]

Uthaman, T., T. Chua and S. Ang (2015), "Older nurses: A literature review on challenges, factors in early retirement and workforce retention", *Proceedings of Singapore Healthcare*, Vol. 25/1, pp. 50-55, http://dx.doi.org/10.1177/2010105815610138. [50]

Vadean, F. and S. Allan (2017), *The Effects of Minimum Wage Policy on the Long-term Care Sector*, The Economics of Social and Health Care Research Unit, Canterbury, http://www.pssru.ac.uk. [39]

Wendsche, J. et al. (2016), "High job demands and low job control increase nurses' professional leaving intentions: the role of care setting and profit orientation", *Research in nursing & health*, Vol. 39/5, pp. 353-363, http://dx.doi.org/10.1002/nur.21729. [36]

Williams, C. (2018), *Elements of a Preventative Approach towards Undeclared Work: an Evaluation of Service Vouchers and Awareness Raising Campaigns*, European Commission, Brussels. [52]

Wortley, V. and L. Grierson-Hill (2003), "Developing a successful self-rostering shift system", *Nursing Standard*, Vol. 17/42, pp. 40-42, http://dx.doi.org/10.7748/ns2003.07.17.42.40.c3413. [49]

Annex 4.A. Country abbreviations

Country abbreviations used in this chapter are listed in Annex Table 4.A.1.

Annex Table 4.A.1. Abbreviations used for countries in Figures 4.5 and 4.13

AU	Australia
AT	Austria
BE	Belgium
BG	Bulgaria
HR	Croatia
CY	Cyprus
CZ	Czech Republic
DK	Denmark
EE	Estonia
FI	Finland
FR	France
DE	Germany
GR	Greece
HU	Hungary
IE	Ireland
IT	Italy
LU	Luxembourg
MT	Malta
NL	Netherlands
NO	Norway
PL	Poland
PT	Portugal
RO	Romania
SK	Slovak Republic
SI	Slovenia
ES	Spain
SE	Sweden
CH	Switzerland
UK	United Kingdom

Notes

[1] Tenure is defined by the number of years LTC workers spend with their employers.

[2] A zero-hours contract is a type of contract between an employer and a worker in which the employer is not obliged to provide any minimum working hours.

[3] Shift work refers to work comprising recurring periods in which different groups of workers do the same jobs in relay.

5 Improving care pathways for elderly people

This chapter explores recent policy developments to improve co-ordination between the long-term care (LTC) and health care sectors, and their effect on the LTC workforce. In the coming years, LTC services will be more people-centred and organised nearer to communities; they will also require closer interaction with health services and family caregivers, as elderly people develop more complex needs and suffer more chronic diseases and other disabilities. The chapter discusses how countries are trying to provide more integrated care between hospital and home care, and what this means for workers in terms of their skills and care models. It also discusses the changes towards more teamwork and case management to provide LTC co-ordinated services at the community level. Finally, it highlights changes to leverage the help of family carers by increasing co-ordination with formal LTC workers and supporting family carers.

5.1. More integrated care is needed

In the future, LTC services should be more people-centred and organised closer to communities. Ensuring good care co-ordination is particularly important for elderly people. Support with activities of daily living (ADL) – such as bathing and dressing – and instrumental activities of daily living (IADL) – such as cooking and cleaning – will not be enough. Elderly individuals will also require attention to their complex medical needs for management of chronic conditions. This requires sustained efforts by care recipients and their families to understand and navigate the information and help needed within a fragmented health and care system. In addition, frail elderly people do not only want to see their remaining days maximised – they also want better quality of life in their later years.

Countries rated care co-ordination between health and social care workers as the most important policy in their LTC workforce agendas. Approximately one-third of OECD countries have policies in place to support better co-ordination of services provided by caregivers and to promote more integrated care (Figure 5.1). The majority of these policies aim to strengthen integration between health and social care services. Another important set of policies refers to initiatives promoting co-ordination between formal and informal workers. Informal caregivers – such as families, friends, neighbours and volunteers – represent an important proportion of care providers.

Figure 5.1. Co-ordination is the number one policy in countries' workforce agendas

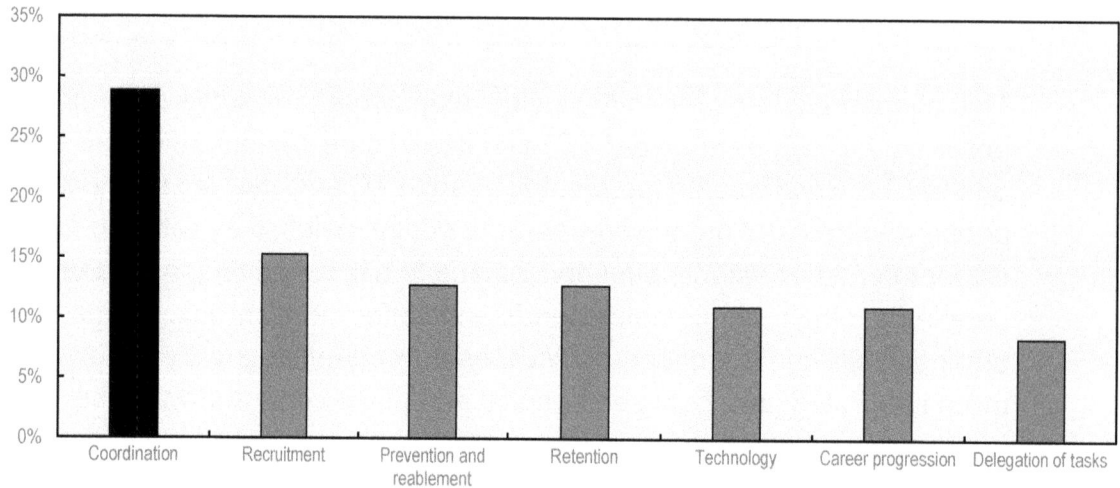

Source: OECD Long-term care workforce questionnaire, 2018.

With population ageing, a growing share of elderly people are using acute hospital beds and needing both health and LTC services to manage their chronic conditions and activity limitations. Failure to provide more integrated care pathways for elderly people can push up hospital costs through unnecessarily long hospital stays because of delayed discharges (Suzuki, forthcoming[1]; Osterman, 2017[2]) and, after discharge, may result in hospital readmission (Fuji, Abbott and Norris, 2013[3]). Evidence from pilot programmes shows that integrated teams of health and social care workers led in some cases to reduced emergency care bed use and delayed transfers (World Bank, 2016[4]); meanwhile, use of residential and nursing homes fell and there was an increase in use of home care services (Thistlethwaite, 2011[5]). Lack of appropriate care support at home can also increase societal costs by placing a heavy burden on informal carers. Indirect costs of informal care include forgone employment or worse health for informal carers. The United States estimated the economic value of informal caregivers at about USD 350 billion in 2006 – the income forgone by caregivers due to time spent caregiving (Gibson and Houser, 2007[6]). In New Zealand, this value represented USD 10.8 billion or 5% of GDP in 2013 (Grimmon, 2014[7]).

In response, countries are implementing a number of programmes that support co-ordinated LTC services closer to home. Care co-ordination – i.e. system-wide efforts and/or formal policies to ensure that elderly people get people-centred services – can improve outcomes and avoid care fragmentation that may lead to safety issues and increases in costs. For instance, integrated care services for frail elderly people in Canada reduced the costs of institutional and home care and of acute hospitalisations (Béland et al., 2006[8]). Such integrated community care systems require new health and social integrated pathways, an expanded role for LTC professionals working in teams monitoring chronic conditions and better integration and support of informal carers.

Widespread evidence on the effectiveness of integrated care on outcomes other than quality of care is still inconclusive and depends on many organisational and training factors. Numerous obstacles hinder workers' and caregivers' ability to provide co-ordinated services at the community level. In the majority of countries, LTC funding is fragmented, and when care is funded from multiple institutional silos and different levels of government, it tends to inspire cost shifting instead of shared care provision by workers. In addition, regulations hinder workers from delivering services in an effective manner, when and where needed, and can confine what professionals can do or delegate to their peers.

Section 5.2 discusses measures to improve co-ordination between LTC at home and acute and hospital care. Section 5.3 explores how professionals are finding new ways of working together to deliver such co-ordination. Options for better integration and support of informal carers are discussed in Section 5.4.

Key findings

- Close to one-third of OECD countries ranked LTC co-ordination as the number one policy challenge within their workforce agendas. Elderly people want care services that satisfy their needs and preferences: care that is organised, co-ordinated and delivered closer to home in their community. However, elderly people – many of whom endure several chronic conditions – require attention from multiple providers across fragmented and poorly co-ordinated health and social care systems.

- Countries are developing integrated health and care pathways to avoid unnecessarily long hospitalisations for elderly people. For instance, Australia, Canada, the United Kingdom, France, Portugal and Spain are implementing mobile hospital-at-home services, either as follow-up hospital-level care at home after discharge of a dependent elderly person from a short hospital stay, or as a preventive way to avoid hospital admission. Some countries, such as Belgium, Australia and England, United Kingdom, are also developing geriatric knowledge in hospitals. The rationale is two-fold: to prevent hospitalisation worsening autonomy and to avoid people staying for unnecessarily long periods in hospitals or being readmitted soon after discharge.

- Prompt discharge from hospitals requires appropriate follow-up; "step-down" alternatives can ensure continuity of care at lower cost. There is scope for expanding the role of nurses and personal care workers to perform more duties in monitoring health conditions among elderly people, health coaching and assisting transitions from hospital to homes. In Portugal, for example, trained nurses can perform both care and cure, and received a good level of training, including in hospital-based management of medical conditions.

- There is also need for more geriatric expertise in the community and appropriate referrals between primary care and LTC. Geriatricians (elderly care physicians) in the Netherlands can address complex care needs at home. In England (United Kingdom), multispecialty community providers facilitate recovery at home and enhance home care services, with an enhanced role for community nurses. In Quebec (Canada), care recipients are assessed using a screening tool for autonomy and morbidity and are assigned a case manager, who refers them to LTC home services and co-ordinates with primary care and other services.

- Intermediate care facilities are offered in some countries such as Norway and the United Kingdom, as a model for facilitating better care co-ordination between acute and LTC services. There is evidence that using such intermediate care following hospital discharge may reduce a person's need for further LTC and hospital services.
- Care managers can help alleviate the administrative burden of LTC carers and help co-ordinate their needs and those of care recipients. In the majority of OECD and EU countries, nurses and personal care workers already conduct tasks supporting this role. For transfers from hospital care into the community, the transitional care nurse (TCN) model in the United States has shown positive results. For this to happen, professionals need to be trained in communication skills, leadership roles, ICT skills and more advanced clinical skills.
- In addition to care managers, complex care management requires multidisciplinary teams to help co-design and co-decide care plans. In Portugal and the United States, such teams are part of the health care system to help elderly people with complex needs. More training will be necessary for nurses and personal care workers to work in such teams.
- Given the potential shortage of formal workers in the LTC sector, facilitating collaboration between formal and unpaid family carers – including informal networks and associations – in the team will be essential. Certain OECD countries have started, as part of integrated care, to include carers as part of the care team. In Australia, for instance, family carers have access to shared care planning tools.
- Formal carers will also increasingly be asked to collaborate with family carers, providing skills training and directing family carers to the services available to them. Several OECD countries have improved recognition of family carers and their dual role as workers and carers, but better support is still needed. Without it, family carers are likely to feel overburdened, resulting in increased hospitalisations and emergency visits for their loved ones.
- Respite care, which is designed to offer caregivers a break from their regular duties, is often cited as an important component to ensure that carers can continue to care. Few countries have made access to overnight respite care a right for family carers. Germany offers legal entitlement to a maximum number of respite care and short-term care days per year. There is evidence that education, training and information interventions are effective. Beyond training, carers who spend a substantial amount of time out of the labour force would also benefit from recognition and certification of skills acquired as carers.

5.2. Some countries are developing integrated health and care pathways

Poor co-ordination between different professionals makes it more likely that elderly people go to hospital unnecessarily. This can contribute to unnecessarily long stays but also to a high risk of readmission. People aged 65 and over represent a high proportion of patients in acute care hospitals, and stay longer than younger patients (Suzuki, forthcoming[1]). In addition to longer lengths of stay, older people make up the vast majority of patients experiencing delayed discharge from hospital which are often due to the lack of appropriate care arrangements (Figure 5.2).

Figure 5.2. There are gaps in hospital discharge planning

Percentage of elderly people who experienced a gap in hospital discharge planning, 2016

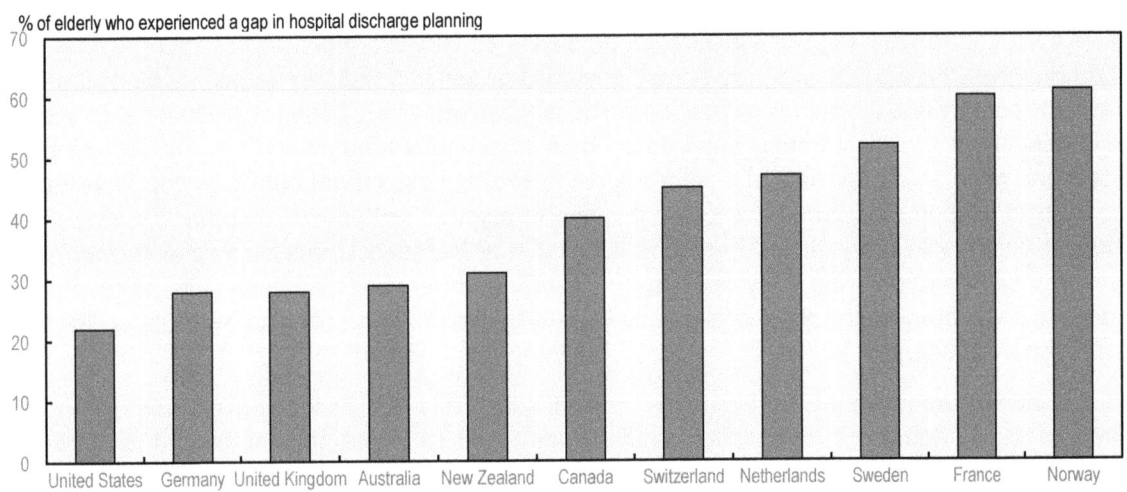

Note: Gaps include: i) not discussing the purpose of taking each of the medications, ii) not having arrangements for follow-up care with a doctor or other health professional and iii) not receiving written information on what to do upon return home and what symptoms to watch for.
Source: 2016 Commonwealth Fund International Health Policy Survey (data refer to 2016).

There is some evidence of the cost-effectiveness of integrated care interventions. Ensuring that more cost-efficient care is provided through better co-ordination may well support controlling costs (Hofmarcher, Oxley and Rusticelli, 2007[9]). The opportunities to save costs through home-based care and nurse-led health promotion for older people at risk of being admitted to an institution are many, but there is almost no evidence supporting an incremental quality of additional years lived gain compared to normal care. Further, findings comparing costs of an integrated care intervention to costs of hospitalisation are also limited. Comprehensive discharge planning has been seen to reduce costs significantly compared to usual care (reductions of USD 359 in non-US trials and USD 536 in US trials) (Nolte and Pitchforth, 2014[10]).

5.2.1. Improving hospital experience and discharge are important to mitigate health problems for elderly people

For frail elderly people, care transitions between hospital and community services are particularly challenging. Lack of appropriate support can take a toll on an elderly person's health. Many older patients – by some estimates, close to half of patients aged 70 and over – may experience functional decline following a hospital stay. Long hospital stays have been associated with the onset of delirium among older patients, a complication further associated with higher risk of poor outcomes, including institutionalisation, dementia and overall mortality (Suzuki, forthcoming[1]). Staying in hospital longer has also been associated with frailty and a higher risk of mortality, compared with older patients who are not frail, and increases the risk that a patient will develop complications, including hospital-acquired infections. Providing some of the acute care at home or improving the hospital experience is important to preserve the health of elderly people.

Mobile hospital-at-home services can be beneficial for frail elderly people

Bringing hospital services close to home is an innovative way countries have found to fulfil elderly needs for specialised care. Hospital-level care can be provided to patients in their own homes, involving technical care of a more or less complex or intensive nature, without which hospitalisation would be required. This model applies in one of two cases: as follow-up hospital-level care at home after discharge from a short hospital stay, or as a preventive way to avoid hospital admission when acute care beds are in short supply.

Mobile hospital-at-home services can offer a wide range of health care services: short-term medical treatments in response to acute clinical situations, continuous care in the case of chronic illnesses, palliative care and rehabilitation or functional therapies – all services identical to those provided at the hospital. However, their scope will vary across countries depending on the characteristics of the elderly people in the country and the supply of hospital services (Chevreul et al., 2004[11]). In Canada, for instance, home care services provide complex services such as intravenous therapy and dialysis, replacing acute hospital care while also providing LTC services. In Australia, hospital-at-home services have received strong political support, and laws have been changed to ensure that "private" insurance elderly persons can benefit from them. In the United Kingdom, hospital-at-home services are also quite diverse, varying according to objective (allowing early discharge or avoiding admission), pathology, clinical responsibility (allocated to hospital specialist or general practitioner (GP)) and provision of social services or lack thereof (Chevreul et al., 2004[11]).

Hospital-at-home care may save costs, improve patient satisfaction and reduce the probability of hospital-acquired infections and length of hospitalisation. Those cared for in the scheme tended to have higher satisfaction levels than those cared for in hospital (Shepperd et al., 2016[12]). By some accounts, pilots of the model have helped achieve savings of 30% per admission, for similar outcomes and fewer complications (Klein, Hostetter and McCarthy, 2016[13]). However, evidence on effectiveness and safety is mixed. Literature shows different results around the effect of hospital-at-home care on readmissions and significant differences in mortality (Farfan-Portet et al., 2015[14]). Given the demand for acute beds compared to the number available, hospital-at-home care can also be used as a preventive care model to avoid unnecessary hospital admissions. While previous evidence on the resulting avoidable hospitalisation was mixed, and hospital-at-home care may not have any effect on health outcomes per se, a more recent review shows it can increase the chances of living at home for six months.

Such services require strong co-ordination between the hospital team and health and LTC professionals in the community. For instance, in Portugal, in preparation for hospital discharge, a social worker from the care team conducts an evaluation of the patient's house and assesses the availability of an informal caregiver. Meanwhile, the hospital team (nurses, doctors, pharmacists, social workers and a nutritionist) assesses the patient thoroughly before discharge and provides a dossier including team contact details – available 24/7 – to take home. On the day of discharge, the patient receives a visit from a nurse; the following day, a home visit from the physician. Once settled in at home, follow-up is managed by nurses and personal carers attached to the primary care health centre, who co-ordinate care with the hospital.

There is often insufficient workforce capacity for hospital-at-home care to satisfy demand. The development of hospital-at-home options has been slow, relating in part to insufficient information for health professionals about the potential benefits and value added for patients. In France, health care professionals perceive it as a less attractive sector, with a higher workload and lower remuneration.

Adequate implementation of hospital-at-home care requires adaptations of skills to provide complex care in the home environment. In particular, if this is done by doctors or nurses from hospitals or primary care, such professionals will need to gain new expertise – this requires both new modules during baseline training and continuing education (such as basic training in palliative care, dementia and pharmacological intervention for nurses). Beyond acute care needs, development of hospital-at-home care is also linked to co-ordination with palliative care and end-of-life care services (Farfan-Portet et al., 2015[14]). Physician resistance and time constraints can represent a further barrier. Doctors at times still try to avoid referring patients for home care services as they want to ensure their patients are appropriately cared for. They may also hesitate to refer to such services as it takes time to make a comprehensive screening assessment – it is simpler just to admit patients to hospital (Klein, Hostetter and McCarthy, 2016[13]).

Geriatric knowledge in hospitals delays health deterioration for elderly people

Evidence shows that comprehensive assessment of elderly patients in hospitals can be of significant benefit (Oliver, Foot and Humphries, 2014[15]), but hospitals are not always well equipped to provide frail elderly people with high-quality care. This is particularly problematic for people with dementia, for instance. Many of the behavioural challenges of dementia, which can be exacerbated by distress at being in hospital, can be difficult for hospital staff to manage effectively.

With ageing populations, hospitals are also adapting departments and service lines to meet the needs of ageing patients. In this type of department, nurses are trained in geriatric illnesses and comorbidities. Alongside physicians, the care team includes a geriatric nurse navigator, a social worker, physical therapists and pharmacists when needed. All senior patients are screened for several geriatric conditions – dementia, delirium, dietary problems, depression and risk for falls. A patient identified as vulnerable to any of those conditions receives a thorough work-up and appropriate referrals (Flood and Allen, 2013[16]). Evaluations of special geriatric care units in Australia and Germany suggest that the care received can help to reduce negative outcomes of hospitalisation, including adverse events such as falls and reductions in capacity to perform ADL, though they may not reduce the length of stay in hospital (OECD, 2018[17]) (Deschodt et al., 2016[18]). Mobile interdisciplinary geriatric consultation teams are also used as an alternative to specific units for elderly people.

Belgium has long experience of hospital care for geriatric patients, starting in 1985. Regulations specify that each acute hospital must have either a care programme for geriatric patients or an established a collaboration agreement with another acute hospital offering such programme. Such programmes specify that any patient over 75 needs to be screened using a validated screening tool; if deemed at risk, the multidisciplinary team is consulted. Care programmes for geriatric care in Belgian hospitals are structured around five main components: a geriatric unit, an inpatient geriatric consultation team, an external geriatric consultation function, geriatric ambulatory consultations and geriatric day hospitals.

Another good practice example comes from England, United Kingdom. Many older people are admitted to hospital due to hip fractures, at an average age of 84. This outcome is often associated with frailty, bone fragility and multiple other comorbidities. While evidence-based treatment may be available, mortality at 12 months post admission is around 20%. To tackle this issue, in 2007 standards for management of patients with hip fracture and guidelines were drafted. A national hip fracture database was implemented in 2008, linking it to a national best practice in 2009. By 2013, 30-day mortality had fallen from 10% to 6%, the average overall length of hospital stay had been reduced, and an increased number of patients were leaving hospital having received comprehensive assessments and good preventive interventions (Oliver, Foot and Humphries, 2014[15]).

A number of countries have developed innovative new staff positions and teams working in hospitals to deal specifically with patients exhibiting symptoms of dementia. In Australia, the Dementia Behaviour Management Advisory Service is available in acute hospital settings to help deal with people with dementia exhibiting behavioural and psychiatric symptoms. In Ireland, a dementia nurse specialist role has been developed in acute hospital settings to serve as a link between hospital and community-based services. A similar role has been introduced in hospitals in Slovenia. Specialist mental health liaison teams in the United Kingdom also help to advise hospital staff on recognising and responding to delirium and dementia (OECD, 2018[17]).

One issue potentially impairing the performance of these programmes is the lack of geriatricians. In Belgium, only 28 physicians started geriatric training between 2010 and 2013, well below the minimum number of 80 places planned during those years, and this shortage is expected to worsen in future. There are fewer than four certified geriatricians in the United States per 10 000 75-year-old individuals. In addition, a career in geriatrics is chosen by less than 1% of US medical school graduates (Sorbero, 2012[19]). To tackle this, policy measures are being considered, such as imposing minimum enrolment in geriatric training and increasing the attractiveness of this speciality (for example, by increasing the number of training places or rewards) (Deschodt et al., 2015[20]).

Proper planning for hospital discharge needs to be well supported to avoid readmission. This often requires a skilled multidisciplinary team that, together with the patient and family, discusses needs and agrees on a post-hospitalisation plan. In Sweden, before an elderly patient can be discharged from hospital (to go home or to a lower-acuity care setting), a physician from the hospital and a case worker from the municipal social services agency must jointly develop a plan to ensure the patient will receive follow-up services. This has enabled the country to reduce the number of patients kept in the hospital once they no longer need high-acuity treatment. In the Netherlands, a recent pilot programme has been developed where community nurses are placed in hospitals to conduct triage and check which patients are eligible for hospital care. If it is not required, the nurses redirect the patient to the right service in the community. When there is a need to attend hospital, the elderly are accompanied by professional aide.

For transfers from hospital care into the community, the transitional care nurse (TCN) model in the United States has shown positive results. An advanced practice nurse or registered nurse supports comprehensive in-hospital planning and home follow-up for patients with multiple chronic diseases and complex therapeutic regimes, through which hospitalised patients receive 4-12 months of post-hospitalisation care. The TCN aims at long-term positive outcomes, ensuring that both patients and family caregivers are equipped with the knowledge and skills to deal with health issues. United States-based research used randomised controlled trials to show that this model improves acutely ill older adults' experiences of care, quality of life, patient safety and health outcomes (Occelli et al., 2016[21]) (Zhang et al., 2017[22]).

The TCN role is different from that of a nurse. In addition to typical nursing skills, the TCN has the competencies to act as a care manager and patient advocate, to manage complex cases and palliative care, to engage actively with family caregivers and to ensure inter-disciplinary care. The TCN does not work in isolation but collaborates with different physician specialists, other nurses, social workers and discharge planners, to name a few of the actors within the health care team. Usually, weekly clinical case conferencing sessions take place with a team of multidisciplinary experts for support in addressing the most complex issues (Box 5.1).

Box 5.1. A successful co-ordination model for complex patients, led by nurses

The TCN – usually an advanced practice nurse – has primary responsibility for ensuring care management of the elderly person throughout episodes of acute illness to avoid deterioration of health status and frequent hospital visits. A patient admitted to hospital is evaluated within 24-48 hours, based on screening and risk assessment. If the patient is eligible, a TCN will be in charge of providing individualised care, based on a tested protocol involving four areas of action: hospital visits, a series of post-discharge home visits, accompanying the patient on first visits to physicians and ensuring continuity of care post-transitional care. Randomised controlled trials on the TCN show significant results for avoidance of hospital readmission and emergency room visits, as well as reductions in total health care costs.

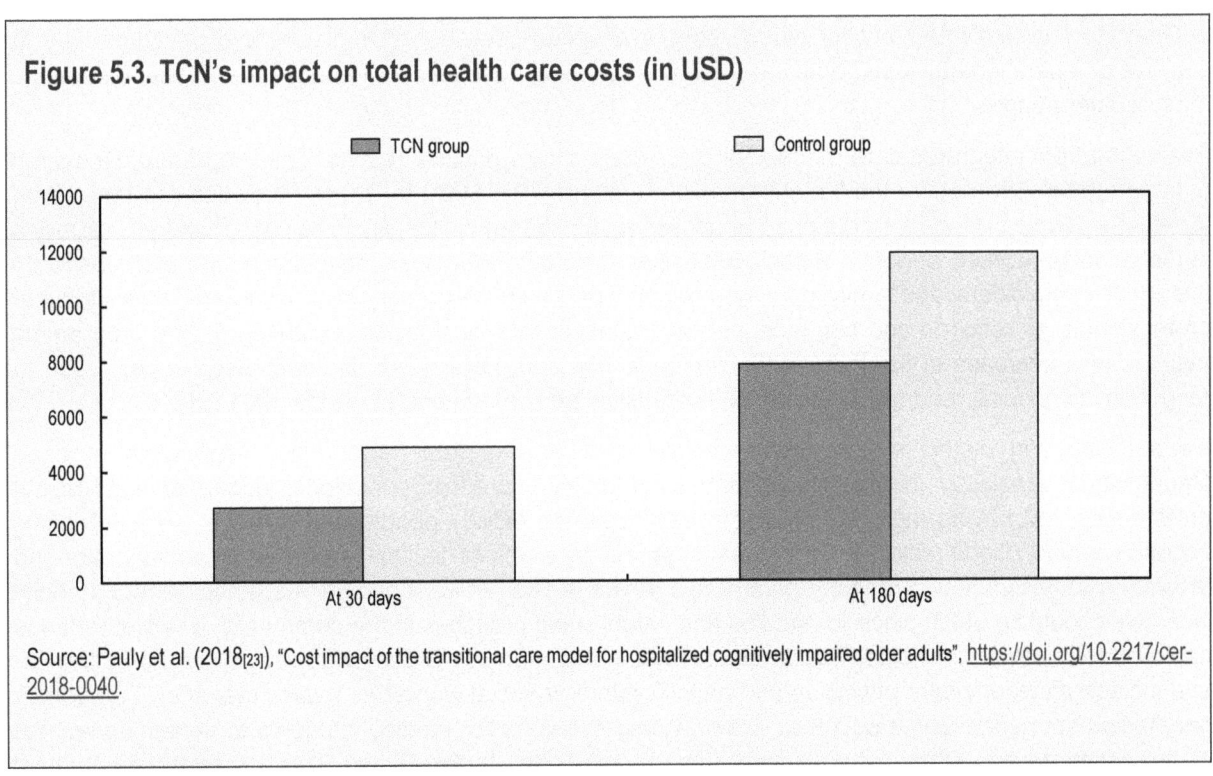

Figure 5.3. TCN's impact on total health care costs (in USD)

Source: Pauly et al. (2018[23]), "Cost impact of the transitional care model for hospitalized cognitively impaired older adults", https://doi.org/10.2217/cer-2018-0040.

5.2.2. Increasing geriatric expertise in the community will smooth care pathways

In addition to co-ordination at the hospital level, good discharge planning requires appropriate care at home or in the community, or sufficient intermediate care options to avoid a risk of hospital readmission in the future. Elderly patients with complex needs that span health and LTC may require an intensity of support that goes beyond what primary care physicians can deliver. For elderly people to stay at home as long as possible and prevent unnecessary hospital (re)admissions, more geriatric expertise in the community is needed. Hospital admission may follow any number of safety incidents, some of which could be avoided. It is estimated that the total cost of avoidable admissions to hospitals from LTC facilities in 2016 was almost USD 18 billion[1], according to an analysis using data from 25 OECD countries. This figure is equivalent to 2.5% of all spending on hospital inpatient care or 4.4% of all spending on LTC (de Bienassis, Llena Nozal and Klazinga, forthcoming[24]).

Several countries are enhancing the collaboration between professionals

A single access point for frail elderly people and co-ordination of services across acute, primary and LTC is important to provide appropriate follow-up for those with complex needs. The World Health Organization (WHO) has proposed the Integrated Care for Older People (ICOPE) approach: a people-centred approach to care that develops a continuum of care services for elderly people, ranging from prevention to rehabilitation (WHO, 2015[25]). This includes shared decision-making and goal setting; support for self-management; multidisciplinary teams; unified information or data-sharing systems; community linkages or integration; and supportive leadership, governance and financing mechanisms.

Several countries and regions have moved ahead in the integration of services or are at different stages of development in different parts of the country. In Scotland, United Kingdom, work has been under way since 2016 to integrate services across health and social care. The Czech Republic has started to integrate health and social care services in the Pardubice region to support individuals with reduced self-sufficiency. Saxony in Germany has introduced standard assessments and treatment pathways for geriatric patients with chronic conditions (EU, 2017[26]). Technological solutions and "continuity nurses" are used in Valencia in Spain to facilitate treatment for elderly people. Sweden uses quality registers and benchmarking to improve co-operation between home care, primary care and hospital care to better co-ordinate care of the most ill older people.

Evaluation from integrated care models for the elderly shows positive results. The Program of Research to Integrate the Services for the Maintenance of Autonomy (PRISMA) in Quebec provides integrated care for elderly people through a single point of access and a shared clinical file. The case manager, usually a nurse or social worker, performs a basic assessment for autonomy loss, develops a care plan based on the needs of the elderly and family input, co-ordinates care with the primary care physicians, refers to other professionals as required and conducts periodic re-assessments (MacAdam, 2015[27]). The programme resulted in a decrease in the level of functional decline and there were also decreases in costs due to reductions in hospital readmissions and institutionalisation (Béland and Hollander, 2011[28]).

Geriatricians and district or community nurses can be important actors in co-ordination of care. Geriatricians specialise in treating patients with multiple chronic conditions, understanding patient preferences and having the competency to deal with frail elderly people and those at a risk of losing cognitive and functional abilities. Shortages of geriatricians reflect declining numbers of primary care and medical students choosing to study geriatrics. There is a need to incentive such specialisation. Financial incentives could be put in place for studies and establishing practices in the community. The Netherlands has tried to develop more elderly care expertise in the community. Elderly care teams are led by the GP and include an elderly care physician and an LTC nurse or social worker as a case manager. To address geriatrician shortages, some countries are providing exposure for medical students to geriatric medicine or promoting greater scope for advanced nurse practitioners. In the United States, the Medical Student Training in Aging Research is an example of such a programme. Nurse practitioners in Canada, the United States and the Netherlands have been effective in the care of older people and have improved physical function and reduced falls and hospital admission (Chavez, Dwyer and Ramelet, 2018[29]). In England, United Kingdom, district nurses operate in partnership with LTC services to delay and reduce the need for care and support, while also helping elderly people to recover from ill health and manage long-term conditions.

Increasing the expertise of LTC workers to detect health risks and manage health conditions appears promising

The United States has a programme to enhance the LTC workforce: the Health Resources and Services Administration Geriatrics Workforce Enhancement Program. This training programme seeks to integrate geriatrics and primary care models, to address gaps in health care for older adults, to promote age-friendly health systems and dementia-friendly communities, and to address the social determinants of health.

Nurses who are LTC workers can be a key element of enhanced integration between health and LTC services. For instance, LTC home care nurses in the Netherlands are part of the Transitional Care Bridge programme, which is used by 50% of hospitals to provide a smooth post-hospitalisation transition. They are also case managers as part of SamenOud or Embrace model, and provide advice on health conditions, housing adaptation and both health and social care.

Some specialists argue that personal care workers could also be trained in the necessary skills to observe health conditions, offer health coaching and assist in transitions from hospital to home (Osterman, 2017[2]). Personal care workers have the opportunity to observe the living environment, as well as slight changes in medical conditions or functioning that could be important for teams deciding on therapeutic interventions. As such, they can be key partners in the co-ordination of care. They also have the opportunity to observe and shape the home environment, such as by detecting and removing allergens, fall risks and social isolation. There are, of course, pros and cons to task delegation and risks that personal care workers are not well prepared for such roles (see Chapter 3).

Upskilling of personal care workers has been tried in several pilots across the United States with positive results. Additional training includes clinical topics to understand patients' health conditions, navigating transitions in care and supporting health-promoting behaviours. In New York, for the Mount Sinai Hospital Home Care Collaboration Solutions, personal care workers were trained as health coaches in a pilot programme to help improve patient transitions from hospital and to solve caregiving challenges; they also served as links to interdisciplinary teams. Evaluation suggests that the programme may improve patients' performance of health maintenance behaviours, such as diet and exercise, and their ability to manage symptoms, as well as reducing the number of emergency visits (Russell and Kurowski, 2015[30]). The Care Connections Senior Aide programme run by the Professional Healthcare Institute led to an 8% reduction in the rate of emergency department visits (Stone and Bryant, 2019[31]). The Enhanced Home Care pilot programme in California trained personal care workers in medication management, mental health nutrition and physical skills, resulting in better health results – in particular, a 40% improvement in medication compliance and a reduction in patients' unhealthy days (Service Employees International Union, 2014[32]).

Increased staffing of intermediate care facilities is reducing LTC needs and hospital readmissions

In many cases, frail elderly people may no longer require the intensity of care they receive in acute hospital care, but may nevertheless require a level of support they cannot obtain if discharged directly to home. In these cases, intermediate care facilities can offer an important "step-down" alternative to hospitalisation. Intermediate care can also help maintain elderly people's autonomy, focusing on rehabilitation and delivered by a combination of professional groups. Intermediate care beds are available in hospital and community hospital settings, nursing homes, residential rehabilitation units and, more recently, in day hospitals and at home.

There is evidence that using intermediate care following a hospital admission may reduce patients' need for further LTC and hospital services. Intermediate care facilities are intended to reduce avoidable hospital admissions while reducing length of hospital stay (OECD, 2014[33]). In Norway, a study of intermediate care use following hospital discharge found that patients who were transferred to intermediate care (rather than staying in hospital) required fewer days in nursing homes and less health care support at home (Herfjord et al., 2014[34])

There is significant cross-country variation in availability, and countries have moved to increase the capacity of intermediate and step-down care facilities. The 2012 Co-ordination Reform in Norway mandated that all municipalities develop intermediate care units by 2016 (OECD, 2014[33]), providing federal funding to support this. All municipalities have 24-hour care services to provide intermediate, short-term care, although capacities vary across municipalities. Availability of intermediate care facilities is also relatively widespread in the Netherlands, and has been credited with improved patient flow through hospitals and reduced hospital readmission rates (van der Brug, 2017[35]). However, a lack of standardisation means that relative capacity, settings and services can differ (OECD, 2014[33]).

In other countries, intermediate care facilities are not yet sufficient. In Scotland, United Kingdom, intermediate care facilities have been identified as an important approach to delivering care closer to home and reducing delayed discharge from hospital, although the development of new intermediate care beds has progressed more slowly than expected. In Sweden, waiting times to access beds in intermediate care are considered a major driver of delayed discharge from hospital.

Increasing beds in intermediate care facilities requires ensuring that intermediate care teams include staff from a broad range of disciplines. Trained nurses need to perform both care and cure and receive a good level of training, including hospital-based management of medical conditions. In addition, staffing needs include specialists for rehabilitation such as physiotherapists, occupational therapists, speech therapists and rehabilitation assistants, as well as nutritionists/dieticians psychologists and social workers. In addition to recruiting the right staff mix, the workforce needs to have skills to support people to optimise recovery and regain as much independence as possible. Intermediate care staff will need training to be able to recognise and respond to chronic conditions such as diabetes, mental health and neurological conditions, to support needs in the areas of nutrition and hydration, and to evaluate deterioration in the care recipient's health or circumstances.

In Portugal, a major reform in 2006 contributed to preventing hospital stays and reducing their length (see Box 5.2). Following the reform, the number of public institution beds more than quadrupled to reach 8 400 beds in 2016 in convalescent units, rehabilitation units, maintenance units and palliative care units, up from 1 808 beds in 2007. A similar increase was observed for treatment places, as they went up from 1 660 in 2008 to 6 264 treatment places in 2016 (Lopes, Mateus and Hernandez-Quevedo, 2018[36]). These increases suggest that the reform filled a gap in the coverage of LTC by creating multiple types of care taking into account different care needs and freeing up hospital beds.

Box 5.2. National networks ensure co-ordination between home care and acute care services

In Portugal, in 2006, a major reform took place to create a network providing integrated LTC services: the National Network for Long-term Integrated Care. This aims to integrate health and social care as a way to prevent long stays in hospitals for elderly people, and to have both medical and social services provided under the same umbrella. The network provides integrated LTC at home and in institutions, as well as three types of intermediary care: convalescence beds for intensive rehabilitation for up to 30 days, funded entirely via the Ministry of Health; medium-term beds for between 31 and 90 days, funded by both the Ministry of Health and Ministry of Labour and Social Solidarity; and long-stay beds for care beyond 90 days, funded by both ministries, but with a greater contribution from the latter. In the future, the network will also provide day services to promote autonomy.

Source: 2018 OECD Long-term care interviews.

5.3. LTC workers will benefit from additional skills for integrated care

The lack of collaboration among different stakeholders can also become a burden for patients and families, who are left to manage the schedules of nurses and different specialists (Suzuki, forthcoming[1]). An increased role for case managers and greater integration of LTC workers with other health and social care professionals through use of multidisciplinary teams are avenues to help elderly people navigate the system better. Both require enhanced training for LTC workers and provide opportunities for specialisation and career development.

5.3.1. Case managers improve care pathways for the elderly

Case managers can help alleviate the administrative burden of LTC carers and help co-ordinate their needs and those of care recipient (Box 5.3). A case manager playing the role of a co-ordinator between different health and social services can simplify follow-up procedures significantly for both patient and informal caregivers. Effective case management can reduce the utilisation of hospital-based services, enable a cost-effective approach to cases and improve care outcomes (Ross, Curry and Goodwin, 2011[37]; Roland et al., 2012[38]). With case management, there was an increased use of home and health services which increase the probability of detecting deterioration before the need for acute hospital admission (Eklund and Wilhemson, 2009[39]). Surveys conducted in several countries have shown that case management supports care continuity and can reduce the need for institutionalisation by up to 50% (Paat and Merilain, 2010[40]).

> **Box 5.3. What is it case management and what does a case manager do?**
>
> Case management refers to the service co-ordinating the various system components to achieve a successful outcome. It entails assessment of a person's LTC needs and is followed by appropriate recommendations for care, monitoring and follow-up. Case management's primary goal is service provision for the elderly, not management of the system or its resources. This includes responsibility for referral, consultation, prescription of therapy, admission to hospital, follow-up care and (where necessary) prepayment approval of referred services. It includes responsibility for relocating, co-ordinating and monitoring all medical care on behalf of a patient. Case management essentially aims to limit health costs by reducing the need for hospitalisation and the use of emergency services by high-risk individuals. It is normally organised by case management doctors or nurses, often in consultation with an insurer.
>
> Source: OECD Long-term care questionnaire and missions, 2018.

Case management of LTC for elderly people works differently across countries.

- In Austria, for instance, carers can enrol in local support centres, which put them in contact with a district nurse who assesses the carer's needs and directs them towards appropriate entities and services. Administrative and co-operative tasks are the primary focus of these institutions, but the services also act as brokers and contacts between the elderly and formal services. The aim is to avoid gaps between health and social care provision and empower carers with knowledge and skills to face the difficulties of caring duties.
- Japan created a new profession of LTC managers -which requires a license and a qualification exam- to co-ordinate provision of health and social services care needs for elderly individuals. Care managers carry primary responsibility for ensuring co-ordination of care for elderly individuals with complex needs, and are a first point of contact for such patients and their families. The profession is now highly systematised, with clear qualification criteria and need to renew their licence every five years to assure the quality of services. The role, competencies and responsibilities of care managers are clearly recognised as an important part of the solution to providing better-quality health and social care. Care managers in Japan come from a mix of professional backgrounds (including nurses, dentists and social workers) and their professional association, which has around 25 000 members, offers training, seminars and publications.
- In the Netherlands, the case manager helps care recipients who are no longer independent and have complex care needs. The role of case manager is still being developed, and is currently only implemented to aid those suffering from dementia but is planned to expand to other groups with LTC needs. Main tasks include counselling before and after diagnosis, mapping care needs of the elderly, providing information and advice on diagnosis, prognosis and consequences, co-ordinating care by offering information on processes, motivating elderly people who avoid care, and providing emotional and practical support.

Several countries use case managers to co-ordinate transitions within and between community settings and hospitals. In the large majority of OECD and EU countries, nurses and personal care workers already conduct tasks supporting this role (see Chapter 3). Evidence supports the use of nurses as case managers, as they can improve clinical outcomes and reduce costs. Nurses can co-ordinate care interventions (e.g. via telephone) to monitor conditions of those at risk of hospitalisation and to facilitate communication between and with other health professionals and informal caregivers (Kim, Marek and Coenen, 2016[41])

Case management requires that professionals hold a specific set of skills. Case managers need sound clinical training to identify health needs and design care plans, in consultation with other professionals.

The new bachelor's degree for nurses in the Netherlands incorporates a strong emphasis on enhancing analytical and critical thinking skills, as well as investigative skills. In addition, as part of the care plan, more countries require case managers to improve their skills in educating patients in self-management (Horntvedt et al., 2018[42]). Evidence-based practice is imperative to ensure patient safety. In addition, five core case management activities are assessment, planning, linking, monitoring and advocacy. They are very important to ensure information transfer between different caregivers.

In a few countries, nurses have received specific training in case management. While the module and competency set in the curriculum will depend on the type of case management, some of the areas most commonly found include communication and teamwork skills. Communication skills are an important element in ensuring satisfaction with services and that care is effective. Communication needs to be effective with other providers, but also with the elderly. The case manager needs to oversee follow-up consultations and focus on the care recipient and the family. Elderly people are sensitive to establishing a bond and trust with their case manager. This is particularly the case for patients suffering from multiple comorbidities, who display a need for case managers who help them deal with their emotional needs (Hjelm et al., 2015[43]).

In Norway, while case management is not formalised yet, an important financial envelope was allocated in 2018 to improve nurses' skills in communicating with formal and informal caregivers. Around NOK 360 million are being allocated to developing new competences of the workforce, among others. Nursing education is being revamped to increase improve interprofessional communication skills (formal and informal), manage budgets and use new technologies (such as GPS trackers). The goal is to continue to increase nurses' specialisation – around 18% of community nurses are specialised – and allow them to take on leadership roles.

In Germany, the Community-based support for primary care (or AGnES) care model – nurses acting as case managers when visiting elderly patients at home – provides specific training in case management. AGnES professionals can be qualified nurses or other assistants who have accumulated three years of professional experience; they receive training as a Medizinischen Fachangestellten and received an AGnES qualification. To work as case managers they undertake an additional training module on communication and conflict management. AGnES nurses are also trained to deal with inter-professional and inter-sectoral collaboration (i.e. network and system management, co-ordination and control of aids, quality assurance in case management) and basics for taking a leadership role in care: assessing needs, monitoring and evaluating a patient. The training emphasises the importance of dialogue with other professionals, as most tasks of a case manager relate to supporting co-ordination of appointments with specialists, co-ordinating LTC provision and rehabilitation after hospital stays and co-ordinating services with pharmacists.

5.3.2. Multidisciplinary teams are beneficial in LTC

Integrated multidisciplinary teams can help promote autonomy and reablement and therefore support patients to stay home for longer. These teams way of working involves professionals from different disciplines and with a multitude of skills co-design and co-decide care plans and their implementation instead of working alongside with the elderly. This goes beyond traditional teamwork in health and LTC settings in the way that it assumes integrated decision-making among different professionals. Typically, teams are composed of a set of professionals – e.g. nurses, personal care workers and occupational therapists – and professionals working part time – e.g. doctors, nutritionists and social workers.

Evidence of the impact of multidisciplinary teams working on LTC is limited but shows positive results. Research has shown that integrated multidisciplinary teams can contribute to fewer difficulties in IADL, greater self-efficacy, less fear of falling, fewer home hazards and greater use of adaptive strategies. They can reduce deterioration of health and functional ability, improve daily life activities, increase social activities, decrease the length of hospital stays and delay readmission. Interdisciplinary teams can also contribute to patients' satisfaction with care (Socha-Dietrich, forthcoming[44]).

Team composition will depend on a number of factors such as care needs and local contexts. In countries like the Netherlands, composition of these teams is regulated by national policies; in others, like Norway, these are decided at the municipality level. The type of professionals in each team will vary depending on care needs, funding resources and availability of workers. It is, however, relevant that the elderly have a voice in deciding team composition. A high degree of rotation of the team members and the number of individuals see in a day can cause distress and make care recipients feel overwhelmed. Geographical misdistribution of health and social workers is one key challenge faced by LTC providers and governments. Rural areas normally face shortages of most qualified and skilled professionals, who may be reluctant to practise in socio-economically disadvantaged regions due to concerns regarding career, family and lifestyle (OECD, 2016[45]). The unequal distribution of professionals between metropolitan areas and rural/remote areas is one of the biggest workforce challenges in Australia.

There is some positive but still weak evidence of the impact of team training on the performance of multidisciplinary teams. In many instances, it is up to employers to ensure that teams work in an integrated manner (Buljac-Samardžić, 2012[46]). They enforce this by providing tailored theoretical or on-the-job training. Data collection from visits to a few nursing homes and home services companies in Norway, the Netherlands, Portugal and Germany shows that current themes for such training include understanding team dynamics, grasping the structure of multidisciplinary interventions and learning how to communicate in a team.

The United States, for instance, has been successful in operationalising fully integrated inter-professional teams at the primary care level, taking care of elderly patients with complex care needs. A number of managed care organisations have created inter-professional teams including primary care physicians, specialty trained nurses (for example, in diabetes), registered nurses, dieticians, speech therapists and social workers. Some of these teams comprise liaison community health workers responsible for outreach to underserved groups, such as indigenous populations, ethnic minorities or people with financial/housing difficulties. Recent developments within the integrated health systems and organisations show a trend towards further specialisation of inter-professional teams in care for specific groups of high-need patients. For instance, the Commonwealth Care Alliance launched a Senior Care Options programme, which provides primary care to elderly patients with complex needs through teams including geriatric social workers and palliative care clinicians, among the other usual categories of primary care professionals. Other inter-professional teams with a similar focus (for example, Community Aging in Place, which is active in 12 large cities) also include a handyman, who allows the team to make home modifications, helping elderly patients to navigate their homes more safely (Socha-Dietrich, forthcoming[44]).

5.4. Informal carers are also key actors in LTC services

In all OECD countries, both formal and informal caregivers provide LTC. Given the potential shortage of LTC workers, facilitating the work of carers and collaboration between formal and informal carers is essential. A move away from institutional care towards community-based care will require better integration of informal carers – whether family carers or other informal networks and associations – into the care team, and better support and compensation of informal carers so that they do not feel overburdened.

The role of formal care workers cannot be considered in isolation from informal care provision, and appropriate policies need to be in place for both types of worker to provide care that is more effective. Many countries rely heavily on informal carers to provide help to elderly people and are expanding formal care provision. Others are considering enhancing informal care, given financial pressures or difficulties with expanding the formal workforce. At the same time, co-ordination between formal and informal carers ranks low as a priority for countries. Less than half of OECD countries (45%) have implemented policies to strengthen co-ordination between formal and informal LTC workers.

This section analyses challenges that arise in co-ordinating informal and formal care workers. It suggests appropriate policy solutions to improve co-ordination, mainly in the area of incorporating informal carers as part of the care team and policies to improve the skills of informal carers and compensate them. Without better support, informal carers may be unable to sustain their care efforts, are more likely to have health problems themselves and may resort to emergency hospitalisation for their loved ones.

5.4.1. Changes in guidelines and incentives for formal carers can foster collaboration with informal carers

An average of 30% of people age 65 years and over receive both formal and informal care across OECD countries, ranging from as low as 13% in Slovenia to as high as 46% in Belgium. Care is shared between paid health care professionals and unpaid family caregivers (Figure 5.4). Coexistence of formal and informal care is more common in situations of greater need when both types of care become complementary (Litwin and Attias-Donfut, 2008[47]).

Figure 5.4. Receiving informal care alone is predominant but 30% of elderly people receive both formal and informal care

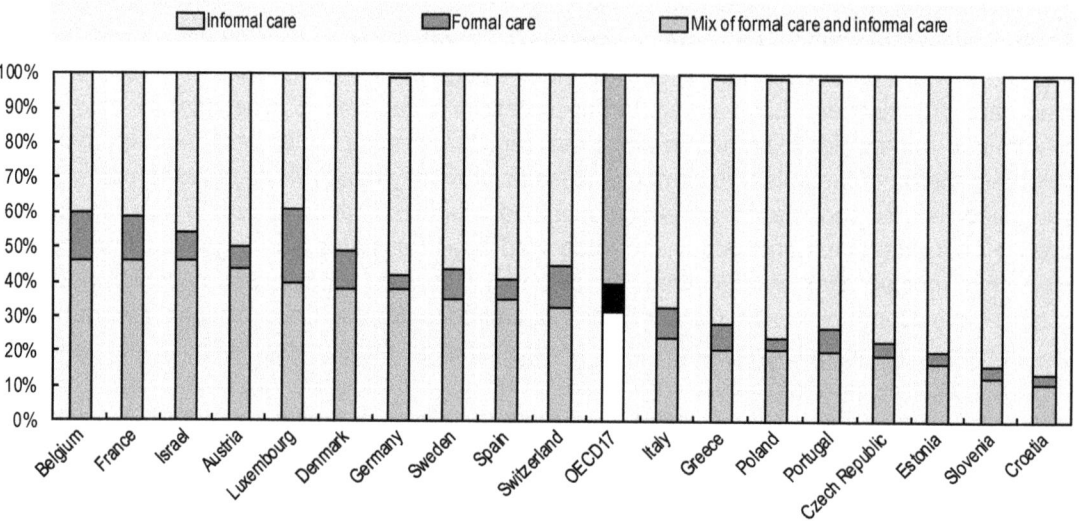

Source: OECD calculations based on the Survey of Health and Retirement Survey in Europe, wave 6 (data refer to 2015). The OECD average is unweighted.

Both types of care can either substitute for or complement each other, depending on the country and availability of various forms of formal care. Findings from the United States suggest that increased paid home care primarily went to people who were already receiving a greater amount of informal care from their adult children (Liu, Manton and Aragon, 2000[48]; Langa et al., 2001[49]). In Europe, informal care tends to be a substitute for formal home care and paid domestic help, and more informal care exists in countries where there is a lack of formal care (Van Houtven and Norton, 2004[50]; Bonsang, 2009[51]; Bolin, Lindgren and Lundborg, 2008[52]).

Formal and informal carers work in parallel and perform different tasks

Informal and formal caregivers are often dissatisfied with their collaboration. Formal caregivers may fail to recognise the contribution of informal carers and do not view them as partners in a shared care arrangement. This can result in informal carers being excluded from treatment decisions and care planning. In turn, formal care workers complain about being watched or asked to perform tasks that are beyond their duties (Sims-Gould et al., 2015[53]). This affects the satisfaction and turnover of formal caregivers (Carpentier and Grenier, 2012[54]).

There is scope for clarifying tasks and strengthening collaboration from the outset. Informal caregivers can provide help with IADL, while they may find provision of help with ADL – especially certain ADL such as hygiene, incontinence and cognitive impairments – more difficult, requiring help from formal carers.

Informal carers perform a variety of tasks, although the core of their activities is help with IADL or household care and emotional support. The majority of informal carers are heavily involved with practical care tasks or household care work: important IADL, such as shopping, cooking and doing laundry. Another task that falls to informal carers is administrative help, such as paying the bills. Large numbers of informal carers have a key role in providing company and emotional support, such as "keeping an eye" on the care recipient and making sure they are safe. In contrast, fewer informal carers perform personal care tasks and administer medication (Wanless, 2006[55]).

Roles and responsibilities of informal caregivers will become more complex and demanding. With delayed institutionalisation and higher numbers of elderly people staying at home with complex needs, especially with dementia, informal caregivers will have growing responsibilities and are likely to provide more tasks such as personal care and specialised medical care, including injections. It is also likely that they will become surrogate decision-makers for relatives who have suffered from physical or mental decline (Arber and Venn, 2011[56]). More frequent interaction should lead to a different collaboration, in which formal carers are trying not to fill gaps but to support informal carers in performing their tasks (Janse et al., 2018[57]).

Training and guidelines for formal care workers can improve collaboration with informal carers and efficiency in delivery

Collaborating with informal caregivers will require professionals to adopt a different way of working, in many instances. The current focus is mainly on the care recipient for whom they care, and not on the informal carers of the care recipient, even though they are an invaluable source of information about the needs of an elderly person. There is therefore a strong rationale to recognise the role and tasks performed by both formal and informal carers.

A way forward in the collaboration would be to include a training module for professional carers on how to work with informal carers. Research from the Netherlands concludes that such a module should be included in the curricula of allied health, nursing and social work education, and that similar training courses could be developed for the continuing education of personal care workers (Hengelaar et al., 2018[58]). Other forms of training suggested in Canada include case management conferences or in-service training sessions involving families, workers and managers, to gain shared understanding of the scope of the role and clear mechanisms for communication and conflict resolution (Sims-Gould et al., 2015[53]).

Regular communication between formal and informal carers is not always facilitated by current service provision. Professional care has a great deal to offer informal carers, such as advice, guidance, skills training and sharing of knowledge. Equally, professional carers benefit from good communications with the family caregiver. Rapid staff turnover and having different care providers with insufficient relays between them are obstacles to smooth collaboration. A permanent contact person, such as a case manager, might improve collaboration (Stephan et al., 2015[59]).

Informal carers are an indispensable but vulnerable link in the care chain, and more countries are seeking to give them stronger input into care. This includes consulting informal caregivers during creation of the care plan and directing them to available services (Jorgensen et al., 2010[60]). In the United Kingdom and Sweden, for instance, informal carers are entitled to a carers' assessment separate from the care recipient, and should be eligible for appropriate support services afterwards. In Finland, the law specifies that the informal carer must be able to provide care as certified by a GP through a health check. The new Care Plan in Norway notes that agreements made with family members and volunteers should be recorded in the case files and individual plans, both to co-ordinate these efforts with public care services and to assess relevant measures relating to training, guidance and relief from the caregiving burden.

Certain countries have started, as part of integrated care, to include informal carers as part of the care team. In Australia, for instance, informal carers have access to shared care planning tools. In Flanders, Belgium, the Informal Care Plan was adopted by the Flemish Parliament on 1 February 2017. The informal caregiver becomes a partner in the care and support plan, and professional care providers are encouraged to involve informal caregivers and respect their role in the care process and, where necessary, in care co-ordination. This will be further reinforced by planned modifications to the decrees on primary care, mental health care, local social policy and residential care, which should include the principle that the informal caregiver is a fully fledged partner in care.

5.4.2. Training and emotional support will help informal carers to perform their tasks better

Informal carers are the backbone of the system in many countries, yet they receive little training and psychological support, which results in lower quality of care. Psychosocial interventions have a positive impact on carers' well-being and mental health (Larkin, Henwood and Milne, 2019[61]).

Many informal carers request skill-building and LTC knowledge training

Because caregivers often experience anxiety and insecurity, and feel unprepared for their role, education and skills training can improve caregiver confidence. According to Eurocarers, training in the following skills is particularly useful: disease-specific knowledge; skills required to maintain the health status of the patient and, if possible, facilitate rehabilitation; skills to deal with management of symptoms; skills related to daily life activities; and management of emergency situations (Eurocarers, 2015[62]). Some practical nursing skills – mainly managing and administering medication, pain management and moving and handling techniques without suffering strain – are also needed.

Availability of training services is fragmented across OECD countries, and is often provided by civil society. Take-up tends to be low because training is not necessarily available nearby, there is a lack of information and carers do not always have the time to attend (Eurocarers, 2015[62]). One fruitful avenue is including formal care workers in the delivery of training, which can also help them understand better the challenges faced by carers (Johannessen, Engedal and Thorsen, 2016[63]; Eurocarers, 2015[62]). A training programme that is flexible for informal carers and contains a mixture of face-to-face learning and e-learning might also help.

More training and certification for informal carers will not only help them to improve the quality of care but will also assist with transferability of skills. For those carers who are interested in pursuing employment in the health and community services sectors, given the variety of skills they may have developed, it is important that they are able to supplement gaps and standardise their knowledge and ability.

Psychosocial interventions and counselling have also proved to have a positive impact on carers' capacity to deliver care. Addressing emotional strain by providing coping strategies such as self-care, stress management, problem-solving and decision-making guidance are fruitful avenues to reduce caregiver stress and improve quality of care (Brimblecombe et al., 2018[64]). Building carer resilience with techniques for coping with demands, relaxation and reducing isolation through peer support are also valuable interventions (Larkin, Henwood and Milne, 2019[61]; Brimblecombe et al., 2018[64]). Examples of such interventions include, for instance, the municipal learning and mastery centres in Norway, which offer mastery courses to close family members to help them cope with their everyday lives.

Improved carer well-being strengthens their ability to care

The association between informal caring and poor health outcomes is well documented across studies (Thomas et al., 2015[65]; Stansfeld et al., 2014[66]). Caregivers are much more likely to report poorer subjective quality of life than similar adults who do not care for family or friends (Thomas et al., 2015[65]). Further, caregiver burden and ill health have also been associated with worse health outcomes for their care recipients. Higher caregiver burden has also been associated with a higher prevalence of falls among care recipients (Vaughon et al., 2018[67]).

Respite care, which is designed to offer caregivers a break from their regular duties, is often cited as an important component to ensure that carers can continue to care. Some respite care services are designed to offer short-term, often regular, breaks in care. These often included day care services delivered through municipalities and community organisations, or in-home care services. In addition to such day services, some countries offer caregivers the opportunity to take longer breaks from caring by offering temporary placements in residential care services, such as local nursing homes. Emergency respite care services, which offer caregivers respite at short notice, are less regularly available, although a number of countries have recognised the need to develop these programmes.

While many countries have overnight respite care services, their availability can vary greatly by municipality or local community. Overnight respite care is commonly provided by offering temporary residence in local nursing homes or other LTC institutions. Many municipalities have developed agreements with local nursing homes to use a designated number of beds for respite care, but availability can vary substantially by community. Co-ordination with formal carers is important to avoid the condition of care recipients, especially those with dementia, suffering a setback when they are taken away from their familiar environment.

Because of the high cost of providing respite services, some countries have determined legal maximums for the number of days carers may receive overnight respite care services. In New Zealand, respite care is funded to a maximum of 28 days per year, while in Israel, no more than two weeks are reimbursed. Few countries have made access to overnight respite care a right for informal carers, although Germany offers legal entitlement of six weeks per calendar year for respite care and eight weeks for short-term care, for which families can be reimbursed up to a fixed amount.

Innovative respite care services are also necessary to include either holiday breaks or mobile respite services at home. In Austria, a holiday respite care programme for people with dementia and their families integrates external care for people with dementia and training for carers into a holiday for the family. The municipality of Lyon is currently experimenting with respite care at home, although it tends to target mostly carers of people with disabilities. Mobile respite teams evaluate informal carers' needs and health, and provide appropriate solutions to reduce burnout, collaborating with health professionals and associations.

Although carers show satisfaction with breaks, there is little quantitative evidence of improvements to carers' emotional well-being and the cost-effectiveness of respite. Several meta-analyses show no evidence of the impact of respite on physical and mental health (Brimblecombe et al., 2018[64]). On the other hand, other research shows that respite care enabled 50% of carers to have more time for themselves, and that the health of those without access to respite care deteriorated more rapidly (Yeandle and Wigfield, 2012[68]). Part of the lack of evidence may be due to the lack of high-quality research in this area and the short-term services, which only offer temporary relief.

5.4.3. Compensating carers well and addressing their double burden will ensure more sustainable care

Individuals do not provide care in isolation from the other roles and responsibilities in their lives. Estimates from the Survey of Health and Retirement in Europe show that informal carers are less likely to work when providing care to a spouse. Across Europe, 45% of men aged 50-64 work if they are caring for their spouse, compared with 60% of those who are not carers; the equivalent figures are 34% and 52% for women. Quality of care requires reducing the double burden and stress of combining work and care by providing more flexibility at work – not only care leave but also the right to reduced working hours and flexi-time.

An effective contribution for informal carers also necessitates cushioning lifetime income losses. This could be done through either appropriate compensation when carers leave work or recognition of the role of carers with entitlements to pension rights and subsidies for social security contributions.

Informal carers need to balance work and caring responsibilities

Balancing the dual responsibilities of working and caring is difficult, but leave and flexible work can help. Informal carers in OECD countries have a 20% higher prevalence of mental health problems than those who do not provide care (Colombo et al., 2011[69]) and also tend to have worse physical health. Intensity and duration of care tend to lead to worse outcomes. Informal care also reduces the likelihood of being in paid employment because of the hours of work, and leads to higher chances of sickness absence. Care leave tends to limit the negative impact of caring on employment, especially in combination with flexible working conditions (Brimblecombe et al., 2018[64]).

Across OECD countries, there is growing commitment to support informal carers combining work and caring. Three-quarters of countries (30 countries) provide some rights to leave to care for a family member – either paid or unpaid – up from two-thirds of countries 10 years ago (Table 5.1). Currently, 19 countries offer some form of paid leave for caring, and four introduced paid care leave in the past decade.

However, in most countries offering paid leave for informal carers, it is only available for a limited duration – in most cases less than two weeks. Paid leave is also sometimes tied to an employee's sick leave allowance. Both Israel and New Zealand deduct time spent caring for sick family members from the carer's own allotted sick leave. In the Netherlands and Spain, employers are allowed to refuse requests for care leave if there is a strong business case for doing so. A number of countries have criteria based on employer size (Ontario, Canada, and the United States) or employment history (Canada, Ireland, New Zealand, the United States) that can exclude some carers from eligibility.

Care leave is still seldom used, through lack of awareness or fear of sending a negative signal to the employer, or because it is not adapted to the needs of the employee. Use of formal care leave arrangements is often limited, and caregivers prefer to use holidays or sick leave, or make individual arrangements with their supervisors (Colombo et al., 2011[69]; Oldenkamp et al., 2018[70]). Carers are often unaware of leave options, particularly those with lower education levels, and the opportunities available do not always match carers' needs. Formal care leave arrangements are more often used in cases of high intensity and burden of care, but when caring responsibilities are prolonged, they may be insufficient. While unpaid leave is often much longer, carers may be unable to afford such periods without income.

Programmes that allow for more work flexibility, including reducing hours and teleworking, may be better suited to supporting carers. Flexible working hours are critical to sustain the combination of work and caring, lower the chance of reduced working hours and increase employment prospects (Arksey and Glendinning, 2007[71]). In the United Kingdom (England), for example, all employees – including carers – may request a flexible working arrangement after an initial 26-week qualifying period. In Germany, a family care leave scheme was recently introduced for employees needing to support a relative with LTC needs. Employees may take up to six months off full-time work, or elect to work part time. Three months of leave is provided when caring for relatives at the end of life. In addition to the leave provided, employees have the opportunity to access interest-free loans (conditional on employer size) to help support them while their income is reduced.

Table 5.1. More countries have leave entitlements to care for the sick than ten years ago

Country	Pension credits	Leave for carers	Paid leave available	Duration per year
Australia	–	Yes	Yes (100% of earnings)	10 days
Austria	Yes	Yes	Yes (100% of earnings)	1 week
Belgium	No	Yes	Yes (flat rate)	12 months per episode
Canada	–	Yes	Yes (for family members at risk of dying in the next 26 weeks; for employees who have worked ≥600 hours in the past year; 55% of earnings) Yes, family caregiver benefit for adults	Up to 26 weeks up to 15 weeks
Chile	–	–	–	–
Croatia		Yes	Yes (for spouse; 70% of earnings)	20 days per episode
Czech Republic	Yes	Yes	Yes (60% of earnings)	9 days
Cyprus	No	Yes	–	7 days
Denmark	Yes	–	–	
Estonia	–	Yes	Yes (80% of earnings)	7 days per episode
Finland	Yes	Yes	Unpaid but can depend on collective agreements	
France	No	Yes	Paid for terminal illness (payment for 3 weeks)	3 months
Germany	Yes	Yes	No but can receive short-term carer grant	6 months
Greece	No	Yes	–	6 days
Hungary	No	–	–	–
Iceland	–	–	–	–
Ireland	Yes	Yes	Yes (for close family member, when employee has worked for ≥12 months)	3 days
Israel	–	Yes	Yes (for spouse or parent)	6 days
Italy	Yes	Yes	Yes (100% of earnings)	2 days over their working life
Japan	–	Yes	Yes (40% of earnings)	93 days over their lifetime
Korea	–	Yes	–	90 days
Latvia	Yes	–	–	–
Lithuania	Yes	Yes	–	–
Luxembourg	Yes	–	–	–
Mexico	–	–	–	–
Netherlands	No	Yes	Yes (although employers can refuse "on serious business grounds"; 70% of earnings)	10 days
New Zealand	–	Yes	Yes (for employees who have worked for ≥26 weeks; 100% of earnings)	5 days taken from sick leave
Norway	Yes	Yes	–	10 days per episode
Poland	Yes	Yes	Yes (80% of earnings)	14 days
Portugal	–	Yes	–	15 days
Romania	–	No	–	–
Slovak Republic	–	Yes	Yes (55% of earnings)	10 days
Slovenia	Yes	Yes	Yes (for co-resident family members; 80% of earnings)	7 days (maximum 6 months if severely ill)
Spain	No	Yes	Yes (although employers can refuse on "serious business grounds"; 100% of earnings)	2 days
Sweden	No	Yes	Yes (80% of earnings)	100 days
Switzerland	–	Yes	–	–
Turkey	–	–	–	–
United Kingdom	Yes	Yes	–	–
United States	–	Yes	–	12 weeks

Source: OECD Family Database 2016 for leave; information on pension credits from Hamilton and Thomson (2017[72]), "Recognising unpaid care in private pension schemes", https://doi.org/10.1017/S1474746416000312.

In designing care leave for the future, countries need to balance the rights of working carers with eligibility conditions. Identification of who is the primary carer and the number of hours of caring are important when establishing entitlements to prevent an abuse of care leave. Similarly, a fine balance needs to be found between the amount of compensation and the length of leave to prevent the risk of early retirement or falling into a long period of inactivity, which would limit re-employment options.

Career loss compensation provides a forward-looking vision for carers

The majority of OECD and EU countries (two-thirds) provide care recipients with cash benefits for the person in need of care to support informal care, rather than supporting the informal carer directly (Table 5.2). While some countries require that care recipients make a formal contract with their caring relatives, most countries do not control what care recipients do with those cash benefits. A smaller number of countries support the informal carer directly financially – for example, Austria and the Netherlands. Finland and Belgium (Flanders) support informal carers in both ways, while Flanders and France support only care by adult children (care by spouses is not directly financially supported).

Table 5.2. Most countries have cash benefits for informal care

No support	Support the care recipient	Support the informal carer
Sweden	Belgium (Flanders)	Australia
Japan	Bulgaria	Austria
France (spouse)	Croatia	Belgium (Flanders)
Belgium (spouse)	Czech Republic	Canada (Nova Scotia)
Lithuania	England	Estonia
	Germany	Finland
	Finland	France
	Iceland	Hungary
	Israel	Ireland
	Italy	Netherlands
	Korea	Slovakia
	Latvia	
	Luxembourg	
	Netherlands	
	Poland	
	Portugal	
	Spain	
	Slovenia	
	United States	

Source: OECD Long-term care questionnaire.

Cash benefits for the care recipient include a number of benefits and drawbacks, especially from the point of view of informal carers. Cash benefits are used in several countries as a way to provide choice and flexibility for recipients and encourage care by a relative, which is often a preferred option. Such benefits avoid difficulties in identifying carers, which simplifies eligibility requirements and makes the financial contribution depend on needs. On the other hand, the benefit does not always go to the carer, leaving them dependent, and trapping informal caregivers in a low-paid role.

Carers are at risk of financial penalties with respect to accumulated retirement income for their second-tier pension (i.e. mandatory, contributory public or private savings for income replacement in old age) because of lower workforce participation. OECD countries have created "carer credits" for those with interrupted workforce histories, which take the form of an amount of time credited to the carer's working record. To avoid those with fewer years of contributions receiving a lower pension, the government provides a credit to their contribution record or reduces the required balance for a full contribution record. Carer credits can also be in the form of a financial credit to the pension account.

The social protection rights of informal carers for pension credits have improved by making credits more generous in value or duration and extending the rights. In Germany and Luxembourg, an increasing number of caregivers benefit from pension contributions. In Germany the value of the credit depends on the type of benefits and the constituting care level. It may reach 100% of the average wage, and caregivers are entitled to payment of pension contributions if they are not gainfully employed for more than 30 hours of care; they are also covered by unemployment and accident insurance. In Finland, France and the United Kingdom, credits have become easier to access (Hamilton and Thomson, 2017[72]). There is still a challenge in improving retirement income for women on low pay and those in precarious work, and in compensating those who work part time for care reasons with top-up credits, for instance. In addition, with the growing importance of occupational pensions, carer credits in mandatory private pension schemes will be needed because credits tend to be available for childcare only, with a few exceptions. Only in one country – the United Kingdom – do employers continue to contribute to the occupational pension on behalf on an employee during periods of care. In Sweden, while this is not mandatory, employers are encouraged to do so and most comply (OECD, 2011[73]).

Cash benefits and pension credits can alleviate poverty for families, but there are several reasons why governments would prefer to limit the generosity of cash benefits to carers. First, the benefit rarely constitutes remuneration for carers' full efforts and does not typically cover the full cost of care. It is rather a recognition that providing care involves costs for carers and compensation for the opportunity costs of caring – that is, for reduced working hours. Second, high compensation risks trapping carers in low-paid roles, with few incentives to participate in the formal labour market. Appropriate compensation for carers needs to be balanced against the potential side-effects on the labour supply of carers, acting as a disincentive to gainful employment. Previous analysis showed that carers' allowances can discourage work for low-skilled workers, especially if they are means-tested (Colombo et al., 2011[69]).

5.5. Conclusion

Improved co-ordination will require appropriate financial incentives and information-sharing mechanisms. Payment systems for complex patients need to be redesigned so that they reduce barriers to collaboration. Current funding mechanisms and payment incentives often exacerbate the problems of fragmented care. Integrated LTC budgets may also help to overcome co-ordination issues if decision-making power on funding allocation is spread across different levels of government and different ministries. In Portugal, the integrated care network receives funding from both the Ministry of Health and the Ministry of Social Protection. Funding is set for all professionals who are either part of local health units providing care at home or intermediate care facilities. In Scotland, United Kingdom, integration authorities are responsible for the governance, planning and resourcing of social care, primary and community health care and unscheduled hospital care for adults. It is important that workers treating an elderly person with complex needs are able to share important data about that patient in a timely way. A single electronic record, as used in Quebec for PRISMA for all the patient's medical care, will also facilitate the process.

The elderly would also benefit from a closer coordination across formal and informal carers. Part of this would necessitate a broader outlook in the care plans to include informal carers and ensure a sharing of tasks. In addition, informal carers will need a range of services to improve their wellbeing, compensate from their costs out of work and training options to enhance their roles as carers.

References

Arber, S. and S. Venn (2011), "Caregiving at night: Understanding the impact on carers", *Journal of Aging Studies*, Vol. 25/2, pp. 155-165, http://dx.doi.org/10.1016/j.jaging.2010.08.020. [56]

Arksey, H. and C. Glendinning (2007), "Combining work and care: carers' decision-making in the context of competing policy pressures", *Social Policy & Administration*, Vol. 42/1, pp. 1-18, http://dx.doi.org/10.1111/j.1467-9515.2007.00587.x. [71]

Béland, F. et al. (2006), "Integrated services for frail elders (SIPA): a trial of a model for Canada", *Canadian Journal on Aging / La Revue canadienne du vieillissement*, Vol. 25/1, pp. 25-42, http://dx.doi.org/10.1353/cja.2006.0019. [8]

Béland, F. and M. Hollander (2011), "Integrated models of care delivery for the frail elderly: international perspectives", *Gaceta Sanitaria*, Vol. 25/2, pp. 138-146, https://doi.org/10.1016/j.gaceta.2011.09.003. [28]

Bolin, K., B. Lindgren and P. Lundborg (2008), "Informal and formal care among single-living elderly in Europe", *Health Economics*, Vol. 17/3, pp. 393-409, http://dx.doi.org/10.1002/hec.1275. [52]

Bonsang, E. (2009), "Does informal care from children to their elderly parents substitute for formal care in Europe?", *Journal of Health Economics*, Vol. 28/1, pp. 143-154, http://dx.doi.org/10.1016/j.jhealeco.2008.09.002. [51]

Brimblecombe, N. et al. (2018), "Review of the international evidence on support for unpaid carers", *Journal of Long-term Care*, pp. 25-40, http://eprints.lse.ac.uk/id/eprint/87978. [64]

Buljac-Samardžić, M. (2012), *Healthy Teams: Analyzing and Improving Team Performance in Long-term Care*, Erasmus University, Rotterdam, https://www.eur.nl/sites/corporate/files/Proefschrift_Martina_Buljac_0.pdf. [46]

Carpentier, N. and A. Grenier (2012), "Successful linkage between formal and informal care systems", *Qualitative Health Research*, Vol. 22/10, pp. 1330-1344, http://dx.doi.org/10.1177/1049732312451870. [54]

Chavez, K., A. Dwyer and A. Ramelet (2018), "International practice settings, interventions and outcomes of nurse practitioners in geriatric care: a scoping review", *International Journal of Nursing Studies*, Vol. 78, pp. 61-75, http://dx.doi.org/10.1016/j.ijnurstu.2017.09.010. [29]

Chevreul, K. et al. (2004), *The Development of Hospital Care at Home: an Investigation of Australian, British and Canadian Experiences*, Institute for Research and Information in Health Economics, Paris, https://www.irdes.fr/EspaceAnglais/Publications/IrdesPublications/QES091.pdf. [11]

Colombo, F. et al. (2011), *Help Wanted? Providing and Paying for Long-Term Care*, OECD Health Policy Studies, OECD Publishing, Paris, http://dx.doi.org/10.1787/9789264097759-en. [69]

de Bienassis, K., A. Llena Nozal and N. Klazinga (forthcoming), "The Economics of Patient Safety Part III: Long-Term Care", *OECD Health Working Papers*, OECD Publishing, Paris. [24]

Deschodt, M. et al. (2015), *Comprehensive Geriatric Care in Hospitals: the Role of Inpatient Geriatric Consultation Teams – Synthesis*, Belgian Health Care Knowledge Centre, Brussels, https://kce.fgov.be/sites/default/files/atoms/files/KCE_245Cs_geriatric_care_in_hospitals_Synthesis.pdf. [20]

Deschodt, M. et al. (2016), "Structure and processes of interdisciplinary geriatric consultation teams in acute care hospitals: A scoping review", *International Journal of Nursing Studies*, Vol. 55, pp. 98-114, http://dx.doi.org/10.1016/j.ijnurstu.2015.09.015. [18]

Eklund, K. and K. Wilhemson (2009), "Outcomes of coordinated and integrated interventions targeting frail elderly people: a systematic review of randomised controlled trials", *Health and Social Care in the community*, Vol. 17/5, pp. 447-458, https://doi.org/10.1111/j.1365-2524.2009.00844.x. [39]

EU (2017), *Tools and Methodology to Assess Integrated Care in Europe*, Publications Office of the European Union, Luxembourg, https://ec.europa.eu/health/sites/health/files/systems_performance_assessment/docs/2017_blocks_en_0.pdf. [26]

Eurocarers (2015), *Informal Carers' Skills and Training – A Tool for Recognition and Empowerment*, Eurocarers, Brussels, https://eurocarers.org/publications/informal-carers-skills-and-training-a-tool-for-recognition-and-empowerment/. [62]

Farfan-Portet, M. et al. (2015), *Implementation of Hospital at Home: Orientations for Belgium*, Belgian Health Care Knowledge Centre, Brussels, https://kce.fgov.be/sites/default/files/atoms/files/KCE_250_implementation_hospital_at_home_Report.pdf. [14]

Flood and Allen (2013), "ACE units improve complex patient management", *Today's Geriatric Medicine*, Vol. 6/5, p. 28, http://www.todaysgeriatricmedicine.com/archive/090913p28.shtml (accessed on 6 May 2019). [16]

Fuji, K., A. Abbott and J. Norris (2013), "Exploring care transitions from patient, caregiver, and health-care provider perspectives", *Clinical Nursing Research*, Vol. 22/3, pp. 258-74, http://dx.doi.org/10.1177/1054773812465084. [3]

Gibson, M. and A. Houser (2007), *Valuing the Invaluable: a New Look at the Economic Value of Family Caregiving*, AARP Public Policy Institute, Washington DC, https://assets.aarp.org/rgcenter/il/ib82_caregiving.pdf. [6]

Grimmon, D. (2014), *The Economic Value and Impacts of Informal Care in New Zealand*, Infometrics, Wellington, https://cdn.auckland.ac.nz/assets/auckland/about-us/equity-at-the-university/equity-information-staff/information-for-carers/The%20economic%20value%20of%20informal%20care%20in%20New%20Zealand%20Final%20copy.pdf. [7]

Hamilton, M. and C. Thomson (2017), "Recognising unpaid care in private pension schemes", *Social Policy and Society*, Vol. 16/4, pp. 517-534, https://doi.org/10.1017/S1474746416000312. [72]

Hengelaar, A. et al. (2018), "Exploring the collaboration between formal and informal care from the professional perspective. A thematic synthesis", *Health Social Care Community*, Vol. 26/4, pp. 474-485, http://dx.doi.org/10.1111/hsc.12503. [58]

Herfjord, J. et al. (2014), "Intermediate care in nursing home after hospital admission: a randomized controlled trial with one year follow-up.", *BMC Research Notes*, Vol. 7, p. 889, http://dx.doi.org/10.1186/1756-0500-7-889. [34]

Hjelm, M. et al. (2015), "The work of case managers as experienced by older persons (75+) with multi-morbidity – a focused ethnography.", *BMC Geriatrics*, Vol. 15, p. 168, http://dx.doi.org/10.1186/s12877-015-0172-3. [43]

Hofmarcher, M., H. Oxley and E. Rusticelli (2007), "Improved health system performance through better care coordination", *OECD Health Working Papers*, No. 30, OECD Publishing, Paris, https://dx.doi.org/10.1787/246446201766. [9]

Horntvedt, M. et al. (2018), "Strategies for teaching evidence-based practice in nursing education: a thematic literature review", *BMC Medical Education*, Vol. 18/1, p. 172, http://dx.doi.org/10.1186/s12909-018-1278-z. [42]

Janse, B. et al. (2018), "Formal and informal care for community-dwelling frail elderly people over time: a comparison of integrated and usual care in the Netherlands.", *Health and Social Care in the Community*, Vol. 26/2, pp. 280-290, http://dx.doi.org/10.1111/hsc.12516. [57]

Johannessen, A., K. Engedal and K. Thorsen (2016), "Family carers of people with young-onset dementia: their experiences with the supporter service", *Geriatrics*, Vol. 1/4, p. E28, http://dx.doi.org/10.3390/geriatrics1040028. [63]

Jorgensen, D. et al. (2010), "The New Zealand informal caregivers and their unmet needs", *The New Zealand Medical Journal*, Vol. 123/1317. [60]

Kim, T., K. Marek and A. Coenen (2016), "Identifying care coordination interventions provided to community-dwelling older adults using electronic health records", *Computers, informatics, nursing : CIN*, Vol. 34/7, pp. 303-311, http://dx.doi.org/10.1097/CIN.0000000000000232. [41]

Klein, S., M. Hostetter and D. McCarthy (2016), *The Hospital at Home Model: Bringing Hospital-Level Care to the Patient*, The Commonwealth Fund, New York, https://www.commonwealthfund.org/publications/newsletter-article/hospital-home-programs-improve-outcomes-lower-costs-face-resistance. [13]

Langa, K. et al. (2001), "National estimates of the quantity and cost of informal caregiving for the elderly with dementia", *Journal of General Internal Medicine*, Vol. 16/11, pp. 770-778, http://dx.doi.org/10.1111/j.1525-1497.2001.10123.x. [49]

Larkin, M., M. Henwood and A. Milne (2019), "Carer-related research and knowledge: findings from a scoping review", *Health and Social Care in the Community*, Vol. 27/1, pp. 55-67, http://dx.doi.org/10.1111/hsc.12586. [61]

Litwin, H. and C. Attias-Donfut (2008), "The inter-relationship between formal and informal care: a study in France and Israel", *Ageing and Society*, Vol. 29/1, pp. 71-91, http://dx.doi.org/10.1017/s0144686x08007666. [47]

Liu, K., K. Manton and C. Aragon (2000), "Changes in Home Care Use by Disabled Elderly Persons: 1982-1994", *The Journals of Gerontology Series B: Psychological Sciences and Social Sciences*, Vol. 55/4, pp. S245-S253, http://dx.doi.org/10.1093/geronb/55.4.s245. [48]

Lopes, H., C. Mateus and C. Hernandez-Quevedo (2018), "Ten years after the creation of the Portuguese National Network for Long-Term Care in 2006: achievements and challenges", *Health Policy*, Vol. 2010-216/3, p. 122, https://doi.org/10.1016/j.healthpol.2018.01.001. [36]

MacAdam, M. (2015), "PRISMA: Program of Research to Integrate the Services for the Maintenance of Autonomy. A system-level integration model in Quebec", *International Journal of Integrated Care*, Vol. 15/6, http://doi.org/10.5334/ijic.2246. [27]

Nolte, E. and E. Pitchforth (2014), *What is the evidence on the economic impacts of integrated care?*, WHO Regional Office for Europe, Copenhagen, http://www.euro.who.int/en/about-us/partners/observatory/publications/policy-briefs-and-summaries/what-is-the-evidence-on-the-economic-impacts-of-integrated-care. [10]

Occelli, P. et al. (2016), "Impact of a transition nurse program on the prevention of thirty-day hospital readmissions of elderly patients discharged from short-stay units", *BMC Geriatrics*, Vol. 16, p. 57, https://dx.doi.org/10.1186/s12877-016-0233-2. [21]

OECD (2018), *Care Needed: Improving the Lives of People with Dementia*, OECD Health Policy Studies, OECD Publishing, Paris, https://dx.doi.org/10.1787/9789264085107-en. [17]

OECD (2016), *Health Workforce Policies in OECD Countries: Right Jobs, Right Skills, Right Places*, OECD Health Policy Studies, OECD Publishing, Paris, https://dx.doi.org/10.1787/9789264239517-en. [45]

OECD (2014), *OECD Reviews of Health Care Quality: Norway 2014: Raising Standards*, OECD Reviews of Health Care Quality, OECD Publishing, Paris, https://dx.doi.org/10.1787/9789264208469-en. [33]

OECD (2011), *Pensions at a Glance 2011: Retirement-income Systems in OECD and G20 Countries*, OECD Publishing, Paris, https://dx.doi.org/10.1787/pension_glance-2011-en. [73]

Oldenkamp, M. et al. (2018), "Combining informal care and paid work: The use of work arrangements by working adult-child caregivers in the Netherlands", *Health and Social Care*, Vol. 26/1, pp. e122-e131, http://dx.doi.org/ 10.1111/hsc.12485. [70]

Oliver, D., C. Foot and R. Humphries (2014), *Making our Health and Care Systems Fit for an Ageing Population*, The King's Fund, London, https://www.kingsfund.org.uk/publications/making-our-health-and-care-systems-fit-ageing-population. [15]

Osterman, P. (2017), *Who Will Care for Us? Long-term Care and the Long-term Workforce*, Russell Sage Foundation, New York, http://www.jstor.org/stable/10.7758/9781610448673. [2]

Paat, G. and M. Merilain (2010), *Long-term Care in Estonia*, CEPS, Brussels, https://www.ceps.eu/ceps-publications/long-term-care-estonia. [40]

Pauly, M. et al. (2018), "Cost impact of the transitional care model for hospitalized cognitively impaired older adults", *J Comp Eff Res*, Vol. 7/9, pp. 913-922, http://dx.doi.org/10.2217/cer-2018-0040. [23]

Roland, M. et al. (2012), "Case management for at-risk elderly patients in the English integrated care pilots: observational study of staff and patient experience and secondary care utilisation", *International Journal of Integrated Care*, Vol. 12/5, http://doi.org/10.5334/ijic.850. [38]

Ross, S., N. Curry and N. Goodwin (2011), *Case Management: What it is and How it can Best Be Implemented*, The King's Fund, London, https://www.kingsfund.org.uk/publications/case-management. [37]

Russell, D. and D. Kurowski (2015), *Evaluating a Collaborative Health Coaching Partnership for High-Risk Heart Failure Patients*, United Hospital Fund 26th Annual Symposium on Health Care Services in New York: Research and Practice, https://www.crainsnewyork.com/assets/pdf/CN10076184.PDF. [30]

Service Employees International Union (2014), *St John's Enhanced Home Care Pilot Program*, https://phinational.org/resource/st-johns-enhanced-home-care-pilot-program/. [32]

Shepperd, S. et al. (2016), "Admission avoidance hospital at home", *Cochrane Database of Systematic Reviews*, http://dx.doi.org/10.1002/14651858.cd007491.pub2. [12]

Sims-Gould, J. et al. (2015), "Home support workers perceptions of family members of their older clients: a qualitative study", *BMC Geriatrics*, Vol. 15/165, p. 165, http://dx.doi.org/10.1186/s12877-015-0163-4. [53]

Socha-Dietrich, K. (forthcoming), *Interprofessional teams in primary care: Patients' and health professionals' experience*, OECD, Paris. [44]

Sorbero, M. (2012), *Addressing the Geriatrician Shortage May Help Reduce Costs Without Compromising Quality*, Rand Corporation, Santa Monica, https://www.rand.org/blog/2012/08/addressing-the-geriatrician-shortage-may-help-reduce.html (accessed on 3 June 2019). [19]

Stansfeld, S. et al. (2014), "Stressors and common mental disorder in informal carers – An analysis of the English Adult Psychiatric Morbidity Survey 2007", *Social Science & Medicine*, Vol. 120, pp. 190-198, http://dx.doi.org/10.1016/j.socscimed.2014.09.025. [66]

Stephan, A. et al. (2015), "Successful collaboration in dementia care from the perspectives of healthcare professionals and informal carers in Germany: results from a focus group study", *BMC Health Services Research*, Vol. 15/1, http://dx.doi.org/10.1186/s12913-015-0875-3. [59]

Stone, R. and N. Bryant (2019), "The future of the home care workforce: training and supporting aides as members of home-based care teams", *Journal of the American Geriatrics Society*, Vol. 67/S2, pp. S444-S448, http://dx.doi.org/10.1111/jgs.15846. [31]

Suzuki, E. (forthcoming), *Delayed hospital discharge*, OECD, Paris. [1]

Thistlethwaite, P. (2011), *Integrating Health and Social Care in Torbay: Improving Care for Mrs. Smith*, The King's Fund, London, https://www.kingsfund.org.uk/publications/integrating-health-and-social-care-torbay. [5]

Thomas, G. et al. (2015), "Informal carers' health-related quality of life and patient experience in primary care: evidence from 195,364 carers in England responding to a national survey", *BMC Family Practice*, Vol. 16/1, http://dx.doi.org/10.1186/s12875-015-0277-y. [65]

van der Brug (2017), *Readmission Rates: What can we Learn from the Netherlands?*, Nuffield Trust, London, https://www.nuffieldtrust.org.uk/news-item/readmission-rates-what-can-we-learn-from-the-netherlands. [35]

Van Houtven, C. and E. Norton (2004), "Informal care and health care use of older adults", *Journal of Health Economics*, Vol. 23/6, pp. 1159-1180, http://dx.doi.org/10.1016/j.jhealeco.2004.04.008. [50]

Vaughon, W. et al. (2018), "Association between falls and caregiving tasks among informal caregivers: Canadian Community Health Survey data", *Canadian Journal on Aging / La Revue canadienne du vieillissement*, Vol. 37/1, pp. 70-75, http://dx.doi.org/10.1017/s0714980817000496. [67]

Wanless, D. (2006), *Securing Good Care for Older People Taking a Long-term View*, King's Fund. London, https://www.kingsfund.org.uk/sites/default/files/field/field_publication_file/securing-good-care-for-older-people-wanless-2006.pdf. [55]

WHO (2015), *World Report on Ageing and Health*, World Health Organization, Geneva, https://www.who.int/ageing/events/world-report-2015-launch/en/. [25]

World Bank (2016), *Deepening Health Reform in China: Building High-Quality and Value-Based Service Delivery*. [4]

Yeandle, S. and A. Wigfield (2012), *Training and Supporting Carers: The National Evaluation of the Caring with Confidence Programme*, CIRCLE, https://essl.leeds.ac.uk/sociology-research-expertise/dir-record/research-projects/873/evaluation-of-the-caring-with-confidence-programme. [68]

Zhang, P. et al. (2017), "Effects of a nurse-led transitional care program on clinical outcomes, health-related knowledge, physical and mental health status among Chinese patients with coronary artery disease: a randomized controlled trial", *International Journal of Nursing Studies*, Vol. 74, pp. 34-43, http://dx.doi.org/10.1016/j.ijnurstu.2017.04.004. [22]

Note

[1] USD 17 740.5, Millions, Current prices, current PPPs.

6 Shortfall in innovation: how technology, skill mix and self-care can change long-term care

This chapter discusses innovative solutions to help long-term care (LTC) workers achieve more by increasing their productivity and increasing prevention effort to delay a worsening of LTC needs. Such policies are important to allow LTC workforce focusing on essential care and make the best use of their skills. The chapter discusses three important axes of action – use of technologies, improving the skill mix and helping elderly people to age healthily – and their implications for the current LTC workforce. The analysis finds that, while such policies hold the promise of improved outcomes, workforce barriers in terms of skills, allocation of tasks and worker engagement also need to be addressed.

6.1. Increasing productivity and delaying long-term care needs will increase quality of care

With population ageing, the demand for care services is expected to increase. In addition, the cost of providing LTC is rising, in part because of growing demand from ageing populations but also because labour-intensive services in a growing economy tend to see falling productivity (often referred to as "Baumol's cost disease"). With continued pressure on demand for workers, policies that can improve LTC worker productivity may make it easier to meet the needs of ageing populations with a limited workforce.

In the light of shortages faced in the sector, there is an urgent need to find innovative ways to narrow the gap between LTC supply and demand and to improve LTC worker productivity. One method may be to help LTC professionals to work in smarter ways, ensuring that the same number of professionals are able to do more and deliver better care services. This could free professionals' time from tasks that it is possible to automate, allowing them to focus on the activities that are most important for the people in need of care. Importantly, this may also help to promote better quality of care. Better use can be made of workers' time in three ways: by promoting smarter use of technology, by improving the workforce skill mix and by helping elderly people age well.

Promoting productivity gains in the LTC sector is not a straightforward exercise, as it is a highly labour-intensive sector. Many of the tasks carried out by health and social workers are difficult to standardise and need to be delivered by a person. Productivity in the care sector is known to be rather low. Estimates for the United Kingdom reveal that the residential and social care sector ranks second to last in absolute levels of labour productivity (Forth and Aznar, 2018[1]). Recent evidence, however, suggests that there is room to do better: the recent Topol review (NHS, 2019[2]) notes that with the use of tele-consultation between nursing homes, residential homes and experienced clinicians, approximately 38% of general practitioner (GP) referrals could be prevented, and ambulance conveyances decreased by up to 40%.

There is significant variation in how countries rank the topic of LTC workforce productivity in their workforce agendas. In 60% of cases – including Austria, Belgium, Estonia and Germany – improving the productivity of LTC workers is a medium to high priority. In the remainder – including Luxembourg, Cyprus and Bulgaria – this issue is placed at medium/low priority (Figure 6.1). This variation may well be related to countries' differing national priorities, but it may also be driven by the implicit idea that increasing the productivity of LTC workers is challenging.

Figure 6.1. Productivity ranks as a medium/high priority for the majority of countries

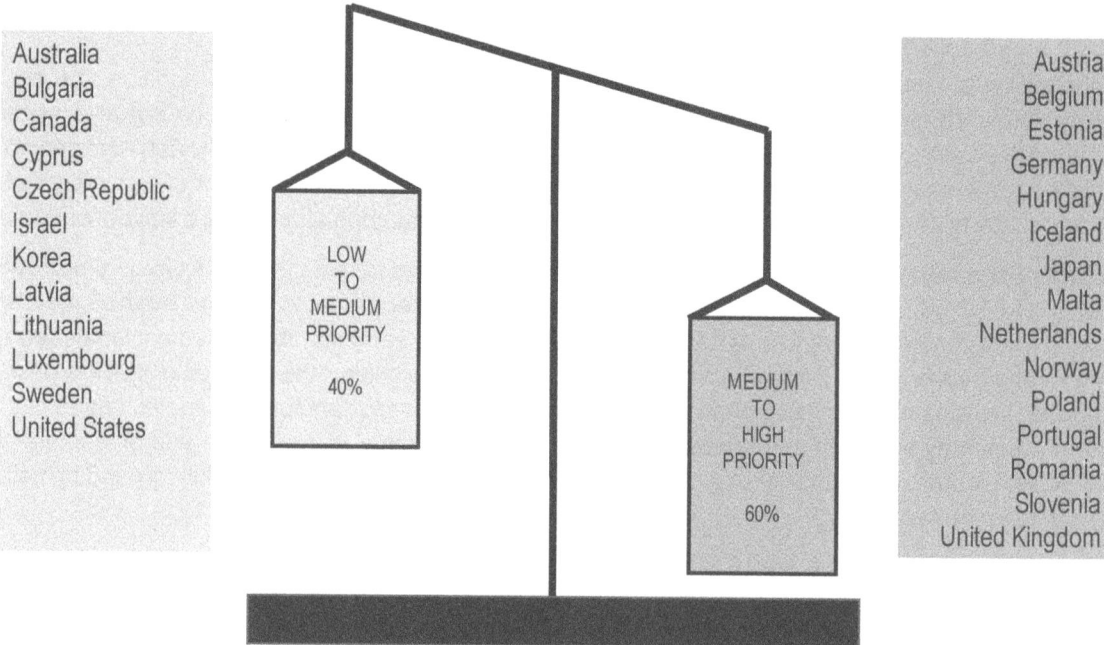

Note: Answers to "On a scale of 1 (low) to 5 (high), please indicate the level of priority of workforce issues within the LTC policy agenda". OECD countries not listed in this chart did not answer this question in the OECD Long-term care workforce questionnaire, 2018.
Source: OECD Long-term care workforce questionnaire, 2018.

This chapter discusses policy options that support nurses and personal caregivers in provision of high-quality care while making the best use of their time. Several options discussed are based on national-level approaches, but it also includes bottom-up initiatives and ongoing pilots, for which evaluations are scarce. Conclusions are therefore tentative, as this is a field for which robust research is rapidly evolving but not yet consolidated. Section 6.2 explains policies in the area of technology, Section 6.3 investigates the area of improving the skill mix and Section 6.4 examines healthy ageing and reablement.

Key findings

- New technologies can help improve work processes and reduce LTC workload – for instance, by helping to share care plans and reducing the amount of repetitive and physically demanding tasks. Many providers already use or are looking for ways to implement simple technologies such as smartphones, alarm systems, sensors and GPS monitors in nursing homes or for home care delivery. More complex technological devices – such as companionship robots or self-sufficient smart homes – are showing positive results in labs and making their way into care settings in Japan and northern European countries.
- To help achieve this, however, LTC workers need to make the best use of these technologies. Carers need to become more digitally and technologically savvy. In Norway, a new nationwide strategy has been introduced to improve the digital skills of care workers during initial education, but given the speed at which new technologies are evolving, there is also a need to upskill and reskill the current workforce. Employers are playing a key role in this through in-house training and using digital champions, as in the case of the United Kingdom.

- There is also a need to reduce LTC workers' resistance to new technologies. Their buy-in could be attained by raising awareness of LTC sector innovations, such as distributing evidence on how new technologies can help them perform work in smarter ways. In countries such as the United Kingdom and Germany, nurses are now able to identify elderly people's needs that could be solved using technology, and are developing competencies to help engineer devices that may improve care provision. In several countries, innovation incubators and hubs are bringing together tech experts and health and social professionals to develop useful care technologies jointly.

- One-third of OECD countries make use of task delegation between LTC professionals, but the range and nature of tasks formally delegated to care professionals vary. Nurses can be allowed to perform a variety of medical actions delegated by doctors (e.g. in Israel) or the tasks they are allowed to undertake may be limited to a few actions like sewing complex wounds and injections (e.g. in the Netherlands). When allowed, task delegation raises the need for additional training for LTC workers.

- Two main factors contribute to the promotion of task delegation in LTC. First, it is often developed when there is a shortage of care providers. Second, the increasing use of new technologies in care for elderly people provides more opportunities. For instance, the democratisation of digital aides allows personal care workers to perform tasks such as taking temperature or blood pressure (as in Israel).

- Investing in healthy ageing not only helps elderly people enjoy a better quality of life but also postpones the need for LTC. Evidence suggests that much more needs to be done to ensure that the LTC workforce is competent to assess elderly people's needs. In Norway, for instance, the government designed a standardised form for home assessments. In several OECD countries, nurses can receive advanced education or training that improve their clinical judgement and management competencies, preparing them to conduct comprehensive diagnosis of elderly people's needs.

- Improving LTC workers' communication skills and knowledge about health literacy can strengthen prevention policies designed for elderly people. At least one-third of OECD populations may have low levels of health literacy, and elderly people represent a high-risk group. A number of countries such as the United States and Canada have guidelines on how to speak to people with certain illnesses, such as dementia, hearing impairment or memory loss. However, data on how these tools effectively support both LTC workers and care recipients are limited. Training LTC workers to became aware of recipients' health knowledge needs, which has been shown to have positive results in France, would improve their experience of care, as well as increasing the impact of counselling about lifestyle behaviours and strengthening the connection between physicians and frail elderly people.

- More and more countries are investing in rehabilitation or reablement to help older individuals recover their autonomy. Such policies usually target frail elderly people who live in the community, and there is increasing evidence of their cost-effectiveness and overall positive impact. The Danish Fredericia model of reablement, for example, has shown positive results with people recovering functional ability and reducing their care needs significantly. A few countries are increasing the number of occupational therapists (OTs) and physiotherapists to help perform this type of activity, focusing on better, more people-centred use of resources. However, for such initiatives to be successful, countries may need more aligned incentives.

6.2. Technologies can help LTC professionals improve their productivity

New technologies hold enormous potential to support LTC workers, particularly when it comes to improving communication with and monitoring of elderly people in need of care, helping to record and process their data and improving professionals' working conditions. The current lack of a uniform electronic record that connects health and social care may be creating inefficiencies. In the United Kingdom, it is estimated that 15-70% of a care worker's time is spent on administrative tasks (NHS, 2019[2]). In the Netherlands, around one-third of nurses' time is spent on administrative reporting, such as filling in forms for insurance companies, council departments and similar.

In the long run, the use of technology in the care sector may help save costs and improve care quality and safety. A report in the United Kingdom has shown that 30% of social care tasks could be automated. Technologies such as telecare have also reduced hospital admissions and length in hospital stay for the elderly. For instance, the Advanced Telecare service in the Limousin Region in France achieved a reduced number of falls among the elderly at home and reduced hospitalisation (Carretero, 2015[3]).

There is increased evidence that technological services and devices are improving the independence of older people at home and increasing carers' productivity (Carretero, 2015[3]). Wearable devices with advanced algorithms can also support remote monitoring in home care, and may reduce time spent by workers in promoting self-care practices. Home devices (like intelligent fridges) and medication dispensers can promote self-care and allow better management of elderly people's basic need. Silent alarm systems that replace noisy ones, intelligent systems filtering information to identify truly urgent needs and home devices (like intelligent fridges) can allow better management of elderly people's needs and professionals' time.

6.2.1. Innovative technologies are slowly but firmly making their way into LTC

The fourth industrial revolution is there and increasingly affecting all areas of our lives and the LTC sector is no exception to this transformation. Nursing homes, home care services and other community services are slowly embracing technology as a way to support their staff in service delivery, but also improve their residents' wellness and engagement. The range of tools varies from simple and easy to access technologies, such as smartphones, alarm systems, sensors and GPS monitors, up to more complex devices such as surveillance and companionship robots or comprehensive technologies such as self-sufficient smart homes.

Most technologies in use have low entry costs and are easy to access

The majority of technologies currently used in LTC are those that carry low marginal costs of production and that are easily available. These include, for instance, alarm systems, cameras and sensors to detect movement. The degree of penetration of these devices varies considerably across and within countries. Unsurprisingly, private nursing homes and home care service entities or those receiving more public funding support are those where pockets of innovation are more prevalent. To a lesser extent, countries are also exploring more complex technologies. These include humanoid robots that replace or supplement LTC workers and fully fledged smart homes that support independent living.

The technologies available for LTC can grouped into four clusters (Figure 6.2).

Figure 6.2. Four categories of technology are available to support LTC workers

Assistive technologies: devices that allow a caregiver to perform a task or that increase ease and safety for the patient
- Personal alarm button service at home (used in Estonia). This is a government-funded service that allows elderly people to feel safe at home. It takes an average of 30 minutes for a professional to arrive at a person's home when needed.
- Tablets and smartphones are starting to make their way into nursing homes. They are used in numerous ways, such as monitoring care recipients at a distance or registering patient data.

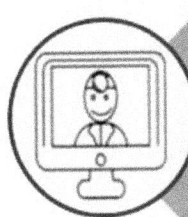

Remote care and disease management technologies: software to monitoring diseases or home adjustment treatment
- Helix (used in Australia) is a cloud-based clinical software solution providing the flexibility to offer care in different settings. It allows professionals to access records, bookings, consultations, payments and more via a laptop, desktop or tablet, and soon via mobile phone.
- Spider (used in Norway) is a software logistics programme that facilitates organising home services more effectively by informing users of the exact time professionals will arrive at their home.

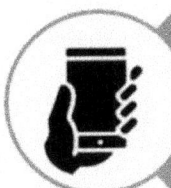

Self-management technologies: devices that create social circles of support and help connect with family, peers and the community
- CanAssist (used in Canada) is a programme from the University of Victoria, partly funded by the Canadian federal government, that develops customised technologies to prevent or delay the need for residential care services. Innovative tools for self-management include CanApp – an application that supports elderly people with cognitive challenges by breaking down any task into a sequence of easy-to-follow photos – and the Aphasia Education App, which helps care providers learn how to interact with individuals with aphasia.

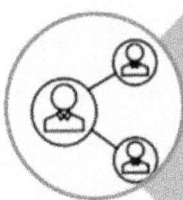

Social technologies: services that enable elderly people to take control of personal health and care management
- The Health Care Home Model (used in Australia) uses telehealth services as a way to support elderly people with managing chronic conditions and participating in care plan development.
- Giraff (used in Sweden) is a home telehealth care platform that allows care workers to enter the home of a patient virtually through the internet and conduct a secure visit. It allows family, friends and professional caregivers to create a network of care for elderly people living at home.

Source: OECD long-term care questionnaire and interviews, 2018.

According to data collected, in the large majority of countries, assistive technologies are being used in LTC care provision. Assistive technologies include sensors used at home or installed in nursing homes, which are connected to smartphones, for instance. They help professionals monitor care recipients, thus freeing up their time. When used in nursing homes, the devices can take some pressure off staff. They allow communication across teams (e.g. between a nursing home and a hospital), support autonomy of care providers and enable nurses to cover several care recipient homes. The use of remote care and self-management technologies is also quite common. These include, for instance, interactive programmes to work on psychomotor skills for elderly people (as used in Germany) or special gyms where elderly people can exercise and socialise.

To a more limited extent – in one-third of the countries – social technologies are also being used as a way to connect health professionals with each other or with users. In Norway, for instance, a social media messaging app similar to WhatsApp connects nurses who work in the same region but have different clients. This helps them share professional advice, which is particularly relevant in home care services. In

France, in the Ille-et-Vilaine region, a new teleprocessing tool was implemented to allow nurses to communicate in real time, to co-ordinate working schedules more easily and to share medical data in a secure way.

LTC jobs are at low risk of automation compared with other sectors

New technologies, such as robots and artificial intelligence (AI), are set to disrupt and automate people's jobs. The LTC sector is no exception to this growing phenomenon. The development of humanoid robots is now quite advanced, and they may take on a more important role in the future of LTC provision. Pepper and Paro, for instance, can read and respond to human interactions and emotions, memorise personality traits, play memory games, send emails and show videos (Box 6.1). They are successfully replacing health and social workers in hospitals and nursing homes, and studies have shown that they help to deal with loneliness and to form social connections with elderly people.

Box 6.1. Some assistive social robots are successfully replacing health and social workers

Pepper

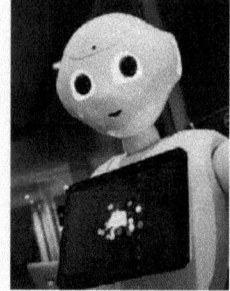

Designed by a Japanese company called Softbanks, Pepper was initially designed as a companion robot. However, it is now being used in different settings such as guiding patients to different hospital departments (as in Belgium) or working as a social care worker in community engagement, awareness-raising and to facilitate other activities.

Paro

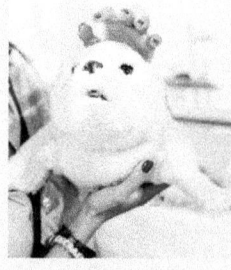

Paro is a therapeutic baby seal robot developed by the National Institute of Advanced Industrial Science and Technology. Its behaviour can be programmed according to patient needs. Initial small-scale studies carried out by the manufacturer have found positive results in encouraging interaction and communication among elderly patients.

Source: Broekens, Heerink and Rosendal (2009[4]), "Assistive social robots in elderly care: A review", https://doi.org/10.4017/gt.2009.08.02.002.00.
Image credits: Pepper: Owen Beard/Unsplash.com; Paro: frantic00/Shutterstock.com.

What robots will mean for LTC jobs is uncertain. The risk of automation of LTC jobs is relatively low compared with other sectors. Evidence suggests that health associate professionals and personal care workers are on a par with information and communication technology (ICT) professionals in terms of shares of jobs at high risk (10%) and significant risk (30%) of automation. These proportions are relatively low compared with the risk for workers in mining, construction, manufacturing and transport or in sales (Figure 6.3).

But this is not set in stone. What will happen to LTC jobs will depend on the rate at which technologies will continue to evolve, but mostly on the speed of diffusion and their adoption. It is likely however that, for the most part, robots and AI will supplement and complement LTC workers jobs rather than replace them fully. This is in many ways good news. Automation of certain tasks has the potential to free up time from nurses and personal carers, allowing them to spend more time on caring tasks that require interpersonal skills, such as communication and teamwork.

Figure 6.3. The likelihood of health and personal care worker positions being automated is low

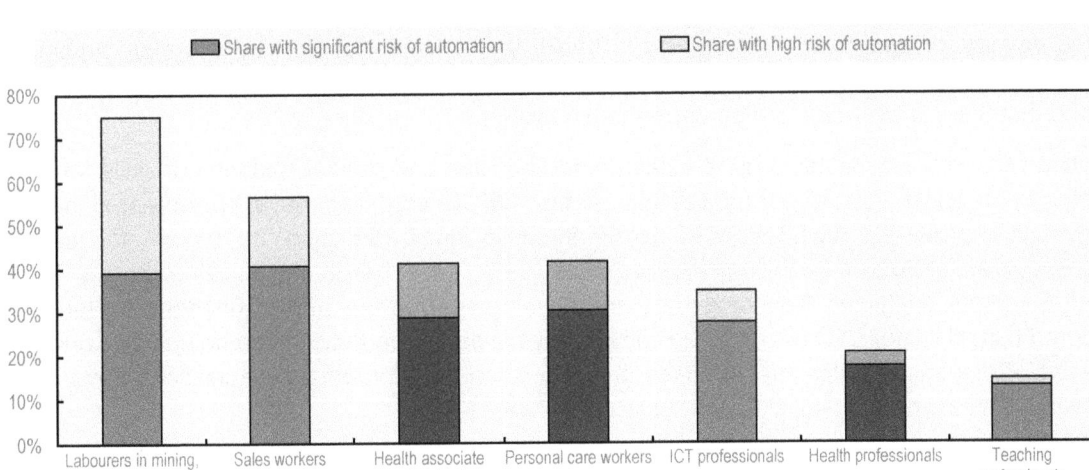

Note: Job automatability for selected occupations, based on European data.
Source: Nedelkoska and Quintini (2018[5]), based on the OECD's Programme for the International Assessment of Adult Competencies (PIAAC) 2012.

More innovation, digitalisation and automation in LTC may also lead to new employment opportunities. These could include jobs for people that are able to bridge knowledge between health and technology development. Making the most of these opportunities and ensuring that the changes result in favourable outcomes will require machine learning engineers and data scientists to work alongside care workers. In the digital age these professions can add much value to non-clinical but very important activities related to system governance and policy decisions. One example is using a range of datasets to generate information on system performance or evidence on the performance of drugs once in clinical use.

6.2.2. Policies need to be in place to ensure that LTC workers reap the benefits of technologies

LTC workers will need support to make the best use of new technologies. This can be achieved in three ways: by improving their digital skills, promoting better understanding of how technologies can support carers' tasks and tailoring regulation.

Increasing professionals' digital skills is a first step

Care workers need to become digitally literate. This refers to an individual's ability to learn, work and develop effectively in a digital workplace and society (NHS, 2017[6]). The advantages of a digitally literate care workforce are numerous. Care workers that are digitally savvy will be able to share data and digital care plans with home and institutional providers. Digital skills can improve decision making, reduce the amount of repetitive and physically demanding tasks and increase flexibility and productivity (Skills for Care, 2016[7]). Improving digital literacy in the sector may help to attract and retain not only care workers but also people with a range of other skills into care. When digitally literate, home care providers can also help care receivers to use apps and connect digitally with their family members and friends. More automation of certain tasks means that workers will have time to take on more complex tasks, such as problem solving in new situations, and will need to have solid literacy, numeracy and problem-solving skills combined with autonomy, co-ordination and collaborative skills, in addition to ICT skills.

LTC workers are not necessarily digitally savvy. The OECD's PIAAC Survey of Adult Skills suggests that more than 50% of the adult population among 28 OECD countries can only perform a simple set of computer tasks, such as writing an email or browsing the web, or have no ICT skills at all (OECD, 2016[8]). In a survey conducted among 200 European care workers, 80% of individuals claimed that they had not received training, or had insufficient training in health technologies. In Norway, a survey among social employers revealed that a large majority of workers do not possess the skills to adequately manage digital tools and that there is over-reliance on paper-based systems.

Promoting care workers' digital skills requires comprehensive and regular updating of skills for handling technologies in initial education and training. A few OECD countries have implemented nationwide strategies to improve the digital skills of care workers in initial education. In Norway, for instance, a competency plan for 2020 is under way to revamp the curriculum of health and social workers, with 12 new learning outcomes, including technology use and development. In the United Kingdom, digital skills are considered core skills for LTC workers, but without specifying the underlying competencies workers need to develop. Compensating for this, charities and other non-governmental organisations have designed frameworks defining core digital skills for social care (Table 6.1).

Given the speed at which new technologies are evolving, there will also be a need to upskill and reskill the current LTC workforce. In a 2016 European-level digital skills survey among adults, 87% of respondents stated that ICT has changed the tasks of personal care workers in the past five years, and 86% believed that this would continue in the next five years. Employers are responsible for fostering a learning environment that ensures the reskilling and upskilling of care workers in ICT. Data from interviews show that carer training is often conducted on an ad hoc basis, depending on the devices and tools used in nursing homes and home care services. Increasing the range of programmes to promote digital literacy based on health conditions and raising awareness of telecare is recommended (Waights, Bamidis and Almeida, 2018[9]). Different methods of learning should also be supported, including informal and social learning. For instance, one successful way of promoting digital skills is using digital champions (as in the United Kingdom). These are staff who are comfortable with technologies and can serve as mentors and knowledge centres for other staff. Digital champions are found to promote learning and provide a range of support to peers (Kispeter, 2018[10]).

Table 6.1. Four core digital skills are needed by care workers in the United Kingdom

Core skills	Reasons they are needed in social care	Examples of use of those digital skills and knowledge
(1) Sharing data	1. to comply with data protection laws 2. to act in service users' best interest 3. to use data and data sharing to safeguard best interests 4. to be a full partner in integration	A. knowing how to share appropriate data safely with colleagues B. knowing how to share data safely with colleagues in other organisations/professions C. knowing how to use password protection safely D. being able to complete digital records accurately E. being able to store information safely F. being able to use insertable and removable storage devices safely G. being able to read, send and receive email communications
(2) Learning and development	1. to support staff development 2. to assess knowledge and skills 3. to monitor learning 4. to create evidence and report learning to monitoring/funding bodies 5. to show evidence of learning to regulators	A. being able to create a log-in and password for a learning account B. being able to print off evidence of completion of learning C. being able to access mobile learning via a tablet or smart phone D. knowing how to record learning digitally for a portfolio E. being able to bookmark a page so it is easy to find again F. using search techniques to locate and select relevant information G. recognising and taking account of currency, relevance, bias and copyright when selecting and using information
(3) Using digital skills in direct care	1. to create business efficiencies 2. to promote self-care 3. to support digital inclusion for service users 4. to conform with commissioner guidelines/wishes regarding assisted living technology	A. knowing how to help someone use their diabetes app B. knowing how to help someone with their falls monitor C. knowing how to help someone access services online (such as claiming benefits, paying rent or booking appointments) D. having the required skills and knowledge to research local activities for a care recipient E. knowing how to set up and support a remote medical consultation for a care recipient
(4) Managing information	1. to ensure efficient internal and external communications 2. to use when tendering for contracts 3. to attract private business 4. to comply with monitoring requirements 5. to create business efficiencies	A. in home care, knowing how to use a remote monitoring system via a smart phone B. in home care/day support, knowing how to update a digital care plan C. in residential or nursing care, knowing how to update digital handover records in a skilled way D. being able to work with files, folders and other means to access, organise, store, label and retrieve information E. being able to follow and demonstrate understanding of the need for safety and security practices F. being able to demonstrate how to create, use and maintain secure passwords G. being able to demonstrate how to minimise the risk of computer viruses

Source: Skills for Care (2016[7]), Core Digital Skills in Social Care, https://www.skillsforcare.org.uk/Documents/Topics/Digital-working/Core-digital-skills-in-social-care.pdf.

LTC workers show resistance to new technologies

LTC workers may take to using new technologies with some degree of resistance. Their concerns often revolve around the depersonalisation of care, fear of losing status and relevance or low awareness of the opportunities and benefits of using new technologies (Ramsey and Montgomery, 2014[11]; Dubois et al., 2013[12]). A scoping review found that nurses and other health and social care workers show worry for care recipients' safety and privacy when using humanoid robots (Papadopoulos, Koulouglioti and Ali, 2018[13]). Some also believe that using technology may shift the art of diagnosing away from LTC workers to algorithms, potentially increasing existing inequalities. Many LTC workers do not trust the data, and this may undermine clinical judgement.

Buy-in from LTC workers may be made possible using a combination of promoting a culture of change and innovation in the LTC sector, providing evidence on how technologies can help LTC workers' daily tasks and making LTC workers co-developers and an integral part of decisions about which technologies to use.

One important element of securing LTC workers' adherence to new technologies is promoting an overall culture of change and innovation in the sector. A few strong local-level initiatives are leading by example. For instance, the Flanders Care programme in Belgium has been set up to respond to the challenges of an ageing population through innovation. Aiming to create a caring and solidarity-based society where everyone gets equal opportunities, this programme has been set up to improve the quality of care through innovation and responsible entrepreneurship. Its focus is on prevention and home care through assistive technologies, monitoring applications, ICT care, diagnostics and imaging. Work practices and employment relations in the sector are also strongly related to the adoption of new technologies. A study found that nursing homes that promoted teamwork and communication adapted faster to the introduction of new systems (Avgar, Tambe and Hitt, 2018[14]). In particular, management allowing staff to experiment and setting up a peer-support system are important for the successful introduction of new technologies.

Interviews also revealed a need to strengthen LTC workers' views on how best to use technologies for the benefit of caregiving provision. Studies show that when staff work in technology-rich environments, they perceive that benefits outweigh potential difficulties with implementation (Ruiz Morilla et al., 2017[15]). When that is not the case, LTC workers fear that new tools and devices may add to their already heavy workload. To smooth the transition, managers need to plan the introduction of technologies carefully and give LTC workers enough time to become acquainted with their use. For instance, nurses can receive training on the advantages of using sensor alarms in home care provision. In countries such as Israel, these alarms are connected to a call centre where a nurse or personal care worker is available to respond to health issues that arise from a multitude of different care recipients. Awareness also needs to be raised on how well-designed AI and other tools can reduce administrative burdens, releasing professionals' time for important care recipient-clinician interaction. In addition, roles could also be developed with responsibility to advise on the opportunities underlying health care technologies and to identify skills gaps among teams of care providers.

Another important way to convince staff to adopt new technologies is to make them co-developers of technological solutions. The current offer of new tools and devices for care service provision is wide and rapidly increasing. In Japan, for instance, the market for personal care robots, which currently stands at around USD 155 million, is projected to grow to USD 3.7 billion by 2035. In Scotland, United Kingdom, the total digital health market – e.g. telehealth, mobile health and wireless health – was estimated at USD 79 billion in 2015 and is expected to reach USD 206 billion by 2020 (Rimpiläinen, Morrison and Rooney, 2014[16]). The number of options is increasing and providers are feeling lost when trying to identify best options for their clients. To solve this issue, a few countries (such as Norway and the United Kingdom) are now training nurses on the basics of technology development and design. The idea is that future nurses will be competent in identifying needs of their clients and help engineers design technological devices that may improve care provision. In several countries – Belgium, France, Germany and Sweden – innovation incubators and hubs are bringing together both technology experts and health and social professionals to help accelerate the identification of care technologies that are most useful. In addition to supporting care adherence and trust in these new devices, these hubs may in future open the possibility for new employment opportunities – for example, for LTC workers who are able to bridge health settings and technological developments.

Workers should be guided on how to use technology better

Technology-enabled care is gaining impetus in several countries; with this comes the need to update and establish regulations on how health and social workers use it. Collection and storage of data on elderly people leaves sensitive information available to hackers. Health and social workers thus need guidance on how to handle, for instance, servers such as email and cloud computing systems in a secure and consistent way to avoid breaches in a care recipient's security. AI is also developing at high speed. Many humanoid robots are now quite advanced, and can change and adapt their behaviour in response to human interaction. There is a need for strong ethical and privacy regulations that help and protect users, particularly care recipients with disabilities.

Most countries have set up guidelines and standards to help LTC workers understand not only the use of new technologies but also ethical and privacy issues concerning how data is collected (Box 6.2).

> **Box 6.2. Standards and regulations on technologies help LTC workers**
>
> In mid-2018, a Concerted Action was implemented in Germany, involving the Ministry of Health, the Ministry of Labour and Social Affairs to recruit more people in LTC. As part of the action, there are concrete proposals for innovative care approaches involving digital solutions to improve the efficiency of nursing care. It prioritised and examined how these approaches can be used in the field, in particular focusing on: using digitisation to design innovative approaches, such as in district networking, telenursing, telecounselling, home assistance systems or eCounselling; using digitisation to relieve nurses, for example, by reducing the bureaucracy of nursing documentation, electronic billing or communicating with doctors and other health professionals, or maintaining and improving the health of employees; involving caregivers in the development of new digital products and applications and introducing them into day-to-day work, while observing ethical principles; and increasing efficiency at the interfaces between nursing and health care (such as discharge from hospital).

To ensure effective use of new technologies in health and social care, countries need stronger regulatory frameworks that are fit for purpose. Stronger frameworks regulating technologies will also help build trust and transparency in their use, not only for caregivers but also for recipients. Elderly people in need of care need to understand issues such as why their data are vital to ensure the right diagnosis and treatment, how the information will be used, the measures in place to secure and protect the data and who is accountable. A survey in the United Kingdom found that only 18% of current AI health and social projects have received regulatory approval, and 78% of respondents felt that regulation was very/extremely important in realising the potential of AI in health and care (NHS, 2018[17]).

Another area that needs attention is the promotion of technology-enabling infrastructure. Across OECD countries, many rural areas do not yet have access to the internet, which makes LTC workers isolated. Further, the use of analogue telephones still prevails in many homes for elderly people. Ensuring connectivity in health and social care means relying on broadband connectivity. If there are variations across and within countries in broadband speeds, this may increase inequalities in access to care and constrain professionals' ability to innovate in their services. In Germany, a series of measures has been implemented to support the integration of medical apps and improve infrastructure. The German Appointment Service and Supply Act, which came into effect in early 2019, required health funds to offer electronic health records by 1 January 2021.

Countries may need to invest more in regulating resources that educate and train care workers in health data provenance, curation, integration and governance, the ethics of AI and autonomous systems and tools, critical appraisal and interpretation of AI and robotics technologies (NHS, 2019[2]). Currently, technological education for care workers remains rather basic.

6.3. Improving the skill mix is another way to improve productivity in LTC

LTC carers need various skills to perform their duties. However, as discussed in Chapter 3, their skills do not always match those required for the job. In addition, automation, AI and other factors are set to disrupt the way labour markets function, and the social and care sector is no exception. Skills mismatches may mean that some LTC workers have acquired more skills than are required for the job, leading to waste of human capital and job dissatisfaction, while others may lack some skills for certain tasks, possibly contributing to lower quality and safety of LTC services (OECD, 2016[18]).

6.3.1. Task delegation is not common in LTC

One-third of OECD countries have implemented task delegation (transferring responsibility for the performance of an activity while retaining accountability for the outcome) between LTC workers since 2011. Task delegation mostly involves administering medication, and the low number of countries implementing it may be explained in part by the organisation of LTC. In many countries, LTC professionals are governed by regulations defining their specific competencies, and are subject to different administrations (such as the ministry of health or ministry of social affairs) and budgets (at the national, regional, departmental or municipal levels). Nurses and personal care workers are usually not in a superior-subordinate relationship and their activities are monitored and sponsored by distinct entities.

In countries that allow it, the range and nature of tasks delegated to care workers vary. Nurses may be permitted to perform a variety of medical actions delegated by doctors (as in Israel), or the boundary of their authorised tasks may be limited to a few actions like sewing complex wounds and giving injections (as in the Netherlands). When allowed, task delegation raises the need for additional training for LTC workers. A study in Sweden showed that some home care assistants administer medication occasionally even their skills or knowledge cannot be appraised (Gransjön Craftman et al., 2015[19]). In the United Kingdom, the Nursing and Midwifery Council states that nurses or nurse associates undertaking delegated tasks must complete the necessary training before carrying out a new role (Nursing and Midwifery Council, 2019[20]). In the United States, medication aides (unlicensed personnel who can administer medication) can be delegated to administer medication in LTC settings (assisted living, nursing homes, adult day care etc.). In a nationwide survey, 21% reported that "they are required to take responsibilities beyond their defined role", which may raise safety issues (Budden, 2012[21]). In all cases, task delegation usually requires strict monitoring of the person receiving care – such as monthly checks of their condition in hospital (Cyprus) – and regular evaluation of the carers' skills and capabilities, which can be done in the form of informal one-to-one practical training or through take-up of a formal training or under specific regulations (United States).

While increased training and monitoring are needed to prevent accidents and medical errors, some countries have developed additional ways of reducing potential errors by staff receiving care task delegation. In Portugal, for instance, personal carers can administer medication in some nursing homes. Pharmacies prepare daily doses of medication, which are already pre-packaged, and explain in a simple way to whom, how and when to administer it. This has been a successful way of delegating tasks from nurses to personal care workers with little margin for potential errors.

Two main factors contribute to the promotion of task delegation in LTC. First, it is often developed when there is a shortage of care providers. In Belgium, an agreement between federal and regional authorities allows personal care workers to perform nursing tasks exceptionally when the elderly person needs them and no other care options are available, but this has not yet been transposed into legislation. Second, the increasing use of new technologies in care for elderly people provides more opportunities for task delegation. For instance, the democratisation of digital aides allows personal care workers to perform tasks such as taking temperature or blood pressure (as in Israel).

A better match between skills, tasks and job roles would be beneficial for LTC workers. This is currently the case in the Netherlands, where legislation was discussed in parliament in 2018 to improve the job profile for nurses and to differentiate the tasks and skills of nurses with university education and those with vocational training (see Box 6.3). Nurses with a university degree (level 5 and 6) receive education to hold managerial roles, including more knowledge concerning their profession, and additional training in soft skills (such as collaboration and communication). Nurses with university education should thus have more responsibility for indicating and organising suitable care, especially in complex situations, using a combination of knowledge and protocols (evidence-based practice), while nurses with vocational training should follow protocols and be involved in less complex care.

> **Box 6.3. Reconfiguring the role of LTC nurses in the Netherlands**
>
> In the Netherlands, nurses with vocational training (level 1) are assistants and work only in nursing homes. They are in charge of cleaning, cooking, hygiene and – to some extent – social activities, but cannot perform medical tasks. They are responsible for providing attention and observing client needs. Nurse assistants (level 2) are also assistants, whose main focus lies in ensuring a good environment for the client by supporting level 3 nurses with tasks related to activities of daily living (e.g. helping elderly people with getting up, dressing, eating). Nurses with a higher level of education (level 3) are independent – in charge of physical care, injections, medication and nursing acts. Nurses with level 4 can also perform toileting and can undertake some risky procedures. This nurse is in charge of judging a situation before referring to a doctor and can co-ordinate cases of a complex situation. They are also independent professionals (as are nurses with level 3), but with higher levels of knowledge about diseases/syndromes and more extensive nursing procedures.

6.3.2. Task delegation has both pros and cons

Task delegation has pros and cons. Prior research explored the impact of task delegation for three geriatric conditions (falls, urinary incontinence and dementia) on the quality of care provided by different professionals: physicians, nurse practitioners, physician assistants, registered nurses, medical assistants and licensed vocational nurses (Lichtenstein et al., 2015[22]). Delegated tasks varied from history taking to referrals. Results show that implementing task delegation within interdisciplinary team management programmes was associated with a higher quality of care for these conditions in community practices.

The delegation of some administrative tasks (such as record-keeping) to personal care workers may also enhance productivity in the LTC workforce. It would help nurses to focus on their core competencies, which are health care provision and care co-ordination. Personal care workers accessing administrative positions could avoid doing physical tasks to pursue a career in care for elderly people. Indeed, workers aged 50 and over often face work-related health issues (such as back problems), and may be better suited to performing some of the administrative tasks currently provided by nurses.

In home-based settings, the delegation of medication administration (pills, eyes-drop etc.) from nurses to personal care workers can lead to better efficacy when, for instance, it reduces unnecessary travel time and allows more time and effort to be dedicated to providing care to elderly people with complex needs. In addition, the Enhanced Home Care pilot programme in California showed that additional training for personal care workers in medication management, mental health and nutrition resulted in lower medication non-compliance rates and improved health (Osterman, 2017[23]). Other evidence from Australia supports the idea that appropriately trained and supervised care workers can help nurses with medicine management in home care settings, particularly for those at low risk of adverse medication errors (Lee, 2015[24]).

However, task delegation may also have drawbacks. Task delegation from doctors to nurses may be difficult. Research has documented that nurses providing LTC can be pressured by doctors when they have to report on the work they do, or may face issues with reaching doctors for urgent matters when tasks are delegated to them (Tjia et al., 2009[25]). Pressure on nurses can also come from the fact that delegation gives them more responsibilities, while they may not necessarily have sufficient training and experience for the most complex cases (such as care recipients with dementia or multiple comorbidities). Consequently, task delegation from primary care providers to nurses may lead to higher risk of burnout (Edwards et al., 2018[26]).

Task delegation from nurses to personal care workers can also raise negative issues. Again, it requires a higher level of training and mentoring. There are concerns about whether personal care workers are able to recognise changes in a patient's condition and to provide the patient with appropriate care (Denton, 2015[27]). Because task delegation is mainly top-down, it can ultimately lead to personal care workers receiving more tasks because they have nobody to delegate to; this can result in increased workload and higher pressure for them.

6.4. Engaging elderly people to help themselves can delay LTC needs

Many countries also invest in activities that help elderly people age well or recover their autonomy when disabled. The former – healthy ageing – consists of a series of programmes optimising opportunities to increase years of good health and autonomy by reducing the number of years of disability. Health and social workers can support healthy ageing by helping with fall prevention programmes, offering education on food nutrition and physical activity, promoting social activities, supporting immunisation and engaging in activities that help prevent cognitive decline. Recovery of autonomy is commonly referred to as reablement or rehabilitation, in which care workers support frail elderly people in regaining some degree of physical or mental autonomy.

Six areas of action can support elderly people to continue to enjoy the quality of life they desire through healthy ageing and rehabilitation services (Figure 6.4).

Figure 6.4. There are six areas of action in which health and social workers can support elderly people to age healthily and remain autonomous

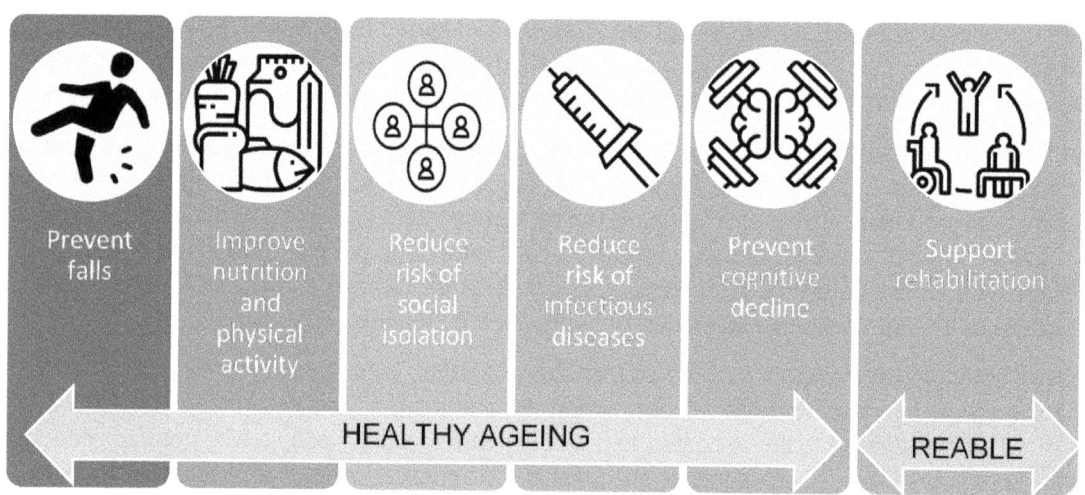

Source: Adapted from the World Health Organization (WHO) Framework on Healthy Ageing.

6.4.1. Prevention measures and rehabilitation activities may ease the growing pressure on LTC

Preventable safety failures are widespread in LTC. The root causes of most safety events can be addressed through improved prevention and safety practices. For instance, elderly people's falls are frequent. WHO estimates show that approximately 28-35% of people aged 65 or over fall each year around the world, and that more than 30 million falls require medical attention every year. Falls among elderly people cost the US health care system roughly USD 34 billion in direct medical costs (National Council for Ageing, 2018[28]). In England, United Kingdom, falls and fractures for those aged 65 and above account for over 4 million bed days per year and fragility fractures cost around GBP 4.4 billion (NHS, 2017[29]). Regular exercise and healthy diet are associated with lower incidence of cardiovascular disease, osteoporosis and bone loss and certain forms of cancer. Studies suggest that exercise alone can reduce falls by 10%; that proportion increases to 25% if the focus is on balance (Oxley, 2009[30]).

Averting cognitive decline helps people continue to take care of daily tasks on their own. With older age, some cognitive abilities – such as conceptual reasoning, memory or processing speed – tend to decline progressively. This results in a variety of symptoms, such as loss of memory and decreased ability to maintain focus or to solve mental tasks. All of this can severely interfere with everyday tasks of daily life; in some cases, a person affected cannot carry on living independently without care. A multi-domain lifestyle intervention showed that simultaneous management of several vascular and lifestyle-related risk factors can benefit cognition among elderly people (Ngandu et al., 2015[31]).

Several safety concerns are present specifically in LTC residences. Health care-associated infections were common in LTC – averaging a prevalence of 3.8% among LTC facility residents in OECD countries in 2016-17 (OECD, 2019[32]). Such infections can lead to increases in morbidity, mortality and health costs for the system. Pressure ulcers – an injury to the skin for due to pressure – are common for the elderly with reduced mobility. Across OECD countries, the prevalence rate of pressure ulcers was 5.35 in LTC institutions (OECD, 2019[32]). Older people also consume more prescribed opioids than the young, despite the adverse effects of these medicines such as dizziness and confusion.

Increased prevention and safety among the elderly will also help increasing the effectiveness of service delivery and postponing disability among the elderly. In the future there will be an increased pressure on LTC spending given population ageing. Projections suggest that LTC spending will continue to grow in the future, even in the best case scenario, in which half of the elderly population ages without disability and mitigates cost growth (Figure 6.5).

Figure 6.5. LTC expenditure will increase, but less so in conjunction with healthy ageing

LTC spending projections – change in spending as % of GDP 2016-70

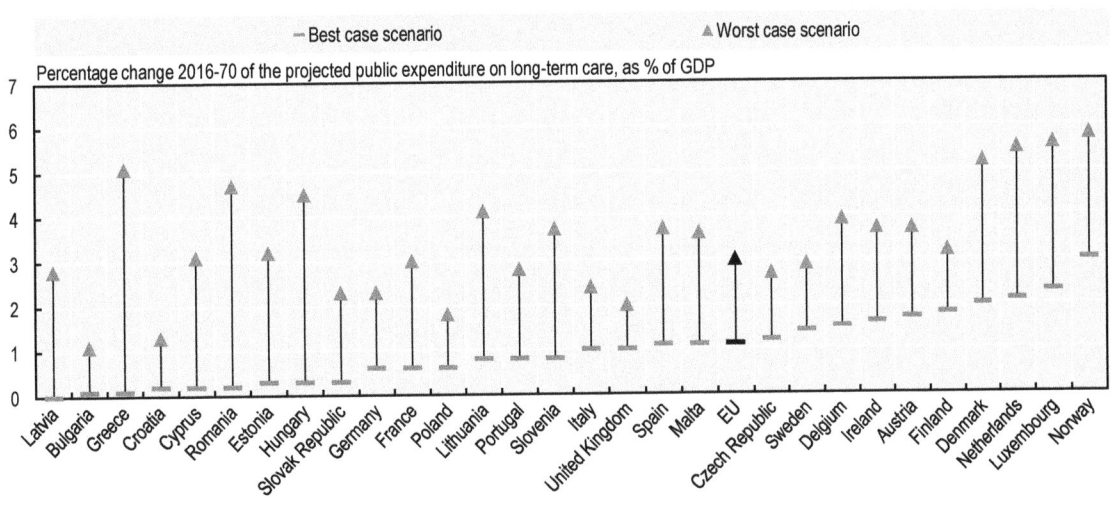

Note: The EU data point is the average, weighted according to GDP, of the 28 countries shown in the chart. In all countries (except Germany, Luxembourg and Poland), the best case scenario is the "healthy ageing" scenario (half of the projected gains in life expectancy are without disability). In all countries, the worst case scenario is the "cost and coverage convergence scenario", which assumes: i) that growing expectations of the populations and the exchange of best practices will lead to an expansion of publicly financed formal care provision into groups of elderly people who previously relied on informal care; and ii) that EU countries in which LTC spending was below the EU28 average in 2016 will encounter an upward cost convergence.
Source: European Commission (2018[33]), *The 2018 Ageing Report*, https://doi.org/10.2765/615631.

6.4.2. Many gaps persist in improving elderly people's well-being

Evidence shows that LTC workers can do more, and do it better. LTC workers play an important role in educating and informing frail elderly people to take better care of their own health, but this is not happening as often as it could. In the LTC sector, data show that, during the past two years, no care professionals discussed physical activity or healthy diet with over 50% of senior citizens in the Netherlands, Sweden, Norway, Switzerland, Germany and the United Kingdom. In France and the United States, the situation is comparatively better (Figure 6.6).

Figure 6.6. Health professionals do not discuss nutrition and physical activity with elderly people

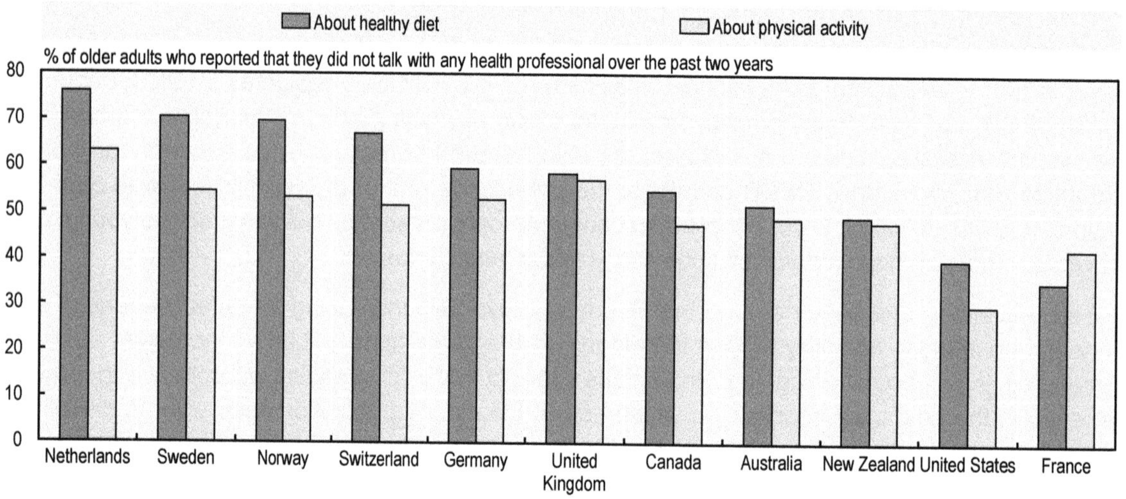

Note: Data show proportion of individuals who answered "no" to the questions "During the past 2 years, has any health professional talked with you about exercise or physical activity?" and "During the past 2 years, has any health professional talked with you about a healthy diet and healthy living?"
Source: 2017 Commonwealth Fund International Health Policy Survey of Older Adults.

Figure 6.7. The proportion of people aged 65 and over receiving flu shots is decreasing in the majority of countries

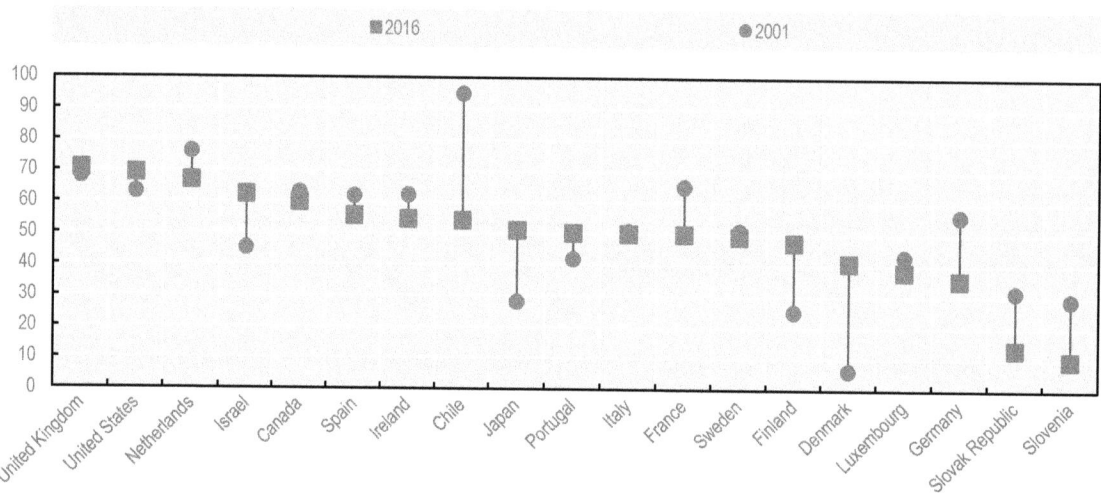

Source: OECD Health Statistics 2018, https://doi.org/10.1787/health-data-en.

Numbers of flu vaccinations among elderly people are also falling. In 11 out of 18 OECD countries, the proportion of elderly people being vaccinated against flu is decreasing (Figure 6.7). In Chile, vaccination rates decreased from 95% in 2001 to 54% in 2016. In France, they fell from 65% to 50% and in Germany, from 56% to 35%. Ignoring this may come at a high cost. When older people get influenza, they become vulnerable to many other serious conditions. Due to their weaker immune systems, people aged 65 years and over are at high risk of developing severe complications following flu, such as pneumonia, heart attacks, strokes or infections. Influenza is associated with increased health care utilisation and thus weighs heavily on health care systems. In the United States, during 2017-18, the influenza virus lead to an estimated 22.7 million medical visits and 959 000 hospitalisations. In Canada, estimates show that each case of flu requiring hospitalisation costs on average CAD 14 612.

6.4.3. Several avenues may keep elderly people healthy and autonomous for longer

In the past decade, a number of countries have increased their focus on prevention and healthy ageing, implementing a number of measures supporting elderly people to age better or regain autonomy. These range from regulations on prevention (e.g. the Prevention Act in Germany) to financial incentives to support home rehabilitation (as in Norway). Several countries have implemented rehabilitation programmes (including the United States, the United Kingdom, Australia, the Netherlands, Norway and Sweden). The province of Saskatchewan in Canada is supporting individuals with chronic complex needs in the community, using multidisciplinary teams to delay admission to LTC.

Japan is developing an integrated community care system that emphasises preventive care and activities to promote longer healthy life expectancy. Since 2005, the Japanese government has opened community-based integrated care centres in every district. The centres are responsible for implementation of preventive care services, outreach and counselling for elderly people in need of care through the use of community health resources networks, and continuous and comprehensive care management support that includes supervision of "care managers" responsible for planning care services provided under LTC insurance (Hatano et al., 2017[34]). The government supports proactive efforts to organise exercise classes and community cafés to increase social participation and reduce isolation. Efforts to promote self-management are also increasing.

In France, healthy ageing is promoted as soon as elderly people retire or before LTC needs develop. Pension insurance schemes finance and implement actions and prevention measures at the regional level. They provide social support to retired people and implement services that mostly target healthy ageing and disability prevention. They have developed workshops to inform and educate retired people about the importance of healthy ageing. A national score – the Aggir scale – has been developed to rank older adults' level of disability. As soon as a person is considerable vulnerable (but not yet disabled), a number of different providers start to co-ordinate activities that help prevent autonomy loss (Box 6.4).

Box 6.4. The Aggir scale and a comprehensive prevention programme helps prevent loss of autonomy among older adults

In France, care services are administered by two entities – the pension insurance schemes and the departmental councils – which are respectively in charge of prevention of loss of autonomy and disability management. A national rule defines eligibility for care and separates vulnerable elderly people from disabled elderly people. Care needs are assessed using a national scale – the Aggir scale – which provides a score ranging from 1 (severe disability) to 6 (non-vulnerable). Elderly people with an Aggir score of 4 and below are considered to be disabled. The score sets the activity of each entity: pension insurance schemes develop disability prevention schemes within the retired population and offer assistance to elderly people who are not yet disabled (with an Aggir score of 5-6), while the departmental councils provide support to disabled elderly people (with an Aggir score of 1-4).

Frailty detection is organised at the regional level within the population with an Aggir score of 5-6. Specific retirement insurance schemes are provided to finance domestic help for elderly people who need help performing basic activities of daily living (using the toilet, washing etc.) and transportation assistance. Financial help is also provided to improve home settings and adapt elderly people's homes to their new needs, and social assistance is provided to manage transitions after difficult events (such as hospitalisation, loss of a partner or sibling).

Workshops on prevention cover a wide range of topics: the benefits of physical activity, brain activation, healthy diet, healthy lifestyle, regular sleep patterns, oral hygiene, fall prevention and risk of social isolation. Based on interactive methods, they include scientific content and practical and engaging advice. Volunteers, social workers or physicians specifically trained on healthy ageing conduct each workshop in a lively and friendly way to encourage retired people to participate and exchange views with each other.

Implementation of such workshops requires comprehensive and multidisciplinary skills training for professionals. Training programmes include distance learning followed by classroom sessions, in which professionals develop a solid knowledge base about good eating habits, physical activity adapted to elderly people and activities promoting wellness for older adults such as relaxation, breathing exercises or intellectual activities.

Regional health education and promotion bodies also organise multiple short courses or one-day training courses on several key topics such as prevention of malnutrition among elderly people, facilitation techniques and communication techniques in health education, project methodology and health promotion evaluation.

Social activity by pension insurance schemes is not limited to prevention workshops: they also aim to avoid social isolation and maintain social bonds. Pension funds can also participate financially to holiday trips for their beneficiaries if they face a fragile economic and social situation. Finally, they support financially the development of adapted housing for elderly people with optimal safety and services, including more than 400 home adaptation projects in 2016.

Preventive home visits to older people in Denmark, mainly by district nurses, are another example of good practice. Assessment have shown the positive effects of preventive home visits on the functional health status of older people. A three-year prospective randomised controlled follow-up study showed that training of home visitors was associated with improved functional ability of older people.

Some countries are also active in the area of healthy ageing by promoting more targeted interventions in one dimension. For instance, in Chile, the Santiago Sano programme brings together professionals from every municipal department into 40 dedicated communities to organise evaluations for elderly people with reduced mobility. It runs three-month workshops focusing on maintaining an independent and healthy lifestyle (OECD, 2019[35]). Public Health England (the executive agency of the Department of Health and Social Care in the United Kingdom) has catering guidance toolkits for those serving food to older people (in residential care), which provides advice for serving food to meet the nutritional needs of this age group in care and other settings. There is also a Workforce Competence Model in Nutrition, which provides a framework that benchmarks competences and underpins standards for expanding the skills of the LTC workforce.

6.4.4. LTC workers can play a stronger role in helping elderly people age well

Three areas of action can help health and social workers support elderly people to age well: giving LTC workers the skills and resources for personalised care assessments and strengthening their role in prevention activities; improving their skills and knowledge of health literacy; and promoting reablement and rehabilitation services.

LTC workers will need to carry out personalised care assessments and support prevention activities

LTC workers can play a major role not only in assessing elderly people's needs but also in guiding their choices and behaviour. They can educate elderly people about the risks of an unhealthy diet, remind them about the schedule for vaccinations and inform them about the importance of being vaccinated. They can also detect changes in a care recipient's cognitive ability and suggest testing to assess whether changes fall within the normal process of ageing and cognitive decline or are pathological.

Traditionally, assessment of an elderly person's needs takes place at the primary care level, usually performed by a GP or a geriatric doctor, but the role of nurses in performing this task is becoming more prominent, given nurses' regular visits to elderly people at home and in their social environment. Evidence suggests that much more needs to be done to ensure that the LTC workforce is competent in assessing elderly people's needs. In several OECD countries, nurses can receive advanced education or training that improve their clinical judgement and management competencies, preparing them for such a role. In eight countries – Australia, Canada, Finland, Ireland, Netherlands, New Zealand, the United Kingdom and the United States – education is available to train as nurse practitioners or advanced practice nurses; these professionals are allowed to work at higher levels of advanced clinical practice.

Countries can strengthen LTC workers' role in health promotion and disability limitation for elderly people by establishing national prevention policies that guide LTC workers on how to help elderly people stay healthy for longer, strengthen professional skills at the primary care level to keep elderly people out of institutions and improve geriatric knowledge among health and social workers working in the community. Nurse practitioners have a strong role to play in healthy ageing (Box 6.5).

> **Box 6.5. Nurse practitioners have successfully provided prevention to elderly people in rural practices in British Columbia**
>
> The nurse practitioner (NP) role has been implemented at different speeds throughout Canada's provinces and territories. In British Columbia, based on an in-depth analysis of three rural collaborative practices where NPs were newly employed, access to care was improved and contributed to enhanced teamwork. NPs spent more time with frail elderly people with chronic conditions and used the extra time for health promotion advice, disease prevention, assessments of complex situations and case management. In addition, NPs often introduced a new, community- and population-based focus to their practices. Activities provided by NPs included outreach activities outside the office for marginalised populations – work not previously done by GPs. These add-on services were appreciated by colleagues and improved physician job satisfaction. Moreover, emergency use and admission rates to hospitals declined *(Roots and MacDonald, 2014[36])*.
>
> Source: Maier, Aiken and Busse (2017[37]) "Nurses in advanced roles in primary care: policy levers for implementation", https://dx.doi.org/10.1787/a8756593-en.

A few countries – including France, Germany and the United Kingdom – have policies in place to guide LTC workers on how to help older adults live longer and healthier lives. These usually take the form of prevention measures as part of LTC policies or plans. For instance, in Germany, the 2015 Prevention Act introduced a new benefit for nursing care funds for prevention and health promotion in inpatient care institutions. The health insurance scheme has developed a guideline with health-promoting offers for this target group. It defines nutrition, physical activity, strengthening of cognitive resources, psychosocial health and violence prevention as necessary fields of action. In the United Kingdom, the NHS Long-term Care Plan outlines interventions to help cut smoking and obesity and to double enrolment in type 2 diabetes prevention programmes.

Finally, countries are also investing in a series of health promotion and disease prevention activities by promoting geriatric knowledge among nurses and personal care workers. As discussed above, many nurses carrying out LTC tasks have not received LTC-specific or geriatric training. To overcome this barrier, some initiatives aim to help LTC workers at the forefront of home care service improve their knowledge of the needs of elderly care recipients. For instance, the Visiting Nurse Service of New York trained personal care workers as health coaches; this led to improvements in self-care maintenance and management of heart failure symptoms, and reduced the number of activities of daily living for which elderly people needed assistance (Osterman, 2017[23]).

LTC workers could benefit from improved communication skills and knowledge of health literacy

At least one-third of OECD populations may have low levels of health literacy, and elderly people represent a high-risk group. Factors such as cognitive decline and lack of understanding of online platforms or digital skills mean that elderly people tend to be less skilled and knowledgeable in how to access, evaluate and apply health information. Literature also suggests that older individuals may feel shame and embarrassment in communicating difficulties with understanding their treatment options, or in raising questions in discussion with doctors (Moreira, 2018[38]). This is worrying, given the high rates of chronic disease that affect this group: good health knowledge to understand and treat long-term conditions is required. Evidence shows that low levels of health literacy are associated with higher risks of elderly mortality, poorer ability to take medication appropriately, lower skills in reading labels and health messages, and poor overall health status for elderly people (Berkman et al., 2011[39]).

LTC workers can support elderly people to improve their health literacy by promoting better communication. Health and social workers can be sensitised to their role in promoting better health literacy by setting up guidelines for better communication or promoting on-the-job training on how to improve communication with elderly people. Several OECD countries make use of guidelines and toolkits to set standards on how health and social care professionals can better communicate with frail elderly people (Table 6.2). A number of countries also have guidelines on how to speak to care recipients with certain illnesses, such as dementia, hearing impairment or memory loss. However, data on how these tools support both LTC workers and elderly people effectively are limited. Countries may need to invest in more campaigns to help LTC workers become sensitive to the impact that effective and simple communication can have on a care recipient's understanding and uptake of health information.

Another complementary option is the use of on-the-job training. Studies suggest that LTC workers' curricula have gaps in creating competency to understand their role in promoting knowledge and understanding of health information. Training LTC workers to become aware of health knowledge needs would improve frail elderly people's satisfaction with information and care, increase the impact of counselling about lifestyle behaviours and strengthen connections between physicians and their patients. Randomised controlled trials have shown that when providers are informed of frail elderly people's health literacy levels, they are more likely to use related strategies. Frail elderly people are also more likely to adhere to colorectal cancer screenings when professionals have received training on how to communicate with people with low health literacy (Moreira, 2018[38]).

Table 6.2. Guidelines and toolkits improve LTC workers' communication with elderly people

Country	Communication policy
Austria	Improving the quality of communication in health care is a national policy towards establishing a patient-centred culture of communication in the Austrian health care system.
Ireland	The Health Service Executive has published national guidelines – *Communicating Clearly for Health Professionals* – which form part of an improvement programme to support staff to communicate clearly and be aware of health literacy issues during their daily work with service users. It provides writing and speaking advice when dealing with care users.
France	*Communiquer pour tous – guide pour une information accessible* is a guide on best practices to provide information in an accessible form to all, particularly those with low levels of health literacy.
United States	The Agency for Healthcare Research and Quality has developed a health literacy universal precautions toolkit with evidence-based guidance on how to improve spoken communication.
Canada	The "Easy Does It! Plain Language and Clear Verbal Communication", developed by the Canadian Public Health Association, is a training manual developed for health providers, carrying advice and stories on how to communicate with care recipients to improve the quality of care.

Source: 2017 OECD Health Literacy survey.

In Canada, a national non-profit organisation supports life-long healthy active ageing through participation, education, research and promotion of information and resources that contribute to overall well-being. It undertakes public education sessions and publishes educational material – communicated in plain language for the public and practitioners – research and study results into the health benefits of active healthy ageing for adults and older adults. It also offers training opportunities through various methods for community leaders throughout Canada, to provide them with the necessary skills and knowledge to facilitate healthy living workshops in their community.

Some countries promote reablement and rehabilitation services

Reablement or rehabilitation usually consists of a short-term intervention (3-12 weeks) in the home of an older person or in a facility designed for that purpose. The focus is on training in daily functions, thus reducing and postponing the need for further care and helping people regain autonomy. There is increasing evidence of the cost-effectiveness and overall positive impact of reablement. The Fredericia model in Denmark helps to reduce care costs significantly (Box 6.6). In Norway, a reablement programme resulted in significantly higher performance and satisfaction of frail elderly people and lowered requests for and duration of home visits, leading to lower overall costs compared with usual care (Kjerstad and Tuntland, 2016[40]). Another reablement programme in the United Kingdom was found to be a cost-effective way to reduce subsequent LTC use, while having a positive impact on both users' and carers' independence and confidence (Glendinning et al., 2010[41]). Research suggests that reablement can boost the morale of carers, as they find an older people's needs are met to a greater degree. Staff also feel more satisfied and are thus less likely to quit their job.

> **Box 6.6. The Fredericia model for reablement in Denmark is cost-effective**
>
> The primary objective of the "Life-long Living" programme in Denmark is to postpone age-related dependence and maintain independent living for as long as possible. First implemented in the Fredericia municipality in 2008, its success led to its integration in the national legislative framework. It is now a model of good practice for all Danish municipalities on how to design empowering and rehabilitative home care services for elderly people.
>
> The aim of the programme is to make a radical change in the way home care is delivered. Passive service delivery and compensatory care are replaced by everyday rehabilitation services, prevention, empowerment and active participation of the care recipient. Rather than focusing on the limitations of elderly people, trained personal carers focus on their resources and stimulate them to maintain or develop their physical abilities. The objective is to help and train older people to regain independence, autonomy and the confidence to perform a wide range of activities perceived as important by the older people themselves, inside their home or within their local community. Under the Life-long Living model, each care recipient has his or her own "citizen plan". Each individual's goals are continually adjusted as the care recipient improves in performing everyday tasks or as motivation changes.
>
> The plans are conducted by multidisciplinary teams and caregivers specifically trained for rehabilitation. Dedicated care teams include 15 "home trainers", 2 OTs, a physical therapist and a nurse. This way of helping older people to regain control over their own lives helps them feel empowered rather than a burden on their community. It allows them to reconnect with their preferred social leisure and physical activities, and to remain active in society.
>
> The results of a project evaluation are promising. First, care recipients who joined the programme significantly improved their physical abilities and now rely less and less on home help from the Elderly Care Department. Second, job satisfaction improved among employees of the Elderly Care Department, as caregivers were more involved in the new working methods and more enthusiastic about the new interaction with senior citizens. The programme also resulted in considerable financial gains: the costs of services provided by the municipality decreased by approximately EUR 170 000 per month – more than EUR 2 million a year. This improved financial performance enables the municipality to provide more care to more people with the same amount of money.
>
> Since 2008, the model has been implemented throughout Denmark. The majority of Danish municipalities replaced their traditional home care services with rehabilitation services as in Fredericia. Other countries, such as Finland, Norway, Sweden, France and the Netherlands are also considering ways to implement similar models.
>
> Source: Kjellberg and Ibsen (2010[42]), "Økonomisk evaluering af Længst Muligt i Eget Liv I Fredericia Kommune [Economic evaluation of Life-long Living in Fredericia municipality]", https://www.vive.dk/da/udgivelser/oekonomisk-evaluering-af-laengst-muligt-i-eget-liv-i-fredericia-kommune-9299/.

The Portuguese National Network for Long-term Integrated Care integrates health and social care as a way to prevent long stays in hospitals for elderly people, with both medical and social services provided under the same umbrella. This was part of a major reform that took place in 2006 to create a network providing integrated LTC services. Two of the three types of institutional care services of the Network include convalescence beds for intensive rehabilitation for up to 30 days and medium-term beds for between 31 and 90 days, where care recipients receive support to regain autonomy. These services are also being developed for use at home, delivered by primary health care centres.

Care workers will be increasingly called on to perform rehabilitation activities in co-ordination with OTs. A few countries are increasing the number of OTs and physiotherapists to help perform this type of activity, focusing on better, more people-centred use of resources. In Norway, the OT profession has grown quickly. In 2011, OTs started to provide services in four Norwegian municipalities. In 2018, they implemented care plans in around 300 municipalities. OTs often have high education levels (a bachelor's or master's degree), but there is no specific reablement certification, so training is organised in workshops. However, for this initiative to be more successful, countries may need further financial support. In Norway, while uptake for reablement is increasing, municipalities complain they do not receive sufficient financial support to develop OT programmes. It is difficult to find financial sponsorship because the priority is currently on nurse recruitment.

6.5. Conclusion

With population ageing, the demand for care services is expected to increase. Closing the gap between supply and demand for LTC workers will require innovative solutions to improve how work is done in this sector.

This chapter outlines some of the innovative ways in which LTC workers can be supported to work in smarter ways, ensuring the same number of professionals are able to do more and deliver better care services. This not only promotes better quality of care but also frees professionals from tasks that it is possible to automate, allowing them to focus on activities that are most important for the people in need of care.

Countries are helping LTC professionals achieve more by increasing their productivity and postponing demand for LTC needs in three ways:

- **Technologies**: this chapter finds that new technologies can help improve work processes and reduce LTC workload. To help achieve this, however, LTC workers need to make the best use of these technologies. Carers need to become more digitally and technology savvy. There is also a need to reduce professionals' resistance to new technologies.
- **Skill mix**: one-third of OECD countries make use of task delegation between LTC professionals. This is often developed when there is a shortage of care providers, but is also promoted due to greater use of technology.
- **Promoting healthy ageing and safety of elderly people**: investing in healthy ageing not only helps elderly people enjoy better quality of life but also postpones the need for LTC. Evidence suggests that much more needs to be done to ensure that the LTC workforce is competent in assessing elderly people's needs – for instance, improving communication skills and knowledge of health literacy can strengthen prevention policies for elderly people. More and more countries are also investing in rehabilitation or reablement to help older individuals recover their autonomy.

References

Avgar, A., P. Tambe and L. Hitt (2018), "Built to learn: how work practices affect employee learning during healthcare information technology implementation", *MIS Quarterly*, Vol. 42/2, pp. 645-659. [14]

Berkman, N. et al. (2011), "Low health literacy and health outcomes: an updated systematic review", *Annals of Internal Medicine*, Vol. 155/2, p. 97, http://dx.doi.org/10.7326/0003-4819-155-2-201107190-00005. [39]

Broekens, J., M. Heerink and H. Rosendal (2009), "Assistive social robots in elderly care: A review", *Gerontology*, Vol. 8, pp. 94-103, http://dx.doi.org/10.4017/gt.2009.08.02.002.00. [4]

Budden, J. (2012), "A national survey of medication aides: education, supervision, and work role by work setting", *Geriatric Nursing*, Vol. 33/6, pp. 454-464, http://dx.doi.org/10.1016/j.gerinurse.2012.05.001. [21]

Carretero, S. (2015), *Technology-enabled Services for Older People Living at Home Independently: Lessons for public long-term care authorities in the EU Member States*. [3]

Denton, M. (2015), "Task shifting in the provision of home and social care in Ontario, Canada: implications for quality of care", *Health and Social Care in the Community*, Vol. 23/5, pp. 485-492. [27]

Dubois, C. et al. (2013), "Why some employees adopt or resist reorganization of work practices in health care: associations between perceived loss of resources, burnout, and attitudes to change.", *International journal of environmental research and public health*, Vol. 11/1, pp. 187-201, http://dx.doi.org/10.3390/ijerph110100187. [12]

Edwards, S. et al. (2018), "Task delegation and burnout trade-offs among primary care providers and nurses in Veterans Affairs Patient Aligned Care Teams (VA PACTs)", *The Journal of the American Board of Family*, Vol. 1/8, pp. 83-93, http://dx.doi.org/10.3122/jabfm.2018.01.170083. [26]

European Commission (2018), *The 2018 Ageing Report*, European Commission, Brussels, http://dx.doi.org/10.2765/615631. [33]

Forth, J. and A. Aznar (2018), *Productivity in the UK's Low-wage Industries*, Joseph Rowntree Foundation, York, http://file:///C:/Users/Rocard_E/Downloads/fourthaznar_-_productivity.pdf. [1]

Glendinning, C. et al. (2010), *Home Care Re-ablement Services: Investigating the longer-term impacts (prospective longitudinal study)*, Social Policy Research Unit, York, https://www.york.ac.uk/inst/spru/research/pdf/Reablement.pdf. [41]

Gransjön Craftman, A. et al. (2015), "Unlicensed personnel administering medications to older persons living at home: a challenge for social and care services", *International Journal of Older People Nursing*, Vol. 10/3, pp. 201-210, http://dx.doi.org/10.1111/opn.12073. [19]

Hatano, Y. et al. (2017), "The vanguard of community-based integrated care in Japan: the effect of a rural town on national policy", *International Journal of Integrated Care*, Vol. 17/2, p. 2, http://doi.org/10.5334/ijic.2451. [34]

Kispeter, E. (2018), *What digital skills do adults need to succeed in the workplace now*, Warwick Institute for Employment Research. [10]

Kjellberg, J. and R. Ibsen (2010), *Økonomisk evaluering af Længst Muligt i Eget Liv I Fredericia Kommune [Economic evaluation of Life-long Living in Fredericia municipality]*, https://www.vive.dk/da/udgivelser/oekonomisk-evaluering-af-laengst-muligt-i-eget-liv-i-fredericia-kommune-9299/. [42]

Kjerstad, E. and H. Tuntland (2016), "Reablement in community-dwelling older adults: a cost-effectiveness analysis alongside a randomized controlled trial", *Health Economics Review*, Vol. 6/1, p. 15, http://dx.doi.org/10.1186/s13561-016-0092-8. [40]

Lee, C. (2015), "Evaluation of a support worker role, within a nurse delegation and supervision model, for provision of medicines support for older people living at home: the Workforce Innovation for Safe and Effective (WISE) Medicines Care study", *BMC Health Services Research*, Vol. 15/460. [24]

Lichtenstein, B. et al. (2015), "Effect of physician delegation to other healthcare providers on the quality of care for geriatric conditions", *Journal of the American Geriatrics Society*, Vol. 63/10, pp. 2164-2170, http://dx.doi.org/10.1111/jgs.13654. [22]

Maier, C., L. Aiken and R. Busse (2017), "Nurses in advanced roles in primary care: policy levers for implementation", *OECD Health Working Papers*, No. 98, OECD Publishing, Paris, https://dx.doi.org/10.1787/a8756593-en. [37]

Moreira, L. (2018), "Health literacy for people-centred care: where do OECD countries stand?", *OECD Health Working Papers*, No. 107, OECD Publishing, Paris, https://dx.doi.org/10.1787/d8494d3a-en. [38]

National Council for Ageing (2018), *Fact Sheet: Falls*, National Council for Aging Care, Washington DC, https://www.aging.com/falls-fact-sheet/. [28]

Nedelkoska, L. and G. Quintini (2018), "Automation, skills use and training", *OECD Social, Employment and Migration Working Papers*, No. 202, OECD Publishing, Paris, https://dx.doi.org/10.1787/2e2f4eea-en. [5]

Ngandu, T. et al. (2015), "A 2 year multidomain intervention of diet, exercise, cognitive training, and vascular risk monitoring versus control to prevent cognitive decline in at-risk elderly people (FINGER): a randomised controlled trial", *The Lancet*, Vol. 385/9984, pp. 2255-2263, http://dx.doi.org/10.1016/s0140-6736(15)60461-5. [31]

NHS (2019), *Preparing the healthcare workforce to deliver the digital future - The Topol Review*, Health Education England, London, https://topol.hee.nhs.uk/wp-content/uploads/HEE-Topol-Review-2019.pdf. [2]

NHS (2018), *Accelerating Artificial Intelligence in Health and Care: Results from a State of the Nation Survey*, The Academic Health Science Network, London, http://ai.ahsnnetwork.com/about/aireport/. [17]

NHS (2017), *Improving Digital Literacy*, NHS England, London, https://www.hee.nhs.uk/sites/default/files/documents/Improving%20Digital%20Literacy%20-%20HEE%20and%20RCN%20report.pdf. [6]

NHS (2017), *NHS RightCare Scenario: the Variation between Sub-optimal and Optimal Pathways*, NHS England, London, https://www.england.nhs.uk/rightcare/wp-content/uploads/sites/40/2017/02/rightcare-susans-story-full-narrative.pdf. [29]

Nursing and Midwifery Council (2019), *Delegation and accountability supplementary information to the NMC Code*, Nursing and Midwifery Council, London, https://www.nmc.org.uk/standards/code/. [20]

OECD (2019), *Health at a Glance 2019: OECD Indicators*, https://doi.org/10.1787/4dd50c09-en. [32]

OECD (2019), *OECD Reviews of Public Health: Chile: A Healthier Tomorrow*, OECD Publishing, Paris, https://dx.doi.org/10.1787/9789264309593-en. [35]

OECD (2016), *Health Workforce Policies in OECD Countries: Right Jobs, Right Skills, Right Places*, OECD Health Policy Studies, OECD Publishing, Paris, https://dx.doi.org/10.1787/9789264239517-en. [18]

OECD (2016), "Skills for a Digital World, Policy brief on the future of work Ministerial Meeting on the Digital Economy Background Report", *OECD Digital Economy Papers*, Vol. 250, https://doi.org/10.1787/5jlwz83z3wnw-en?. [8]

Osterman, P. (2017), *Who Will Care for Us? Long-term Care and the Long-term Workforce*, Russel Sage Foundation, New York, http://www.jstor.org/stable/10.7758/9781610448673. [23]

Oxley, H. (2009), "Policies for healthy ageing: an overview", *OECD Health Working Papers*, No. 42, OECD Publishing, Paris, https://dx.doi.org/10.1787/226757488706. [30]

Papadopoulos, I., C. Koulouglioti and S. Ali (2018), "Views of nurses and other health and social care workers on the use of assistive humanoid and animal-like robots in health and social care: a scoping review", *Contemporary Nurse*, Vol. 54/4-5, pp. 425-442, http://dx.doi.org/10.1080/10376178.2018.1519374. [13]

Ramsey, A. and K. Montgomery (2014), "Technology-based interventions in social work practice: a systematic review of mental health interventions.", *Social Work in Health Care*, Vol. 53/9, pp. 883-99, http://dx.doi.org/10.1080/00981389.2014.925531. [11]

Rimpiläinen, S., C. Morrison and L. Rooney (2014), "Review and analysis of the digital health sector and skills for Scotland : a report by the Digital Health and Care Institute in partnership with Skills Development Scotland – Strathprints", *Social Work in Health Care*, Vol. 53/9, pp. 883-899, https://doi.org/10.17868/63863. [16]

Roots, A. and M. MacDonald (2014), "Outcomes associated with nurse practitioners in collaborative practice with general practitioners in rural settings in Canada: a mixed methods study", *Human Resources for Health*, Vol. 12/69, http://dx.doi.org/doi: 10.1186/1478-4491-12-69. [36]

Ruiz Morilla, M. et al. (2017), "Implementing technology in healthcare: insights from physicians", *BMC Medical Informatics and Decision Making*, Vol. 17/1, p. 92, http://dx.doi.org/10.1186/s12911-017-0489-2. [15]

Skills for Care (2016), *Core Digital Skills in Social Care*, Skills for Care, Leeds, https://www.skillsforcare.org.uk/Documents/Topics/Digital-working/Core-digital-skills-in-social-care.pdf. [7]

Stuart, R., C. Lim and D. Kong (2014), "Reducing inappropriate antibiotic prescribing in the residential care setting: current perspectives", *Clinical Interventions in Aging*, p. 165, http://dx.doi.org/10.2147/cia.s46058. [43]

Tjia, J. et al. (2009), "Nurse-physician communication in the long-term care setting: Perceived barriers and impact on patient safety", *Journal of Patient Safety*, Vol. 5/3, pp. 145-152, http://dx.doi.org/10.1097/PTS.0b013e3181b53f9b. [25]

Waights, V., P. Bamidis and R. Almeida (2018), *Technologies for Care – the Imperative for Upskilling*, Northern Ireland Assembly Knowledge Exchange Seminar Series (KESS), Series 7. 2017-18, http://oro.open.ac.uk/55287/. [9]

www.ingramcontent.com/pod-product-compliance
Ingram Content Group UK Ltd.
Pitfield, Milton Keynes, MK11 3LW, UK
UKHW050413240426
12048UKWH00020B/1490